2nd edition

immunology

The National Medical Series for Independent Study

2nd edition

immunology

Richard M. Hyde

Professor and Vice Chairman
Department of Microbiology and
   Immunology
University of Oklahoma
   Health Sciences Center
Oklahoma City, Oklahoma

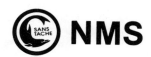 **NMS**

National Medical Series from Williams & Wilkins
Baltimore, Hong Kong, London, Sydney

Harwal Publishing Company, Malvern, Pennsylvania

**Williams
& Wilkins**

Library of Congress Cataloging-in-Publication Data

Hyde, Richard M.
    Immunology / Richard M. Hyde. — 2nd ed.
      p.   cm. — (The National medical series for independent study)
    Rev. ed. of: Immunology / editors, Richard M. Hyde, Robert A.
Patnode. c1987.
    Includes index.
    ISBN 0-683-06230-1 (pbk. : alk. paper)
    1. Immunology—Outlines, syllabi, etc.   2. Immunology—
Examinations, questions, etc.   I. Immunology.   II. Title.
III. Series.
    [DNLM: 1. Allergy and Immunology—examination questions.
2. Allergy and Immunology— outlines.   QW 18 H995i]
QR182.55.H94   1992
616.07'9076—dc20
DNLM/DLC
for Library of Congress

91-21623
CIP

ISBN 0-683-06230-1

©1992 Williams & Wilkins, Baltimore, Maryland

10 9 8 7 6 5 4 3 2 1

Contents

Preface

This text was developed as a syllabus to be used in an immunology course taught to second-year medical students. This second edition has been modified considerably, both in light of new developments in this rapidly moving field and with valued feedback from students and colleagues. In particular, the chapters on the immune response and immunologic mechanisms of tissue damage have been dramatically revised to include information on the cytokines and membrane receptors that are pivotal in these events.

The text first presents a review of native immunity, immunogenicity, the mechanisms and products of immune responses, and practical considerations of immunization and laboratory procedures employed in the diagnosis of disease. The remaining chapters are concerned with defects in native and acquired immunities, with diseases in which the immune system has turned on inappropriately and is autoreactive, and with transplantation and tumor immunology.

This book presents a concise coverage of the fundamentals of immunology in a readily understandable manner. The material is presented in outline format, with key points emphasized by boldface. Complex material is presented in figures and tables to give the student useful summaries. Clinical relevance is stressed, both in the text and in the study questions and explanations.

Richard M. Hyde

Acknowledgments

I would like to express my appreciation to Jim Harris of Harwal Publishing Company, who developed the concept for this series, and to Jane Velker, Managing Editor, for her guidance and support during the preparation of this text. The assistance of Gloria Hamilton in manuscript editing is also acknowledged. Appreciation is extended to Wieslawa Langenfeld for development of the illustrations in the text.

Many colleagues have contributed to the preparation of this book. Dr. D. Rex Billington served as the catalyst for the preparation of the original manuscript; he contributed innumerable ideas on organization and format and was invaluable in my efforts to evaluate the teaching effectiveness of the text. Valuable advice on content was obtained from Drs. William A. Cain, Samuel R. Oleinick, Frank Waxman, and John Harley.

This book is dedicated to the many students, both past and present, who contributed to its preparation through their penetrating questions, thoughtful comments, and constructive criticisms.

To the Reader

Since 1984, the *National Medical Series for Independent Study* has been helping medical students meet the challenge of education and clinical training. In today's climate of burgeoning information and complex clinical issues, a medical career is more demanding than ever. Increasingly, medical training must prepare physicians to seek and synthesize necessary information and to apply that information successfully.

The *National Medical Series* is designed to provide a logical framework for organizing, learning, reviewing, and applying the conceptual and factual information covered in basic and clinical sciences. Each book includes a comprehensive outline of the essential content of a discipline, with up to 500 study questions. The combination of an outlined text and tools for self-evaluation allows easy retrieval of salient information.

All study questions are accompanied by the correct answer, a paragraph-length explanation, and specific reference to the text where the topic is discussed. Study questions that follow each chapter use the current National Board format to reinforce the chapter content. Study questions appearing at the end of the text in the Comprehensive Exam vary in format depending on the book. Wherever possible, Comprehensive Exam questions are presented as clinical cases or scenarios intended to simulate real-life application of medical knowledge. The goal of this exam is to challenge the student to draw from information presented throughout the book.

All of the books in the *National Medical Series* are constantly being updated and revised. The authors and editors devote considerable time and effort to ensure that the information required by all medical school curricula is included. Strict editorial attention is given to accuracy, organization, and consistency. Further shaping of the series occurs in response to biannual discussions held with a panel of medical student advisors drawn from schools throughout the United States. At these meetings, the editorial staff considers the needs of medical students to learn how the *National Medical Series* can serve them better. In this regard, the Harwal staff welcomes all comments and suggestions.

Innate and Adaptive Immunity

I. INTRODUCTION

A. Overview

1. **Immunity (resistance)** is the summation of all the naturally occurring defense mechanisms that protect an individual from infectious diseases.

2. There are two types of immunity: **nonspecific immunity** is innate; **specific immunity** is developed as a result of experiences with a variety of immunogens such as vaccines, microbes that colonize the body, and macromolecules in the diet. **Nonspecific (innate) immunity** is discussed in this chapter; **specific (acquired, or adaptive) immunity** comprises much of the rest of this book. Examples of these two types of resistance mechanisms are presented in Table 1-1.

3. When there is an imbalance in any of the systems involved in natural immunity, the host has trouble with "opportunistic" bacteria. When the defenses of the host are diminished, these opportunists, which are organisms not ordinarily considered pathogenic, can produce disease.

B. Nonspecific (innate) immunity

1. The physiologic mechanisms of nonspecific immunity are present throughout the animal kingdom as inherent, or innate, qualities of the species.

2. These mechanisms do not exhibit specificity. That is, they are not dependent on specific recognition of a foreign material: a single defense barrier will afford protection against many different potential pathogens.

C. Specific (acquired, or adaptive) immunity

1. The specific immunologic response that follows exposure to a particular infectious agent induces lymphocytes to proliferate, mature, secrete antibodies, and "remember" that particular agent. (This is the **primary immune response**.) On further contact with that same agent, increased resistance then develops through the abundant production of specific antibodies or sensitized lymphocytes. (This is the **secondary**, or **anamnestic, immune response**.)

2. Thus, specific immunity has **four essential characteristics:**
   a. An **induction phase,** which is the time interval that follows the first exposure to an antigen, during which precommitted lymphocytes proliferate and mature into antibody-secreting plasma cells or into specifically reactive T cells that will secrete various mediators (lymphokines and cytotoxins) upon subsequent contact with the antigen
   b. The ability to **distinguish self from foreignness**
   c. **Specificity,** which is the selectivity shown by antibodies and lymphocytes of the specific immune system in reacting only with **matching (homologous) antigens**
   d. **Immunologic memory,** which allows antibodies and sensitized lymphocytes to remember their homologous antigen and react with it later

3. Specific immunity may be acquired by natural or artificial processes.
   a. Examples of **naturally acquired immunity** include the immunity that develops during convalescence from an infection and the placental passage of antibody from mother to fetus.
   b. Examples of **artificially acquired immunity** include vaccination or injection of gamma globulin for the induction of an immune state.

Table 1-1. Resistance Mechanisms

Type of Resistance	Examples
Nonspecific	Mucous membranes
	Phagocytic cells
	Enzymes in secretions
	Interferon
Specific	
Naturally acquired	Placental transfer of antibody (passive)
	Recovery from disease (active)
Artificially acquired	Administration of antitoxin (passive)
	Vaccination (active)

4. Specific immune responses are mediated by two interrelated and interdependent **mechanisms**.
   a. **Humoral immunity** primarily involves **b**ursa- or **b**one marrow–derived **(B) lymphocytes, or B cells**.
      (1) The B cell expresses specific immunoglobulin on its surface.
      (2) When this surface immunoglobulin interacts with its matching (homologous) antigen, the B cell is triggered to proliferate and differentiate into plasma cells, which excrete vast quantities of immunoglobulin.
         (a) This immunoglobulin is specific for the same antigen that originally triggered the B cell.
         (b) Immunoglobulins, as proteins in the plasma fraction of the blood, comprise the **humoral** (i.e., **soluble**) component of the specific immune system.
   b. **Cell-mediated (cellular) immunity** primarily involves **t**hymus-derived **(T) lymphocytes, or T cells**.
      (1) The T cell expresses on its surface a receptor molecule that is structurally similar to an immunoglobulin and is similarly specific for its particular homologous antigen.
      (2) When the T cell receptor contacts its homologous antigen, this stimulates proliferation and differentiation of the T cell and its progeny.
         (a) The end product of this developmental process is a variety of T cell subsets with different functions.
         (b) These cells, which reside in the peripheral blood and lymphoid tissues, comprise the **cellular** (i.e., T cell–mediated) component of the specific immune system.
   c. As immunologic barriers to infection, humoral and cell-mediated responses usually work together to neutralize toxic materials or destroy pathogenic microorganisms.

5. **Terminology.** While the terms "humoral" and "cell-mediated" are usually used to refer to specific immune responses (i.e., involving antibodies or T cells), humoral and cellular responses can also be nonspecific (e.g., involving complement activation or phagocytic cells).

D. **Complement** (see Chapter 4). The complement system is a series of serum proteins that interact sequentially with one another.

1. Activation of the complement cascade can take place by either of two pathways.
   a. The **classic pathway** is activated by antibody complexed with its homologous antigen.
   b. The **alternative (properdin) pathway** is triggered by microorganisms and other materials, usually without the participation of antibody.

2. Once activated, the components of the complement system often work in conjunction with the innate immune system to rid the body of invading microbes.

II. COMPONENTS OF THE NONSPECIFIC IMMUNE SYSTEM

A. **Mechanical barriers to infection.** These contribute to innate immunity by inhibiting the attachment and penetration of infectious agents.

1. **Intact skin** is the first line of defense against infection. Consisting of the keratinized outer layer of dead cells and the successive layers of epidermis, undamaged skin is virtually impenetrable to all but a few organisms.

2. **Mucus** coats the epithelial cells of the mucosa, preventing contact between many pathogens and areas that are not covered by skin. Microorganisms and other particles are trapped in the viscous mucus and are removed by other mechanisms. For example:
   a. **Beating of cilia** on the epithelial cells in the respiratory tract removes contaminating microorganisms that become trapped in the mucus. Injury to this mechanism can be caused by smoking and alcoholism.
   b. **Coughing** and **sneezing** dislodge and help to expel the mucous blanket.

3. **Shedding of cells** that carry microbes provides a mechanical cleansing action.

4. Saliva, tears, perspiration, urine, and other body fluids assist in flushing microbes from the body.

5. Other body functions, such as vomiting and diarrhea, also eliminate pathogenic organisms.

B. Chemical and biochemical inhibitors of infection

1. Numerous substances found in body secretions provide a natural defense against microorganisms that invade the body (Table 1-2).

2. The **acid pH** found in most physiologic secretions prevents colonization by microorganisms.
   a. For example, urine and vaginal secretions, as well as the hydrochloric acid in the stomach, maintain acidic microenvironments.
   b. These environments kill most pathogenic microbes, while promoting the growth of non-pathogenic bacteria (e.g., lactobacilli).

C. Physiologic factors that contribute to innate immunity

1. **Body temperature.** Many organisms do not infect humans because they grow poorly at 37° C.

2. **Oxygen tension,** especially high in the lungs, inhibits growth of anaerobes.

3. **Hormonal balance.** An increase in corticosteroids decreases the inflammatory response and lowers resistance to infection. Thus, persons receiving cortisone for control of autoimmune disease or graft rejection have a heightened susceptibility to infectious agents.

4. **Age.** Persons who are very young (aged 3 years or younger) or very old (aged 75 or older) are much more susceptible to infection because their immune responsiveness is suboptimal.

D. Phagocytosis (Figure 1-1)

Table 1-2. Biological Activities of Secretory Products Important in Innate Immunity

Product	Mechanism of Action
Organic acids	Found at low pH in sebaceous gland secretions; many microbes susceptible to low concentrations
Fatty acids	Interfere with functions of the cell membrane
Saliva	Contains enzymes which damage the microbial cell wall and membrane and cause leakage of cytoplasm; also contains antibodies which opsonize microbes and, with the participation of complement, may lyse cells
Tears	Contain lysozyme, which lyses bacteria, particularly gram-positive bacteria, by destroying the bacterial cell wall
Lactoferrin	Binds iron, interfering with microbial acquisition of this essential metabolite
HCl	Denatures proteins
Bile acids	Interfere with vital functions of the cell membrane
Trypsin	Hydrolyzes proteins of cell membrane and wall
Mucus	Entraps foreign particles; sialic acid content blocks attachment of influenza virus to epithelial cells
Spermine	A pH-dependent polyamine found in sperm and seminal fluid; inhibits growth of gram-positive bacteria

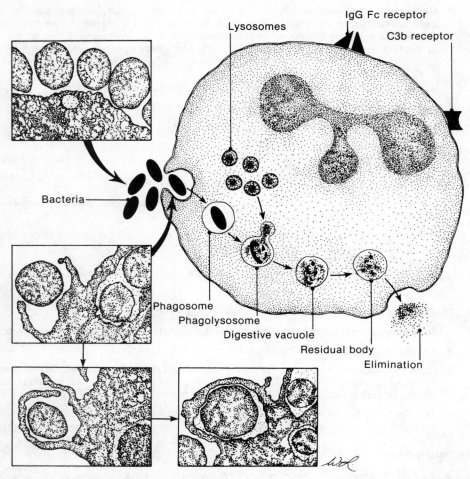

Figure 1-1. The process of phagocytosis. The electron microscopic views (*insets*) demonstrate the phagocytosis of a mycoplasma cell by a neutrophil. *IgG Fc receptor* = receptor for the Fc segment of immunoglobulin G; *C3b receptor* = receptor for complement component C3b.

1. General considerations
   a. Phagocytosis is the process by which particulate substances such as bacteria are ingested by a cell and destroyed.
   b. Phagocytosis is one form of **endocytosis** (the other form is **pinocytosis,** which is the internalization of fluids and solutes).
   c. Phagocytosis requires:
     (1) Energy generated through glucose metabolism
     (2) Synthesis of new cell membrane
     (3) An active cytoplasmic contractile protein system

2. Types of phagocytic cells
   a. Neutrophils (polymorphonuclear leukocytes, PMNs) are granulocytes that circulate in the blood and migrate quickly in response to local invasion by microorganisms.
   b. Monocytes also circulate in the blood but in much lower numbers than PMNs. They migrate to the tissues, where they differentiate into **macrophages,** which reside in all body tissues. For example:
     (1) Kupffer cells of the liver are macrophages.
     (2) Histiocytes in connective tissue are macrophages.
   c. While neutrophils, monocytes, and macrophages are not the only cells that phagocytize, they are the most important.

3. **Movements of phagocytic cells**
   a. **Ameboid movement.** Phagocytic cells migrate in and out of blood vessels and throughout the tissues. The process of cellular emigration from capillaries is called **diapedesis**.
   b. **Chemotaxis.** Phagocytes move toward other cells or organisms by cytoplasmic streaming in response to chemical agents called **chemotaxins** (Table 1-3).
4. **Ingestion and vacuole formation** (see Figure 1-1)
   a. When contact with a particle is made, the phagocytic cell engulfs it, surrounding the particle with a part of its cell membrane.
   b. Once the phagocyte engulfs the particle, the membrane enclosing the particle pinches off and moves into the cytoplasm of the cell, forming a phagocytic vacuole, or **phagosome**.
   c. **Lysosomes,** which are membrane-bound bags of enzymes, fuse with the phagosome to form a **phagolysosome.**
5. **Intracellular destruction.** Inside the phagolysosome, the engulfed material is digested.
   a. Lysosomes contain granules of two types.
      (1) **Primary granules** (also called **azurophilic granules** because they stain dark blue with Wright's stain) comprise 33% of all lysosomal granules. They contain many hydrolytic enzymes, myeloperoxidase, lysozyme, and arginine-rich basic (cationic) proteins.
      (2) **Secondary,** or **specific, granules** comprise 67% of all lysosomal granules. They contain alkaline phosphatase, lactoferrin, and lysozyme.
   b. Secondary granules release their contents into the phagosome first, usually before the vacuole has completely pinched off.
   c. The contents of the secondary granules are partially expelled into the interstitial space; this **reverse endocytosis** process is called **exocytosis,** or regurgitation.
      (1) When this process is accelerated and primary granule contents are also released into the extracellular space, **inflammation** and **tissue destruction** can occur.
      (2) Other mechanisms of phagocyte **degranulation** which can lead to tissue damage include:
         (a) Reverse endocytosis caused by immune complexes deposited on basement membranes (see Chapter 9 IV B)
         (b) Neutrophil cell death
         (c) Perforation of the cell membrane by ingested crystalline substances, such as monosodium urate in patients with gout
   d. The contents of the lysosomal granules are important in breaking down ingested material and in killing microorganisms. The granule contents destroy foreign particles by two mechanisms:
      (1) Certain proteins kill microorganisms by **oxygen-independent mechanisms:**
         (a) **Hydrolytic enzymes** include cathepsin, glycosidase, phosphatase, phospholipase, and arylsulfatase, which degrades the slow-reacting substance of anaphylaxis (SRS-A).

Table 1-3. Factors Chemotactic for Polymorphonuclear Leukocytes (PMNs)

Chemotaxin	Source	Comment
N-Formylmethionine	Bacteria	Activates arachidonic acid metabolism
Endotoxin	Bacteria	Activates the alternative complement pathway
Leukotrienes	Arachidonic acid	Products of the lipoxygenase pathway
C5a	Complement	Also causes degranulation of PMNs
Fibrinopeptides	Fibrinogen	Generated via fibrinolytic pathways
Histamine	Mast cells	Also increases capillary permeability
Platelet-activating factor (PAF)	Mast cells, PMNs	Also aggregates platelets and causes release of serotonin and histamine
Eosinophil chemotactic factor (ECF)	Mast cells	Peptide released on degranulation
Lymphokines	Lymphocytes	Some may also interfere with cell movement (e.g., migration inhibition factor; MIF)

6 *Chapter 1 II D*

      (b) Cationic proteins (not enzymes but basic peptides containing large amounts of arginine in polypeptide form—e.g., nuclear histones) kill microbes by interacting with essential microbial enzymes and transport proteins.

      (c) Lysozyme, a mucopeptidase, attacks bacterial cell walls (see II F 2 g).

      (d) Lactoferrin acts by binding iron (see II F 2 e).

    (2) Other microbicidal compounds are generated by **oxygen-dependent mechanisms** in the respiratory burst that accompanies phagocytosis.

6. Respiratory burst during phagocytosis

    a. Metabolic events during phagocytosis are accompanied by a cellular respiratory burst that produces a number of **toxic oxygen metabolites** (Table 1-4).

    b. In the respiratory burst, the following events take place:

      (1) Oxygen consumption increases.

      (2) Hexose monophosphate shunt (HMPS) activity is stimulated.

      (3) Production of **hydrogen peroxide (H_2O_2)** increases. H_2O_2 is a reactive oxidizing agent that kills microbes.

      (4) Superoxide anion, singlet oxygen, and hydroxyl radicals are produced.

        (a) Superoxide anion is molecular oxygen that has picked up an extra electron.

          (i) Superoxide anion is extremely toxic to bacteria and tissue, but it is very unstable. It is quickly converted to H_2O_2 by the enzyme **superoxide dismutase.**

          (ii) H_2O_2 is still toxic to bacteria but is not as potent. The H_2O_2 is broken down by the enzyme **catalase.**

          (iii) A flaw in the formation of superoxide anion and eventually of H_2O_2 is found in the neutrophils of persons suffering from chronic granulomatous disease (CGD; see Chapter 11 II B 1).

        (b) In **singlet oxygen,** one of the electrons has moved to an orbit of higher energy.

        (c) Hydroxyl radicals are highly unstable oxidizing agents that react with most organic molecules they encounter.

      (5) Myeloperoxidase, in the presence of toxic oxygen metabolites such as H_2O_2, catalyzes toxic peroxidation of a variety of microorganisms. Myeloperoxidase comprises 7% of the weight of neutrophils.

    c. The oxygen-dependent agents can combine and act synergistically, as in reaction 3 of Table 1-4.

      (1) Hypochlorite, the product of the reaction, is more antimicrobial than each of its three components [myeloperoxidase, H_2O_2, and halide (a chloride ion)] alone.

      (2) There are several **mechanisms** whereby such an activated halide could damage microorganisms; for example:

        (a) Halogenation of the bacterial cell wall

        (b) Decarboxylation of amino acids with the resultant production of toxic aldehydes

7. Secreted products. In addition to the intracellular destruction of foreign particles, macrophages also secrete many compounds that have a protective effect in the body. Among these are:

    a. Factors that influence **cell differentiation** (e.g., colony-stimulating factor)

Table 1-4. Production of Toxic Oxygen Metabolites during the Respiratory Burst that Accompanies Phagocytosis

1. Enzymatic generation of superoxide anion

    Glucose + NADP (via the HMPS) → NADPH + pentose phosphate

    NADPH + oxygen + NADPH oxidase → NADP + superoxide anion

2. Spontaneous generation of singlet oxygen, hydrogen peroxide, and hydroxyl radicals

    Superoxide anion + hydrogen ions → hydrogen peroxide + singlet oxygen

    Superoxide anion + hydrogen peroxide → hydroxyl radicals + singlet oxygen

3. Enzymatic generation of halogenating compounds

    Hydrogen peroxide + halide (e.g., a chloride ion) + myeloperoxidase → hypochlorite

HMPS = hexose monophosphate shunt pathway of glycolysis; NADP, NADPH = nicotinamide adenine dinucleotide phosphate and its reduced form, respectively.

   b. Cytotoxic factors [e.g., tumor necrosis factor α (TNF-α; cachectin)]
   c. Hydrolytic enzymes (e.g., proteinases such as collagenase, lipase, and phosphatase)
   d. Endogenous pyrogen (interleukin-1; IL-1)
   e. Complement components C1 to C5, and properdin and factors B, D, I, and H of the alternative pathway
   f. Alpha interferon
   g. Various **plasma proteins** and **coagulation factors**
   h. Oxygen metabolites such as H_2O_2 and superoxide anion
   i. Arachidonic acid metabolites such as prostaglandins, thromboxanes, and leukotrienes

  8. Tests for measuring phagocytic function are described in Chapter 8 IV A.

E. Opsonization

  1. Opsonins are substances that bind to particles and make them more susceptible to phagocytosis.
   a. Phagocytosis can occur in a very simple system. For example, if neutrophils, saline, and bacteria are combined, phagocytosis will occur.
   b. Phagocytosis can be remarkably enhanced in the presence of serum or plasma, however, because the blood constituent contains opsonins.

  2. Opsonins found in serum include the following:
   a. Split products of the complement cascade
     (1) Complement component C3b is the most important complement-derived opsonin; components iC3b and C5b are also active in this process.
     (2) Phagocytic cells possess membrane receptors for these molecules (Table 1-5; see also Figure 1-1).
     (3) Thus, bacteria and other foreign particles with one of these molecules on their surface will have an enhanced interaction with the phagocyte.
   b. Antibodies
     (1) Phagocytic cells have a receptor (see Figure 1-1) for the Fc portion of the IgG molecule (see Chapter 3 Figure 3-1), thus enhancing the strength of interaction between the cell and the antibody-coated (i.e., antibody-opsonized) particle that is being engulfed.
     (2) IgG1 and IgG3 are the most active in this process; IgG2, IgG4, and IgA (see Chapter 3 III A, B) may also be opsonins for phagocytosis.
   c. Other opsonins in serum
     (1) Fibronectin is a glycoprotein that opsonizes and acts like glue to cause neutrophils and their targets to stick together.
     (2) Leukotrienes are derivatives of arachidonic acid; some of the leukotrienes are opsonins. Leukotriene LTB_4 is chemotactic as well.
     (3) Tuftsin, a tetrapeptide split product of an IgG-like molecule called **leukokinin,** is found in the spleen. Tuftsin stimulates chemotactic and phagocytic activities.

F. Humoral factors contributing to nonspecific immunity

  1. Antibody-mediated complement activation in bacteriolysis
   a. Normal serum can kill and lyse gram-negative bacteria.
     (1) This property is probably due to the combined action of antibody and complement, both of which are present in normal serum.

Table 1-5. Phagocytic Cell Receptors for Complement-Derived Opsonins

Receptor	Complement Component Recognized	Function
CR1	C4b, C3b, iC3b	Aids target cell ingestion; allows factor I to cleave C3b to C3dg; important in clearing immune complexes from the body
CR3	iC3b	Aids target cell ingestion; important in cell adherence to surfaces
CR4	iC3b, C3dg	Not well studied but presumed to aid in attachment of phagocyte to target

(2) The activity is destroyed by heating at 56° C for 30 minutes, due to the inactivation of complement.
  b. Bacteriolysis begins with the lytic action of antibody-activated complement on the outer lipopolysaccharide layer of the cell wall (see Chapter 4 III B 4).
   (1) A bacterial cell wall contains two layers: an outer membrane layer of lipoproteins and lipopolysaccharide and an inner layer of mucopeptide (peptidoglycan).
   (2) The antibody and complement disrupt the lipopolysaccharide layer of the cell wall. Complement becomes an esterase, which provides for the majority of this enzymatic activity.
  c. Once the lipopolysaccharide layer is weakened, lysozyme, a mucopeptidase present in serum, can enter and destroy the mucopeptide layer (see II F 2 g).
  d. The end result is the destruction of the bacterial cell.
2. Nonantibody humoral factors contributing to nonspecific immunity
  a. Chemotactic factors attract phagocytes; the chemotaxin C5a is an extremely important split product of C5 generated during complement activation.
  b. Properdin is involved in complement activation by the alternative pathway (see Chapter 4 II C). As a bactericide, properdin is believed to work in conjunction with antibody and complement (plus magnesium ions).
  c. Interferons are proteins produced, usually, by virally infected cells, and they protect other cells in the area. (Although there are other triggers for interferon release, virus infection is the most common and natural one.)
   (1) Types of interferons
    (a) Alpha interferon—secreted by macrophages and other leukocytes—is induced by viruses or synthetic polynucleotides.
    (b) Beta interferon—secreted by fibroblasts—is also induced by viruses or synthetic polynucleotides.
    (c) Gamma interferon—also called **immune interferon**—is secreted by T lymphocytes following stimulation with the specific antigen to which the lymphocyte has been sensitized.
   (2) Protective effects of interferons
    (a) Interferons activate cellular genes, inducing neighboring cells to produce antiviral proteins that interfere with the translation of viral messenger RNA (mRNA).
    (b) Interferons block viral translation by two enzyme-mediated processes.
      (i) Protein kinase transfers a phosphate group from adenosine triphosphate (ATP) to an initiation factor required for protein synthesis. This phosphorylation inactivates the initiation factor, and viral protein synthesis is inhibited.
      (ii) Oligonucleotide polymerase synthesizes adenine trinucleotide. This activates an endonuclease which cleaves mRNA, preventing viral replication.
    (c) Other protective actions of interferons are to:
      (i) Enhance T cell activity
      (ii) Activate macrophages
      (iii) Enhance the expression of major histocompatibility complex (MHC) molecules on cell membranes
      (iv) Increase the cytotoxic action of natural killer (NK) cells
  d. Beta lysin is an antibacterial protein released from blood platelets when they rupture, as in clot formation. It is active primarily against gram-positive bacteria.
  e. Lactoferrin and **transferrin** are iron-binding proteins that compete with bacteria for that essential metabolite.
  f. Lactoperoxidase is found in saliva and milk. Its mechanism of action is similar to that of myeloperoxidase [see II D 6 b (5); Table 1-4].
  g. Lysozyme hydrolyzes the mucopeptide layer of the cell wall of many different bacteria, making the cell susceptible to osmotic lysis. This enzyme is present in serum, tears, saliva, nasal secretions, and other body fluids, as well as in lysosomal granules.

G. Lymphocytic cells contributing to nonspecific immunity. Certain lymphocytic cells are cytotoxic against a variety of targets in the absence of any previous exposure to the targets.

  1. Natural killer cells. These large granular lymphocytes appear to function in immune surveillance (see Chapter 13 III B).
   a. Source and location
    (1) NK cells are innate, or naturally occurring cytotoxic lymphocytes: they are present in the body from the time of birth and are not induced by immunologic insult.

(2) They arise from bone marrow precursors but are of a lineage distinct from that of either T or B cells.

(3) NK cells make up 10% to 15% of the lymphocytes in the peripheral blood and 1% to 2% of the lymphocytes in the spleen. They are absent from the lymph nodes.

b. Functions

(1) NK cells are cytotoxic for tumor cells and virally infected autologous cells.

(2) They also have been reported to play a role in resistance to some bacterial, fungal, and parasitic infections, and to participate in regulation of the immune response through the secretion of lymphokines such as IL-2.

(3) Recent evidence suggests that NK cells, not killer (K) cells, may be responsible for antibody-dependent cell-mediated cytotoxicity (ADCC; see II G 2).

c. Mode of action

(1) NK cells kill their targets by perforating the cell membrane, causing holes to form.

(a) The molecules that are responsible for the pore formation are called **perforins**.

(i) Following intimate cellular contact, perforins are released from granules within the NK cell cytoplasm.

(ii) The perforins insert into the target cell membrane and polymerize, in the presence of calcium ions, forming channels within the cytoplasmic membrane of the target cell.

(b) The end result is depolarization, abnormal ion flux, and essential metabolite leakage from the cytoplasm.

(2) NK cells have a membrane receptor for the Fc portion of antibodies IgG1 and IgG3 [see II G 2 b (2)], but will kill targets in the absence of antibody.

(3) Their target range is broad, and they are not subject to MHC restriction. That is, cytotoxicity by NK cells does not require that the NK cell recognize MHC molecules on the target cells (see Chapter 5 IV D).

(4) NK cells release numerous cytokines during their interaction with the target cells, including alpha and gamma interferons, IL-1 and IL-2, B cell growth factor (IL-4), and lymphotoxin (TNF-β).

(5) The cytotoxic activity of NK cells can be significantly enhanced by exposure to IL-2 and the interferons.

(6) NK cells do not possess antigenic specificity and do not acquire immunologic memory following exposure to virus-infected cells or tumor cells.

2. Antibody-dependent cytotoxic cells. These cells can kill target cells without the participation of complement, if the target cells are coated with specific antibody.

a. Functions. ADCC is thought to play a role in antitumor and antigraft immunity and may be involved in antiviral protection as well.

b. Types of cells

(1) ADCC has been attributed to a unique subset of lymphocytes called **killer (K) cells**.

(2) It has recently been proposed, however, that ADCC is really due to cells that bear the CD16 molecule.

(a) The CD16 molecule is found on NK cells and a subset of T lymphocytes.

(b) CD16 is a membrane receptor for the Fc portion of IgG1 and IgG3, which would explain the mechanism of target recognition and interaction.

(3) In addition to NK cells, macrophages and neutrophils also participate in ADCC.

3. Lymphokine-activated killer (LAK) cells

a. The LAK cell is another naturally occurring cytotoxic cell. It is a quiescent lymphocyte that is induced into an active cytotoxic state by IL-2, a lymphokine.

b. The LAK cell is similar in many ways to the NK cell but has an even broader target cell range.

4. Tumor-infiltrating lymphocytes (TILs) are a type of LAK cell that has been cultured in vitro with IL-2 in the presence of a specific tumor cell. TILs demonstrate enhanced tumoricidal activity when infused back into the donor of the lymphocytes and tumor cells.

STUDY QUESTIONS

Directions: Each of the numbered items or incomplete statements in this section is followed by answers or by completions of the statement. Select the **one** lettered answer or completion that is **best** in each case.

1. Examples of innate resistance processes include

(A) transplacental passage of IgG
(B) response to vaccination
(C) flushing action of tears
(D) recovery from an infection
(E) administration of antitoxin

2. The process by which normal serum enhances phagocytosis is called

(A) chemotaxis
(B) opsonization
(C) proteolysis
(D) bacteriolysis
(E) exocytosis

3. Interferons can best be described as

(A) interfering directly with translation of viral messenger RNA (mRNA)
(B) interfering with viral adsorption onto the cell membrane
(C) inducing the production of antiviral proteins that interfere with translation of viral mRNA
(D) blocking the penetration of viruses into susceptible cells
(E) inducing host cell RNase that hydrolyzes the viral genome

4. The respiratory system is protected from microorganisms by all of the following factors EXCEPT

(A) ciliary propulsion of the mucous blanket upward to the oropharynx
(B) body temperature regulation at 37° C
(C) expulsion of mucus-entrapped microbes by the cough reflex
(D) the low pulmonary oxygen tension
(E) the action of alveolar macrophages

5. Antimicrobial products of the myeloperoxidase system include all of the following EXCEPT

(A) superoxide anions
(B) toxic aldehydes
(C) lysozyme
(D) hypochlorite
(E) hydrogen peroxide

6. All of the following substances are found in the lysosomal granules of phagocytic cells EXCEPT

(A) phosphatases
(B) cationic proteins
(C) mucopeptidase
(D) lactoferrin
(E) endogenous pyrogen

7. Innate immunity can be defined as the

(A) immunity resulting from vaccination
(B) protection acquired via placental passage of maternal antibodies
(C) naturally occurring, nonspecific defense mechanisms that provide protection from infectious agents
(D) resistance to infectious diseases acquired via subclinical infections
(E) resistance to infectious diseases based on specific recognition of the causative agent

8. Characteristics of adaptive immunity include all of the following EXCEPT

(A) induction
(B) specificity
(C) immunologic memory
(D) phagocytosis
(E) recognition of self

9. Macrophage-produced products with antiviral activity include

(A) interferon
(B) lysozyme
(C) both
(D) neither

10. Oxygen-dependent antimicrobial products generated by the macrophage include

(A) hydrogen peroxide
(B) hypochlorite
(C) both
(D) neither

1-C	4-D	7-C	10-C
2-B	5-C	8-D	
3-C	6-E	9-A	

ANSWERS AND EXPLANATIONS

1. The answer is C *[I C 3; II A 4; Table 1-1].*
Innate immune processes are those which are present in the absence of any antigenic exposure. The flushing action of tears is an example. This process is active independent of antigen exposure, and regardless of prior microbial encounters. Transplacental passage of IgG, on the other hand, is a form of naturally acquired passive immunity, in which maternal antibodies, evoked in response to a specific antigenic challenge, cross the placenta and afford the fetus passive protection. This, as well as recovery from disease, is a natural process, but it is not an example of innate immunity. Vaccination is an example of active artificially acquired immunity, and administration of antitoxin is an example of passive artificially acquired immunity.

2. The answer is B *[II E 1].*
Opsonization is the process whereby phagocytosis is enhanced through coating of the foreign particle by an opsonin such as antibody or complement. Chemotaxis is the movement of cells either toward a stimulus (positive chemotaxis) or away from it (negative chemotaxis). Proteolysis is the breakup of protein molecules. Bacteriolysis is the dissolution of bacterial cells; it can occur through enzymatic attack on the cell wall or through the action of antibiotics on cell wall synthesis. Enzymatic proteolysis and bacteriolysis would occur during the digestive phase of phagocytosis that follows the formation of the phagolysosome. Exocytosis, also called reverse endocytosis, occurs when the contents of the lysosomal granules are expelled from the phagocytic vacuole into the extracellular environment.

3. The answer is C *[II F 2 c (2)].*
Interferons induce the cell to produce an oligonucleotide polymerase which synthesizes adenine trinucleotide; this activates an endonuclease in the cell that degrades viral messenger RNA (mRNA). Interferons also induce the host cell to produce other inhibitors of RNA and protein. In addition, interferons activate macrophages and natural killer (NK) cells and increase the expression of class I major histocompatibility complex (MHC) molecules on cell membranes, further amplifying their antiviral activity. There are no antiviral compounds known today that interfere directly with translation of viral mRNA. Certain antiviral agents used in clinical medicine, such as amantadine, inhibit viral adsorption to or penetration of host cells. Antibody is most effective in blocking viral adsorption onto a cell membrane.

4. The answer is D *[II C 2].*
The oxygen tension in the lungs is high, thus inhibiting the growth of anaerobes, whereas low oxygen tension would favor the growth of many human pathogens. Mucus entraps inhaled microorganisms. These are removed from the respiratory tract via the ciliary "escalator," which delivers them to the esophagus, where they are swallowed or expelled from the body by the cough reflex. Body temperature contributes to natural resistance, since many organisms grow poorly at 37° C (e.g., the dermatophytic fungi). The alveolar macrophages (also called dust cells) are the scavenger cells that ingest and dispose of inhaled foreign materials.

5. The answer is C *[II D 5 d (1) (c), 6; Table 1-4].*
Lysozyme is oxygen-independent. It is an enzymatic component of the lysosomal granule that hydrolyzes the mucopeptide (peptidoglycan) layer of the bacterial cell wall. The myeloperoxidase system is an oxygen-dependent system. In the presence of toxic oxygen metabolites such as hydrogen peroxide, myeloperoxidase catalyzes toxic peroxidation of a variety of microorganisms. Antimicrobial products of the myeloperoxidase system, in addition to toxic aldehydes and superoxide anions, include singlet oxygen, hydrogen peroxide, and myeloperoxidase itself, working in concert with halide ions to produce hypochlorite, which is a potent microbicide.

6. The answer is E *[II D 5 d, 7 d].*
Endogenous pyrogen (interleukin-1; IL-1) is not present in lysosomes. It is secreted by macrophages and has a major effect on the T cells of the specific immune system. Lysosomal granules contain many proteins that kill microorganisms via oxygen-independent means, such as phosphatases, cationic proteins, mucopeptidase, and lactoferrin. Other microbicidal compounds are oxygen-dependent, including hydrogen peroxide, superoxide anion, and singlet oxygen. The low pH attained intracellularly is also antimicrobial.

7. The answer is C *[I A, B].*
Innate immunity is a complex system of nonspecific, naturally occurring defense mechanisms that protect individuals from infectious disease. By contrast, acquired (adaptive) immunity is a specific immunologic

response that occurs following accidental exposure (e.g., infection) or deliberate exposure (e.g., a vaccination) to a foreign agent. Adaptive immunity can be acquired actively, such as by subclinical infection, or passively, such as by transplacental passage of antibody to the human fetus.

8. The answer is D *[I C 2].*
Phagocytosis is an innate, not adaptive, process that affords protection against many different pathogens. The four characteristics that are essential to adaptive (acquired) immunity are (1) the presence of an induction phase, (2) the ability to distinguish between self and nonself, (3) immunologic specificity, and (4) immunologic memory. Immunologic memory is the basis of the anamnestic response, wherein a rapid production of antibody to produce a high serum level is achieved upon secondary antigenic exposure.

9. The answer is A *[II F 2 c, g].*
Macrophages produce both lysozyme and alpha interferon. However, lysozyme is an antibacterial agent, not an antiviral agent. Found in the macrophage lysosome, lysozyme causes the breakdown of peptidoglycan in the bacterial cell wall. Interferons are antiviral proteins produced by various cells of the body in response to viral infection or in response to polynucleotides that have been ingested or pinocytosed. The polynucleotides induce the cell to produce proteins that interfere with the replication of viruses. Interferons induce cells to make products which inhibit viral replication. These products include a specific RNase and inhibitors of RNA and protein synthesis.

10. The answer is C *[II D 6 b, c; Table 1-4].*
Digestion of foreign particles within the phagolysosome of the macrophage is accompanied by a respiratory burst that creates a number of microbicidal oxygen-derived free radicals (e.g., superoxide anion). Hydrogen peroxide is a reactive oxidizing microbicidal agent. It is a less potent antimicrobial than hypochlorite, to which it contributes. Hypochlorite killing is an oxygen-dependent process requiring myeloperoxidase enzyme, hydrogen peroxide, and a halide (in this case a chloride ion).

I. DEFINITIONS

A. Antigens. The immune response is characterized by the production of either proteins, called antibodies, or specifically reactive lymphocytes, called T cells, when an animal encounters a foreign macromolecule or cell.

1. The foreign substances that induce an immune response possess two properties.
   a. **Immunogenicity** is the inherent ability of a substance (**immunogen**) to induce a specific immune response, resulting in the formation of antibodies or immune lymphocytes.
   b. **Antigenicity,** or **specific reactivity,** is the property of a substance (**antigen**) that causes it to react specifically with the antibody or lymphocyte that it caused to be produced.

2. The property of antigenicity is extremely important. It is probably the most specific reaction known in biology.

3. Immunogenic substances are always antigenic, whereas antigens are not necessarily immunogenic (e.g., autologous serum proteins).

B. Haptens

1. Haptens are partial antigens. That is:
   a. Haptens are **antigenic:** they can react with immune lymphocytes or antibodies.
   b. However, haptens are **not immunogenic:** they cannot by themselves cause the production of immune lymphocytes or antibodies.

2. Haptens are usually molecules which are too small to be immunogenic.
   a. Examples of haptens are antibiotics, analgesics, and other low-molecular-weight compounds.
   b. **Penicillin,** for example, a clinically important hapten, has a molecular weight of 320 daltons (0.3 kDa).

3. If a hapten is coupled to a larger **carrier molecule,** however, it becomes endowed with immunogenicity.
   a. The carrier molecules may be albumins, globulins, or synthetic polypeptides.
   b. Drugs often couple with carriers in the body and thereby acquire immunogenicity. A classic example in clinical medicine is the **allergic response** of some persons to **penicillin**.
      (1) The penicilloic acid moiety of penicillin, acting as a hapten, can couple with body protein and elicit an immune response.
      (2) The immune response can be harmful, even life-threatening (see Chapter 9 II), thus excluding this antibiotic from use in certain individuals.

C. Epitopes

1. **Definition**
   a. Epitopes (also called **determinant groups,** or **antigenic determinants**) are the sites either on or within the antigen with which antibodies react.
   b. Epitopes and haptens are similar, but while a hapten is artificially added to a molecule, an epitope is an integral part of the native molecule.

2. **Physical properties**
   a. Epitopes are very small (e.g., just four or five amino acid or monosaccharide residues).

   b. The epitopes on an antigen can be **linear** (i.e., continuous within the amino acid sequence of the molecule) or **conformational** (i.e., containing amino acids that end up in the same area on the surface of the protein but are not adjacent in the peptide chain) [Figure 2-1].

   c. Some antibody-binding sites (i.e., epitopes) are on the antigen's **surface** (topographic); others are **internal**.

      (1) Internal epitopes are only expressed after the antigen has been ''processed'' by a phagocytic cell.

      (2) Epitopes are immunoreactive only if their amino acids are spatially accessible due to tertiary protein structure (see V C).

  3. Epitopes and antibody specificity

   a. Epitopes determine the specificity of the antigen molecule and are what induce the antibody response.

   b. Antibodies are specific for epitopes.

   c. Antigens are multivalent; that is, an antigen molecule carries a number of different epitopes —sometimes hundreds of them—some specifying antibody ''A,'' others antibody ''B,'' and so forth. The **valence** of an antigen is equal to the total number of epitopes the antigen possesses.

  4. Molecular changes. Antigen molecules can be artificially manipulated by altering, adding, or taking away epitopes. With each change, antigenicity is altered.

   a. New antigens are produced by altering these epitopes. This can be done by conjugating haptens to the molecule.

   b. Denaturation or hydrolysis of the protein will almost always destroy conformational epitopes.

D. Adjuvants (see also Chapter 6 IV B). Nonspecific stimulation of the immune response can occur via adjuvants (e.g., complete Freund's adjuvant, a mixture of killed mycobacteria and oil).

  1. These substances enhance the immunogenicity of molecules without altering their chemical composition.

  2. The **mechanisms** by which adjuvants exert their biological effects are multiple.

   a. Adjuvants may increase the efficiency of macrophage processing of antigens.

   b. Adjuvants can act as depots and prolong the period of exposure to the immunogen.

   c. Adjuvants may amplify the proliferation of immunologically committed lymphocytes by enhancing the release or the action of lymphokines.

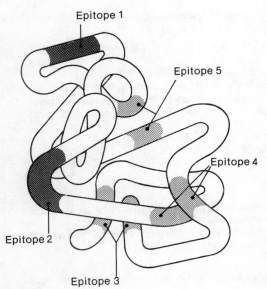

Figure 2-1. Model of epitopes on lysozyme. The *shaded areas* are the specific epitopes. They are composed of chain segments that are either linear (epitopes 1 and 2) or conformational (epitopes 3–5). (Adapted from Klein J: *Immunology: The Science of Self–Nonself Discrimination.* New York, Wiley, 1982, p 356.)

II. PROPERTIES OF IMMUNOGENICITY

A. General considerations. The degree of immunogenicity of a molecule is influenced by several factors. The relationship can be expressed algebraically by the following formula:

$$\text{Immunogenicity} = (\text{foreignness})\,(\text{chemical complexity})\,(\text{molecular size})$$

B. Foreignness

1. An antigen must be foreign or alien to the host with which it makes contact.

2. The greater the phylogenetic difference, the more foreign something becomes. The use of transplant terminology helps to clarify this concept.

   a. **Autologous antigens** are found within the same individual; that is, they are not foreign to that individual. For example, a skin graft from an individual's thigh to his chest is an **autograft,** and is not foreign.

   b. **Syngeneic antigens** are found in genetically identical individuals (e.g., individuals from an inbred strain of mice or identical twins). A graft between members of an inbred strain is a **syngeneic graft** or an **isograft,** and is not foreign.

   c. **Allogeneic antigens (alloantigens)** are found in genetically dissimilar members of the same species. For example, a kidney transplant from mother to daughter is called an **allograft** or a **homograft,** and it is foreign.

   (1) Some alloantigens, called **isoantigens,** are found in some members of a species and not in others.

   (2) The A and B blood group antigens are examples of isoantigens.

   d. **Xenogeneic (heterogeneic) antigens** are found in different species. For example, a transplant of monkey kidneys to humans is called a **heterograft** or **xenograft,** and it is foreign. The term **heterologous** is also sometimes used as a synonym for xenogeneic.

3. **Special types of antigens**

   a. **Heterogenetic (heterophile or heterophil) antigens** are a type of xenogeneic antigen.

   (1) Heterophile antigens occur in different species and have several particular characteristics:

   (a) They are **cross-reacting** (i.e., they combine with antibody induced by a different but closely related antigen).

   (b) They occur in phylogenetically unrelated species.

   (2) The principle of the **cross-reacting heterophile antibody response** has a practical application as it provides the basis for several **clinical tests**.

   (a) The spirochete that causes **syphilis** has a heterophile antigen similar to a hapten called **cardiolipin** that is found in beef heart muscle. This heterophile antigen forms the basis of a diagnostic test for syphilis.

   (b) The heterophile antibody response can also be used in the diagnosis of **infectious mononucleosis** caused by the **Epstein-Barr virus,** as most of the patients have present in their serum an antibody that reacts with sheep red blood cells (SRBCs).

   (c) Serum from patients with **rickettsial** infections agglutinate certain strains of *Proteus vulgaris* (OX19, OX2, OXK). This heterophilic immune response is termed the **Weil-Felix reaction.**

   b. **Sequestered antigens**

   (1) Antibodies are not ordinarily made to autologous brain or cornea protein because these substances do not come in contact with antibody-producing cells since they are inaccessible to antibody-forming lymphoid tissues (i.e., they are "sequestered"). For example, the central nervous system and cornea are devoid of lymphatics, and the cornea is also nonvascularized; both lymphatics and blood vessels are required for an immune response.

   (2) If sequestered antigens are released (i.e., if sequestered tissue is exposed to the antibody-producing lymphoreticular system), then an immune response may result.

   (3) Experimental allergic encephalomyelitis can be produced in animals by injection of homologous or heterologous brain tissue in Freund's adjuvant (see Chapter 6 IV B 1). The antigen is a basic protein in myelin.

4. **Tissue-specific (organ-specific) antigens**

   a. Various organs have in their makeup certain antigens unique to those organs.

   (1) **Thyroid** has an organ-specific antigen, **thyroglobulin.**

(a) Any thyroid from any species contains this unique thyroid antigen.
(b) An immune response to this antigen is seen in patients with Hashimoto's thyroid-itis (see Chapter 10 II I).
(2) **Basic protein** exists in brain tissue regardless of species, and it does not exist in any other organ. Basic protein has been implicated in experimental allergic encephalo-myelitis (see Chapter 10 II E).
(a) A sequence of amino acids in basic protein resembles a sequence in hepatitis B viral polymerase; the viral peptide elicits an immune response that causes inflam-mation of the central nervous system.
(b) This type of immunologic damage due to cross-reacting epitopes is referred to as **antigenic mimicry**.
b. Certain epitopes are found on selected cells. For example, mature thymus-derived lym-phocytes (T cells) bear the CD3 marker in their membranes (see Chapter 5 III B 2 a).

C. Chemical complexity

1. With the exception of pure lipids, most macromolecular organic chemical groupings can be immunogens.
   a. **Proteins.** The majority of immunogens are proteins.
   (1) Proteins are the strongest antigens, because they have the largest array of potential building blocks (amino acids).
   (a) This diversity imparts epitopes of differing specificities to the molecule.
   (b) The total immune response will be the sum of all the individual antibodies that are produced.
   (2) Immunogenicity can be enhanced by adding haptens (i.e., epitopes) to the molecule.
   (3) **Lipoproteins** are a complex type of protein immunogen that exist as part of many cell membranes.
   b. **Polysaccharides**
   (1) Most polysaccharides are haptens or incomplete immunogens.
   (a) They do not possess sufficient chemical diversity for full immunogenicity.
   (b) In addition, they are usually rapidly degraded when they enter a host; thus they are not in contact with the immune apparatus long enough to induce a response.
   (2) However, polysaccharides can be immunogens, occurring in two forms:
   (a) **Pure polysaccharide** substances (e.g., the capsular polysaccharides that are re-sponsible for the protective immune response to the pneumococcus)
   (b) **Lipopolysaccharides** (e.g., the endotoxins that occur within the cell membranes of gram-negative bacteria)
   c. **Glycoproteins**
   (1) The immunogenicity of glycoproteins is best illustrated by the A and B blood group antigens and the Rh antigens.
   (2) The A and B substances are strong immunogens, and the immune response they in-duce is to the carbohydrate epitope of the molecule.
   d. **Polypeptides**
   (1) Polypeptide immunogens include hormones (e.g., insulin, growth hormone) and syn-thetic compounds (e.g., polylysine).
   (2) Polypeptides are usually weakly immunogenic.
   e. **Nucleic acids and nucleoproteins**
   (1) **Nucleic acids** are considered to be nonimmunogenic; however, when single-stranded, they can act as immunogens.
   (2) **Nucleoproteins** are stronger immunogens because the nucleic acid is coupled to pro-tein. In patients with systemic lupus erythematosus (SLE), antibodies to autologous nucleoproteins are produced (see Chapter 10 II B 2 b).
   f. **Lipids.** These are also nonimmunogenic, although a few (e.g., cardiolipin) can function as haptens.

2. Bacterial and mammalian cells are strong immunogens, and present a vast array of different epitopes to the host.

D. Molecular size. Usually, the larger the molecule, the better the immunogen (Table 2-1), although there are exceptions.

Table 2-1. Relationship of Molecular Size to Immunogenicity

Molecule	Size (kDa)	Relative Immunogenicity
Hemocyanin	1000	+ + + +
Gamma globulin	160	+ + +
Diphtheria toxin	58	+ +
Insulin	6	+
Vasopressin	1	+/−
Aspirin	0.18	−

1. As a general rule, molecules below 5 kDa will not be immunogenic. Reasonable immune responses will be induced by molecules like serum albumin (40 kDa).
2. Size is important for several reasons:
   a. The number of epitopes increases proportionately with the size of the protein.
   b. Larger size means that the molecule will be phagocytized.
      (1) Antibodies to most antigens are formed much more efficiently if the antigen is first "processed" by a macrophage (see Chapter 5 IV A 2); this involves phagocytosis of the antigen.
      (2) Antigens that are difficult or impossible to phagocytize are not immunogenic at times.

III. USE OF IMMUNOGENS IN VACCINATION

A. Purpose. The result of active immunization (see Chapter 7 I B; II) is the production of protective antibodies or specifically sensitized lymphocytes.

B. Examples of bacterial immunogens

1. All gram-negative flagellated bacteria (e.g., *Salmonella typhi*) contain two types of antigens to which the host organism makes different antibodies. The two antigens are:
   a. The **H antigens,** referring to the **flagella**
   b. The **O antigens,** referring to the **body** of the organism
2. **Bacterial virulence factors as immunogens**
   a. Any bacterial cell is potentially a good immunogen, since hundreds of different antibodies are formed in response to the bacterial cell.
   b. However, the only protective antibodies are those directed against the cell's **virulence factors,** the factors of the bacterial cell that give it the ability to cause disease.
      (1) The polysaccharides of the **pneumococcal capsule** must be neutralized if the virulence of the pneumococcus is to be overcome, since the capsule is antiphagocytic.
      (2) Protection from **diphtheria and tetanus toxins** can be obtained if antibodies to these toxins are produced, since the toxins are what cause the diseases.
      (3) **Lipopolysaccharide endotoxin** is a major virulence factor for gram-negative bacteria, and antibody against this endotoxin is needed for protection.

IV. BASIS OF ANTIGEN SPECIFICITY. The exquisite sensitivity of the immune response has its basis in molecular differences in antigenic structure. Several examples follow.

A. Differences in position within the molecule

1. This aspect of the specificity of the immune response has been studied in relation to haptens, as illustrated in Figures 2-2 and 2-3.
   a. Haptens can be, for example, side chains of benzene rings, or substituted benzene rings. Attaching these to protein molecules renders them immunogenic; the immune response can then be mounted against both the carrier protein and the hapten.
   b. All of the substituted groups shown in Figure 2-2 are in the para position; however, the para-substituted group is different in each case.
      (1) The immune response generated by any one of the conjugated hapten groups in Figure 2-2 is completely cross-reactive against the others.

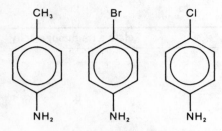

Figure 2-2. Examples of cross-reactive substituted benzene haptens. Antibody raised against any one of the haptens shown will cross-react with the other two haptens. However, a hapten with a carboxyl group in the para position would not react with antibody against the illustrated haptens.

  (2) Apparently, the host can recognize the para position but not the substituent groups (as long as these remain chemically similar).
  c. On the other hand, the host can distinguish between ortho and para positions (see Figure 2-3), and the antibodies formed are not cross-reactive.

2. The extreme specificity of the immune response is used in the identification of several biologically important molecules in human serum (Table 2-2).

B. Differences in glycosidic linkages. A clinically relevant example is provided by the capsular antigens of the pneumococcus, one of the major causes of lobar pneumonia.

1. The pneumococcus has more than 80 different immunologic types of capsular polysaccharide, and an antibody to one type does not react with an antigen of another type.

2. The capsular polysaccharides are structurally different, which accounts for their antigenic differences.
  a. The type II pneumococcal capsule has as its disaccharide building block glucose in $1 \rightarrow 4, 1 \rightarrow 6$ linkages. The antibody directed against pneumococcus type II is directed against this glucose polymer.
  b. This specificity is known because the antibody will react with glucose $1 \rightarrow 4, 1 \rightarrow 6$ linkages regardless of where they are found (e.g., it will react with those found in glycogen).
  c. The reaction is so specific that it can be used to determine if the $1 \rightarrow 4, 1 \rightarrow 6$ linkage exists in unknown polysaccharides.

C. Differences in amino acid residues. Another clinically relevant example of the specificity of the immune response is its ability to distinguish very small changes in compounds, such as the various insulin molecules.

1. Diabetics who use, for example, bovine insulin for maintenance, sometimes become **insulin-tolerant,** and the insulin is no longer effective.

2. Insulin, a weak antigen, has a molecular weight of approximately 6 kDa and is composed of two chains, an A chain and a B chain. Bovine and human insulin vary by three amino acid residues sitting side by side on the A chain.

3. In insulin tolerance, antibodies are formed to these three amino acids and inactivate the molecule.

4. The treatment for this antibody inactivation of the insulin is to switch from beef to pork insulin, since the three amino acids would be different.

V. FORCES OF ANTIGEN–ANTIBODY ATTRACTION.
The antigen–antibody complex is not bound firmly together. It may even dissociate spontaneously. However, the equilibrium is far to the right, with a very large association constant (K_o) of 10^6 to 10^8.

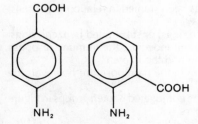

Figure 2-3. Examples of non–cross-reactive substituted benzene haptens. The change from para to ortho substitution produces a new specificity.

Table 2-2. Detection of Hormones in Human Serum Based on Antibody Recognition of Specific Epitopes

Molecular Pair	Structure	Identifying Difference
Digitoxin		

Molecular Pair	Structure	Identifying Difference
Digoxin		Presence of hydroxyl at carbon 12

Molecular Pair	Structure	Identifying Difference
Thyroxine		Presence of iodine at 5′ position

Table 2-2. (Cont.)

Molecular Pair	Structure	Identifying Difference

Triiodothyronine

Corticosterone

Presence of hydroxyl at carbon 11

Deoxycorticosterone

A. **Types of attracting forces.** Various forces act to hold the antigen–antibody complex together.

1. **Van der Waals forces** act because of spatial fit (Figure 2-4). These forces hold antigen to antibody when the two molecules have corresponding shapes (see Figure 2-4A) but are less effective when the correspondence is poorer (see Figure 2-4B).

2. **Coulombic forces** are patterns of complementary electrical charge on the molecule. The electrostatic interactions tend to hold the molecules together (Figure 2-5).

3. Antigen–antibody complexes are probably held together by a mixture of Van der Waals and coulombic forces.

B. **Affinity and avidity**

1. The strength of the attraction between a single epitope and its matching paratope (the antigen-binding site on the antibody molecule) is referred to as the **affinity** of the reaction between the two reactants. Antigen–antibody complexes of low affinity dissociate readily.

2. A related term, **avidity,** refers to the strength of the interaction between multivalent antigens and the population of antibodies which they have induced. Avidity is influenced by the affinity of individual antibodies for their epitopes, the valence of the antigen, and the valence of the antibodies.

C. **Accessibility of the epitope.** Studies using synthetic polypeptides have shown that only those amino acids that are spatially accessible due to **tertiary protein structure** are immunoreactive.

1. Proteins can exist as globular or fibrous proteins or mixtures of the two; the nature of the structure is important.

2. The ability of antibody to bind to antigenic sites can be affected by **altering the tertiary structure**.
   a. The antigenic sites would then no longer be spatially arranged so that antibody–antigen coupling could occur.
   b. **Insulin molecules** provide an illustration.
      (1) As mentioned above (see IV C), insulin is composed of A and B chains. Antibody to either one of these chains can be produced by splitting the chains, purifying them, and injecting them into a foreign host. The host will produce antibody to the particular chain injected.
      (2) If these antibodies are injected back into the animal species that supplied the original insulin, the antibodies will not react with intact insulin molecules.
      (3) The explanation is that the tertiary structure of insulin must be such that the determinant groups on the molecule are accessible.

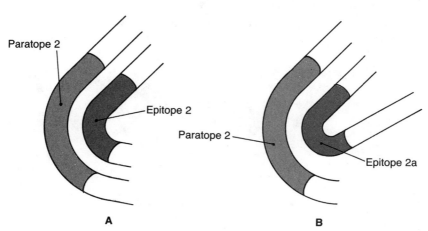

Figure 2-4. Van der Waals forces: influence of spatial fit on antigen–antibody reactions. A significant modification in the shape of epitope 2 of lysozyme (see Figure 2-1) precludes its interaction with the matching antigen-binding site (paratope) of the original antibody molecule.

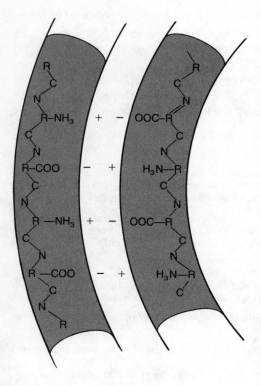

Figure 2-5. Coulombic forces. The pattern of electrical charges influences the interaction between antigen and antibody. As the pattern becomes more complementary, the force of attraction becomes proportionately stronger, and the affinity of the two reactants increases.

VI. THYMUS DEPENDENCE AND IMMUNOGENICITY

A. Most humoral immune responses are **thymus-dependent,** in that there is a need for a thymus-derived "helper" cell in the induction of antibody synthesis (see Chapter 5 IV B 1, F 4).

B. A very small number of responses are **thymus-independent**.

    1. The immunogens in these responses are characterized by having monotonously repeating epitopes. Most are polysaccharides or polymerized proteins such as flagellin.

    2. They induce only IgM antibodies.

    3. There is no anamnestic response on secondary challenge with the same immunogen.

STUDY QUESTIONS

Directions: Each of the numbered items or incomplete statements in this section is followed by answers or by completions of the statement. Select the **one** lettered answer or completion that is **best** in each case.

1. An example of a sequestered antigen is

(A) penicillin
(B) diphtheria toxoid
(C) salmonella O antigens
(D) salmonella H antigens
(E) basic protein of myelin

2. The antigens in thymus-dependent humoral immune responses show which of the following properties? They

(A) induce primarily an IgM response
(B) are mainly polysaccharide in nature
(C) induce an active anamnestic response upon booster injection
(D) are exemplified by the polymerized protein flagellin
(E) are not very common

3. An antigen should possess two properties. These are

(A) chemical simplicity and immunogenicity
(B) allergenicity and immunogenicity
(C) toxicity and allergenicity
(D) toxicity and specific reactivity
(E) immunogenicity and specific reactivity

4. An antigen that occurs in various different species is referred to as

(A) allogeneic
(B) syngeneic
(C) heterogenetic
(D) isogeneic
(E) sequestered

5. The sites in or on antigens with which antibodies react are called

(A) haplotypes
(B) isotopes
(C) epitopes
(D) idiotypes

6. Another name for an antigenic determinant is

(A) immunogen
(B) paratope
(C) carrier
(D) epitope
(E) antigen

7. The degree of immunogenicity is influenced by all of the following EXCEPT

(A) molecular size
(B) degree of foreignness
(C) route of injection
(D) chemical composition
(E) presence of adjuvants

8. In order to be immunoreactive, an epitope must be

(A) part of a globular protein
(B) linear
(C) electronegative
(D) spatially accessible
(E) part of a glycoprotein

9. A substance that can evoke either a humoral or a cell-mediated immune response is termed

(A) an immunogen
(B) a hapten
(C) an epitope
(D) an antigen
(E) an adjuvant

10. The capacity of a molecule to react specifically with a product of induced lymphoid cell differentiation is known as

(A) specificity
(B) antigenicity
(C) affinity
(D) avidity
(E) immunogenicity

1-E	4-C	7-C	10-B
2-C	5-C	8-D	
3-E	6-D	9-A	

11. Antigen–antibody complexes are not bound firmly together, but are held together by

(A) Van der Waals forces
(B) coulombic forces
(C) both
(D) neither

ANSWERS AND EXPLANATIONS

1. The answer is E *[II B 3 b].*
Basic protein of myelin is the only sequestered antigen mentioned in the question. The tissues of the central nervous system are not normally exposed to the immunologic apparatus of the host (i.e., they are "sequestered"). If they become exposed, an autoimmune disease could result. An immune response to the basic protein of the myelin sheath that surrounds neurons is thought to be involved in the autoimmune disease acute disseminated encephalomyelitis. Diphtheria toxoid and salmonella O and H antigens are exogenous antigens; penicillin is a hapten and is also exogenous.

2. The answer is C *[VI A, B].*
Thymus-dependent humoral immune responses do show a lively secondary (anamnestic) response. Most humoral immune responses are thymus-dependent, in that antibody synthesis requires the action of helper T (Th) cells, and these cells in turn require an intact thymus. The antigens that are independent of thymic influence are characterized by the presence of repeating epitopes as are seen in carbohydrates and polymerized proteins such as flagellin. These antigens induce IgM only and fail to induce immunologic memory, so that there is no anamnestic response.

3. The answer is E *[I A 1].*
Antigens must be both immunogenic and specifically reactive. They need not induce allergies (i.e., be allergenic) and need not be toxic, although neither allergenicity nor toxicity would preclude antigenicity.

4. The answer is C *[II B 2 d].*
Heterogenetic, or heterophilic, antigens occur in phylogenetically unrelated species — that is, in widely separated species in the plant or animal kingdoms or both. The Forssman antigen, for example, is found on sheep red blood cells (SRBCs), guinea pig tissues, corn, and certain bacteria. Allogeneic antigens are present in some but not all members of a species. Inbred animals are said to be antigenically syngeneic. Antigens that can generate an immune response in genetically different members of the same species, but not in the member carrying it, are called isogeneic.

5. The answer is C *[I C 1 a].*
The sites on antigens with which antibodies react are called epitopes, or antigenic determinant groups. An epitope comprises approximately three to four amino acids or three to four monosaccharide units. Epitopes are distributed throughout the surface of an antigen and appear in a repeating manner, so that any particular epitope will appear on the antigen surface several times. In addition, a given antigen is likely to have several immunologically different epitopes; for example, bovine serum albumin has seven different immunologically specific epitopes. This array of epitopes is referred to as the epitope mosaic or determinant group mosaic of an antigen. The valence of an antigen is the total number of epitopes on that antigen; that is, the number of antibody molecules with which that particular antigen could potentially react.

6. The answer is D *[I C 1 a].*
The area of an antigen with which an antibody reacts is called an epitope, an antigenic determinant, or a determinant group. Epitopes are usually four to six residues (amino acids or monosaccharides) in size. These areas need not be linear within the molecule: they could be separated residues that come into proximity through folding of the molecular chain. The terms "antigen" and "immunogen" refer to the entire molecule. The paratope is the site on the antibody molecule that combines with an epitope. Carriers are molecules, usually proteins, which impart immunogenicity to haptens that are conjugated to them.

7. The answer is C *[I D 1; II A].*
The route of injection would not affect a molecule's immunogenicity. The relative ability of a molecule to induce an immune response (i.e., its degree of immunogenicity) is influenced by its molecular size, chemical nature, and degree of foreignness. These attributes are not simply additive, nor directly factorial, as a molecule of limited size may be highly immunogenic if it has sufficient complexity. Nonspecific stimulation of the immune response can occur via adjuvants, which can enhance immunogenicity without altering chemical composition. The rate of exposure to the immunogen may influence the amount or type of antibody produced [e.g., local secretory IgA (sIgA) is produced following intestinal exposure] but the innate immunogenicity of the molecule remains the same.

8. The answer is D *[I C 2 c (2); V C]*.
An epitope must be on the outside of a molecule if the antibody is to be able to react with it, otherwise spatial interference would prevent the molecular interaction. Initial surface accessibility is not necessary for immunogenicity, however, as the cell or molecule may be broken down somewhat during phagocytic cell "processing," thus exposing internal antigens or epitopes to the immunologic apparatus of the host.

9. The answer is A *[I A 1 a]*.
Immunogens are substances that are able to induce an immune response. The response may be humoral (resulting in the production of circulating antibodies) or cell-mediated (resulting in the production of specifically sensitized T lymphocytes). An antigen can react specifically with its homologous antibody or lymphocyte, but it may not be able to induce an immune response. A hapten is antigenic, but is not immunogenic unless it is coupled to a carrier molecule. The epitope is the site on the antigen molecule that reacts with specific antibody or lymphocyte. An adjuvant is a substance that intensifies an immune response when administered together with an immunogen.

10. The answer is B *[I A 1 b]*.
Antigenicity is defined as the capacity of a molecule to react with the immunologic product that it induced (i.e., either a humoral antibody or a sensitized lymphocyte). The term "antigenic" is also often used to describe a molecule that can induce an immune response. However, it is more accurate to use the term "immunogenic" to describe molecules that are able to induce immune responses, because some molecules (e.g., haptens) can react but are not able to induce an immune response; that is, they are antigenic but not immunogenic. Affinity and avidity are terms that describe the strength of interaction between antigens and their homologous antibodies.

11. The answer is C *[V A 3]*.
Van der Waals and coulombic forces act to hold together antigen–antibody complexes. Van der Waals forces are active due to spatial fit. The electrostatic interactions of coulombic forces also tend to hold the molecules together. The nature of the structure of globular or fibrous proteins can allow antibody to bind to antigenic sites, although particular changes in the tertiary structure of proteins could change the arrangement of antigenic sites and thus not allow antigen–antibody coupling.

3
Immunoglobulins

I. INTRODUCTION

A. Physiology

1. **Immunoglobulins,** or **antibodies,** are glycoproteins present in the gamma globulin fraction of serum.

2. The concentration of antibodies in the body is equally divided between the intravascular and extravascular (primarily lymphatic) compartments; 25% exchanges each day as the tissues are bathed in plasma proteins.

B. Immunology.
Immunoglobulins are produced by **B lymphocytes (B cells)** or **plasma cells** in response to exposure to an antigen. They react specifically with that antigen in vivo or in vitro and are hence a part of the **adaptive immune response**—specifically, **humoral immunity**.

II. IMMUNOGLOBULIN STRUCTURE

A. Basic unit (monomer)

1. The basic structural unit of an immunoglobulin molecule, called a **monomer,** consists of four polypeptide chains linked covalently by disulfide bonds (Figure 3-1).
   a. **Polypeptide chains** are unbranched polymers composed of amino acids.
   b. The sequence of amino acids in a polypeptide chain is what identifies a given protein and distinguishes it from any other molecule.

2. The four-chain monomeric immunoglobulin structure is composed of two identical **heavy (H)** polypeptide chains and two identical **light (L)** polypeptide chains.

B. Heavy and light chains

1. **H chains**
   a. **Size.** H chains have a molecular weight of 50 to 75 kDa, approximately twice that of L chains, and contain about 400 amino acids, twice the number in L chains.
   b. **Isotypes (classes)**
      (1) Amino acid differences in the carboxy terminal portion of the H chains identify five antigenically distinct H chain isotypes (Table 3-1).
      (2) The H chain isotypes form the basis for the five classes of immunoglobulin molecules (see Table 3-1).
   c. **Subclasses**
      (1) H chain classes γ, α, and μ are subdivided into subclasses of molecules (see Table 3-1). The subdivision is based on the greater similarity of amino acid sequence shown by subclasses of the same class than is shown by different classes.
      (2) The **H chain subclasses** correspond to **immunoglobulin subclasses**: γ_1 corresponds to IgG1; α_1 to IgA1, and so forth.

2. **L chains**
   a. **Size.** L chains have a molecular weight of approximately 23 kDa and are composed of about 200 amino acids.

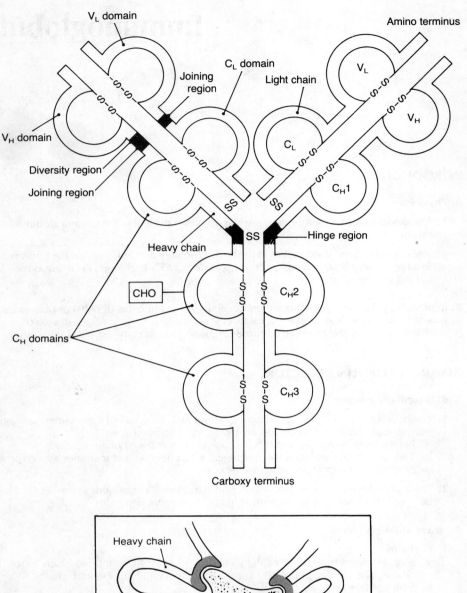

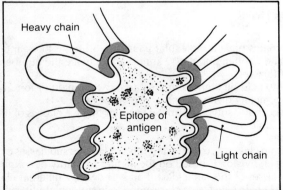

Figure 3-1. Basic unit (monomer) of the IgG molecule, consisting of four polypeptide chains linked covalently by disulfide bonds ($S-S$) with intrachain disulfide linkages as well. The loops correspond to domains within each chain. V = variable domain; C = constant domain; L = light chain; H = heavy chain; CHO = carbohydrate side chain. The *inset* shows the complementarity-determining (hypervariable) regions (CDRs) [*shaded*] and framework regions (FRs) [*open*] of each variable domain in the paratopic region. Similar hypervariable regions are found in the α and β chains of the T cell receptor for antigen.

Table 3-1. Properties of Immunoglobulins

	IgG	IgA	IgM	IgD	IgE
H chain	γ	α	μ	δ	ϵ
H chain subclasses	$\gamma_1, \gamma_2, \gamma_3, \gamma_4$	α_1, α_2	μ_1, μ_2	–	–
H chain allotypes*	Gm (25)	Am (2)			
Molecular weight (kDa)	150	160–400	900	180	190
S value	7	7	19	7	8
J chain	–	+	+	–	–
Carbohydrate (%)	3	7	12	13	11
Serum concentration (mg/dl)	1200	200	120	3	0.05
Serum half-life (days)	21[+]	6	10	3	2
Functions					
Complement activation (classic pathway)	+ +	±	+ + + +	–	–
Opsonization	+ + + +	+	–	–	–
Antiviral activity	+ +	+ + +	–	–	–
Mast cell sensitization	–	–	+	?	+

H chain = heavy chain.
*The number in parentheses = the number of allotypes known. All immunoglobulins have Km L chain allotypes.
[+]IgG3 has a half-life of 7 days.

b. **Types**
(1) L chains are of two types—κ or λ—based on their structural (antigenic) differences.
(2) All immunoglobulin classes have both κ and λ chains. However, a given immunoglobulin molecule may contain either two identical κ chains or two identical λ chains, but never a κ chain and a λ chain combined.
(3) The proportion of κ to λ chains in human immunoglobulin molecules is about 3:2.
(4) There is no isotypic variation in κ chains. However, there are four distinct λ chains, giving rise to four distinct **subtypes** (so called to avoid confusion with the H chain subclasses that distinguish immunoglobulin isotypes). All four λ subtypes are present in each of the immunoglobulin classes.

C. **Bonds. Disulfide ($-S-S-$) bonds** hold together the four polypeptide chains in immunoglobulin molecules, and are of two types.

1. **Interchain bonds** occur between H chains (H−H), between H and L chains (H−L), and between L chains (L−L).
   a. **H−H bonds**
      (1) H−H bonds occur primarily in the hinge region of the immunoglobulin molecule (see II H), but they also occur in the carboxy terminal portion of the H chain.
      (2) They can vary in number from 1 to 15, depending on the class and subclass of the immunoglobulin molecule.
   b. **H−L bonds.** Only one disulfide bond connects H and L chains. H−L bonding occurs in most immunoglobulin molecules; IgA2 lacks an H−L bond.
   c. **L−L bonds.** Single L−L bonds occur in IgA2. L−L bonds can also occur under pathologic conditions [e.g., in Bence Jones protein (see Chapter 9 VI B 1 b)].

2. **Intrachain bonds** occur within an individual chain, and are stronger than interchain bonds.
   a. The number of intrachain disulfide bonds varies:
      (1) L chains have two.
      (2) Human γ, α, and δ H chains have four.
      (3) Human μ and ε H chains have five.
   b. The intrachain bonds divide each immunoglobulin molecule into domains (see II E).

D. **Variable (V) and constant (C) regions**

1. Each H chain and each L chain has a variable region and a constant region.
   a. The **variable region,** which lies in the amino, or N, terminal portion of the molecule, shows a wide variation in amino acid sequence.
   b. The **constant region,** in the carboxy, or C, terminal portion of the molecule, demonstrates an unvarying amino acid sequence, except for minor inherited differences.

2. The variable regions are associated with appropriate constant regions such that:
   a. No variable H chain region will occur in a L chain, and vice versa.
   b. However, a particular variable H chain sequence may occur in more than one H chain class (e.g., γ, α, μ, and so forth).

3. This permits **class switching** (see IV D), which occurs during an immune response, when B cells change their production from IgM, for example, to IgG (see Chapter 5 V A 2).

4. **Hypervariable regions**
   a. Certain areas within the variable regions are highly variable in amino acid sequence (see Figure 3-1 inset).
      (1) These **hypervariable regions,** often called **complementarity-determining regions (CDRs)** or **"hot spots,"** occur at relatively constant amino acid positions in an otherwise relatively invariant molecule.
      (2) They are short polypeptide segments lying near amino acid positions 30, 50, and 95 in the variable regions of both L and H chains.
   b. The CDRs are important in the structure of the antigen-binding site (see II F).
   c. **L chains** have three CDRs [CDR1 (hv1), CDR2 (hv2), and CDR3 (hv3)] and **H chains** have four, although only three of the four have been associated with antibody activity.
   d. There is extreme variability in the amino acids found in the CDR regions.
   e. The intervening peptide sequences, called **framework regions (FRs),** are relatively constant in amino acid sequence.

E. Domains

1. Each immunoglobulin chain consists of a series of globular regions, or **domains,** enclosed by disulfide bonds.
   a. Each **H chain** has four or five domains—one in the variable region (V_H) and three or four in the constant region (C_H1, C_H2, C_H3, and C_H4).
      (1) The γ, α, and δ H chains have four domains (one variable and three constant).
      (2) The μ and ϵ H chains have five domains (one variable and four constant).
   b. Each **L chain** has two domains—one in the variable region (V_L) and one in the constant region (C_L).

2. Domains consist of about 110 amino acid residues.
   a. Peptide loops of 60 to 70 amino acid residues enclosed by intrachain disulfide bonds represent the central portion of each domain.
   b. The amino acid sequences of the loops show a high degree of homology (i.e., the sequences are very similar).

F. Antigen-binding site (paratope)

1. The **paratope** is the area of the immunoglobulin molecule which interacts specifically with the **epitope** of the antigen (see Chapter 2 I C).

2. The paratope is formed by only a very small portion of the entire immunoglobulin molecule.
   a. Folding of the polypeptide chains brings the CDR portions of the V_H and V_L domains into close proximity.
   b. This folding creates a three-dimensional structure which is **complementary to the epitope** (see Figure 3-1).

G. Fragments. Early studies of immunoglobulin structure employed proteolytic (peptide bond–splitting) enzymes, particularly papain and pepsin, to degrade immunoglobulin molecules into definable fragments.

1. **Papain** splits the monomeric basic unit into **three fragments** of approximately equal size at the hinge region (see II H).
   a. Two **Fab** (antigen-binding) fragments each contain an entire L chain and the amino terminal half of the H chain.
      (1) The Fab portion of the H chain is called the **Fd** fragment; it contains the V_H and C_H1 domains.
      (2) A Fab fragment is **monovalent;** that is, it possesses only one antigen-binding site. Therefore, unlike bivalent molecules (see II G 2 b), a Fab fragment cannot facilitate antigen precipitation.

b. One **Fc** (crystallizable) fragment contains the carboxy terminal portion of the H chain.
　(1) This portion of the molecule has several properties:
　　(a) It binds the C1q component of complement (see Chapter 4 II B 2 a).
　　(b) It contains carbohydrate.
　　(c) It dictates whether a given immunoglobulin can, for example, cross the placenta (IgG) or bind to mast cells (IgE).
　　(d) It is responsible for opsonization of bacteria and other cellular elements.
　(2) Phagocytic cells have membrane receptors for the Fc portions of several different immunoglobulins. These **Fc receptors (FcRs)** have the following specificity:
　　(a) **FcγRI** binds the Fc portion of IgG1, IgG3, and IgG4.
　　(b) **FcγRII** binds the Fc portion of all IgG subclasses.
　　(c) **FcγRIII** binds the Fc portion of IgG1 and IgG3.
　　(d) **FcαR**, found on neutrophils, binds IgA.
　　(e) **FcεRI** and **FcεRII**, found on monocytes, mast cells, and basophils, bind IgE.

2. Pepsin digests most of the Fc fragment, leaving one large fragment termed the **F(ab')$_2$ fragment**.
　a. The F(ab')$_2$ fragment consists of two Fab fragments joined by covalent bonds.
　b. The F(ab')$_2$ fragment has two antigen-binding sites; thus it is **bivalent,** possessing the ability to bind and precipitate an antigen.

H. Hinge region. The hinge region is the portion of the H chain between the C_H1 and C_H2 domains (see Figure 3-1).

1. The hinge region is considered a separate domain because it is not homologous to any of the other domains.

2. In this region, interchain disulfide bonds form between the arms of the Fab fragments, preventing them from folding and thus rendering this portion of the molecule highly susceptible to fragmentation by enzymatic attack.
　a. **Papain** cleaves the molecule on one side of the disulfide bonds, acting directly on the hinge region.
　b. **Pepsin** acts on the opposite side of the disulfide bonds, degrading the molecule just below the hinge region.

3. The hinge region is highly flexible and allows for movement of the Fab arms in relation to each other.

I. Carbohydrate moiety. Immunoglobulins are glycoproteins, from 3% to 13% of the immunoglobulin molecule being composed of **oligosaccharides**.

1. The oligosaccharides are **side chains,** and are usually attached to the immunoglobulin at one or more locations in the constant region of H chains (the C_H region).
　a. N-Glycosidic bonds usually link an N-acetylglucosamine in the carbohydrate moiety to an asparagine residue in the polypeptide chain at the C_H region.
　b. Linkage occurs in the Golgi complex via N-acetylglucosamine–asparagine transglycosylase, a transferase enzyme.

2. The **half-life** of antibodies in the circulation (see Table 3-1) depends on the status of the oligosaccharide side chains.
　a. The oligosaccharide side chains terminate in **galactose,** to which **sialic acid** is frequently attached.
　b. When antibodies in the circulation have the sialic acid removed by enzymes such as neuraminidase, they become susceptible to degradation in the liver.
　　(1) The terminal galactose binds to a receptor on hepatocytes and the entire molecule is internalized by the cell.
　　(2) Degradation then occurs due to the proteolytic enzymes in the lysosomes of the cell.

J. J chains. These small proteins connect the two or more basic units in polymeric immunoglobulins (i.e., in IgM and some IgA). They are named **J chains** because of their **joining** function.

1. A J chain is a glycopeptide chain with a molecular weight of approximately 15 kDa.

2. It is covalently linked to the carboxy terminal portions of α and μ H chains.

3. J chain is thought to be involved in the synthesis, polymerization, and/or secretion of IgA and IgM polymers.

4. It is synthesized by B lymphocytes during maturation and is incorporated into polymeric immunoglobulins before they are secreted from the plasma cell.

K. Secretory component (secretory piece) is unique to IgA and is discussed under IgA (see III B 2).

L. The sedimentation coefficient (sedimentation constant) and the S value (Svedberg unit)

1. The **sedimentation coefficient** expresses the rate at which a particle sediments during ultracentrifugation.
   a. The rate depends on the size, shape, and density of the particle, as well as the density and viscosity of the medium and the speed of centrifugation.
   b. Thus the sedimentation coefficient gives an **estimate of molecular weight**.

2. The sedimentation coefficient is expressed in **Svedberg units (S)**.

3. The **S values** of immunoglobulins range from 7S to 19S (see Table 3-1).

III. BIOLOGICAL AND CHEMICAL PROPERTIES OF IMMUNOGLOBULINS.

Immunoglobulins fall into **five classes (isotypes),** based on certain structural differences (see Table 3-1). Each class also has certain unique biological and chemical properties.

A. IgG. IgG is the major immunoglobulin in human serum, accounting for approximately 75% of the total normal serum immunoglobulin pool at a concentration of approximately 1200 mg/dl.

1. **Structure**
   a. IgG is a **monomer** consisting of identical pairs of H and L chains linked by disulfide bridges (see Figure 3-1).
   b. Four **subclasses of IgG** have been identified, based on H chain differences: subclasses IgG1, IgG2, IgG3, and IgG4 correspond to H chains γ_1, γ_2, γ_3, and γ_4.

2. **Biological and chemical properties**
   a. Most IgG subclasses have a molecular weight of 150 kDa and an S value of 7S; IgG3 is slightly larger, at 170 kDa.
   b. Most serum IgG is IgG1.
   c. IgG is the only immunoglobulin that can cross the placenta in humans; therefore, maternal IgG provides most of the protection of the newborn during the first months of life [secretory IgA (sIgA; see III B 2) in colostrum protects the infant's gastrointestinal tract].
   d. IgG molecules are capable of binding complement by the classical pathway (except for IgG4, which activates by the alternative pathway). The binding site for complement component C1q is in the C_H2 domain.
   e. IgG is the major antibody produced in the secondary immune response (see Chapter 5 V A 2 a).
      (1) IgG has a half-life of approximately 21 days (IgG3 has a half-life of only 7 days).
      (2) Effective antitoxic immunity is exclusively IgG.
   f. IgG is the major opsonizing immunoglobulin in phagocytosis (see Chapter 1 II E); neutrophils have receptors for the Fc fragments of IgG1 and IgG3.

B. IgA. IgA is present in two forms: one in the serum and the other in various body secretions.

1. **Serum IgA,** at a concentration of approximately 200 mg/dl, accounts for about 15% to 20% of the total normal serum immunoglobulin pool.
   a. **Structure**
      (1) In humans, over 80% of serum IgA exists in a monomeric form with an S value of 7S.
      (2) The rest exists as dimers, trimers, or tetramers. In these polymeric forms of IgA, the monomeric units are linked by disulfide bonds and J chains.
   b. **Biological and chemical properties**
      (1) IgA does not bind complement via the classic pathway but may do so via the alternative pathway (see Chapter 4 II C).
      (2) IgA has a half-life of 6 days.
      (3) IgA can be inactivated by an IgA protease produced by gonococci, meningococci, pneumococci, and *Haemophilus influenzae*.

2. Secretory IgA (sIgA) is the predominant immunoglobulin in various secretions (saliva; tears; colostrum; bronchial, genitourinary, and intestinal secretions).

  a. Structure

    (1) The sIgA molecule consists of two monomeric units plus J chain and secretory component (Figure 3-2). It has an S value of 11S.

      (a) Secretory component (secretory piece) is a polypeptide chain with a molecular weight of about 70 kDa.

      (b) It is joined to sIgA by disulfide bonds.

      (c) It serves as a receptor for IgA on the surface of epithelial cells lining exocrine glands and is important in the secretion of sIgA.

    (2) The dominant subclass of sIgA is **sIgA2,** the form shown in Figure 3-2. The sIgA2 molecule is unique for its absence of $H-L$ bonds; this subclass instead has $L-L$ bonds.

  b. Biological and chemical properties

    (1) Secretory component is synthesized by exocrine epithelial cells and enables dimeric IgA to pass through the mucosal tissues into the secretions.

      (a) The epithelial cells bear an IgA-specific receptor.

      (b) After binding IgA, the receptor–IgA complex is internalized by endocytosis, transported across the cell cytoplasm, and extruded into the external secretions.

      (c) As the complex is extruded, proteolytic cleavage of the receptor leaves a fragment, the secretory component, attached by a disulfide bond to the IgA dimer.

      (d) Secretory component appears to protect IgA from mammalian proteases.

    (2) Secretory IgA functions in several ways.

      (a) It protects mucosal surfaces by reacting with adhesin molecules on the surface of potential pathogens and interfering with their adherence and colonization.

      (b) It may also opsonize foreign particles, as polymorphonuclear neutrophils (PMNs) have FcαR in their membranes.

C. IgM. IgM represents about 8% to 10% of the total serum immunoglobulins and is present in normal serum at a concentration of approximately 120 mg/dl.

  1. Structure

    a. With an S value of 19S, IgM has a **pentameric** structure (see Figure 3-2) consisting of five monomeric units linked by a J chain and by disulfide bonds at the Fc fragment.

    b. IgM is easily dissociated by reducing agents, forming five monomeric units of 7S IgM.

  2. Biological and chemical properties

    a. IgM is the first antibody that an immunologically committed B lymphocyte can produce. It has a half-life of approximately 10 days.

    (1) IgM will appear in the B cell membrane (followed shortly by IgD) prior to an encounter with its homologous epitope.

    (2) IgM is the predominant antibody in the early (primary) immune response to most antigens.

    (3) IgM is the predominant antibody produced by the fetus. An elevated IgM level in the cord serum of a newborn (normal level, approximately 10 mg/dl) may indicate that the fetus was infected before birth.

    b. IgM is the only antibody made to certain carbohydrate antigens, such as the ABO blood group antigens on human erythrocytes (see Chapter 12 III B).

    c. IgM is the most efficient immunoglobulin at activating complement in lytic reactions.

    d. IgM is not intrinsically opsonic, since phagocytic cells do not possess a receptor for the Fc portion of the μ chain. However, IgM enhances phagocytosis by causing the deposition of the C3b opsonin onto the surface where the IgM antibody resides (see Chapter 4 V B 2 b).

    e. Some IgM is synthesized locally in secretory tissues (e.g., parotid glands). **Secretory IgM,** like sIgA, can bind secretory component.

D. IgD. IgD represents less than 1% of the total immunoglobulin pool and is present in trace amounts in normal serum (approximately 3 to 5 mg/dl).

  1. Structure. IgD exists as a monomer; its S value is 7S.

    a. Structural studies are difficult because of the low serum levels and because IgD is susceptible to enzymatic degradation.

    b. One unique structural feature is the presence of only a single $H-H$ interchain bond, along with two $H-L$ interchain bonds.

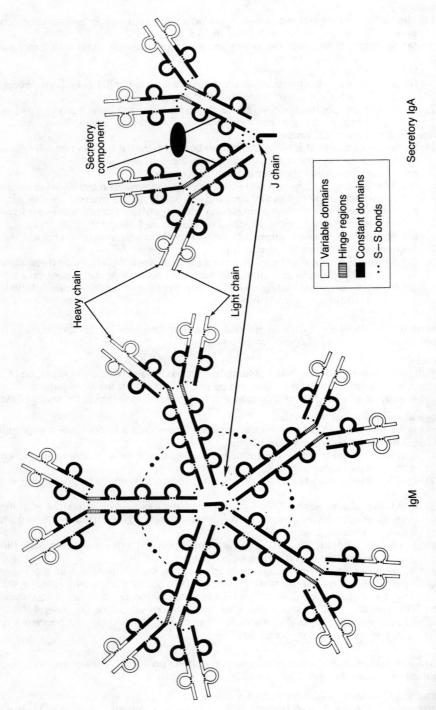

Figure 3-2. Structural models of IgM and secretory IgA (sIgA). IgM has a pentameric structure linked by the J chain at the Fc fragment. The sIgA molecule has a dimeric structure plus J chain plus secretory component. Shown is the dominant IgA2 subclass, which is unique for its absence of a covalent bond between the light (L) and heavy (H) chains. L chains are linked by disulfide bonds.

2. Biological and chemical properties
  a. IgD has a half-life of 2 to 3 days; it is heat- and acid-labile.
  b. There is still controversy over the biological functions of IgD.
    (1) IgD occurs in large quantities on the B cell membrane and may, as an antigen receptor, be involved in B cell activation.
    (2) The molecule may have some antibody activity for penicillin, insulin, and diphtheria toxoid.

E. IgE. IgE is present in trace amounts in normal serum (approximately 0.05 mg/dl), accounting for only 0.004% of total serum immunoglobulins.

  1. Structure. IgE is a monomer with the unusual feature that its fifth domain separates the two interchain H − H bonds.

  2. Biological and chemical properties
    a. IgE has a molecular weight of approximately 190 kDa and an S value of 8S.
    b. IgE is produced by B cells and plasma cells in the spleen, in lymphoid tissue of the tonsils and adenoids, and in the respiratory and gastrointestinal mucosa (see also Chapter 9 II B 3 b). It has a vascular half-life of 2 to 3 days.
    c. IgE production begins in the fetus early in the gestational process; IgE does not cross the placenta.
    d. IgE is associated with immediate hypersensitivity reactions (e.g., atopy and anaphylaxis; see Chapter 9 II).
      (1) IgE is **homocytotropic:** it has an affinity for cells ("cytotropic") of the host species that produced it ("homo").
        (a) This affinity is particularly strong for tissue mast cells and blood basophils.
        (b) Fixation to these cells occurs via the Fc fragment (C_H3 and C_H4 domains).
      (2) Upon combination with certain antigens (called **allergens,** because they generate allergy), IgE antibodies trigger the release of histamine and other mediators of atopic disease from the tissue mast cells.
    e. IgE may also be important in immunity to certain helminthic parasites.
    f. It is unable to activate complement via the classic pathway.
    g. IgE is heat-labile at 56° C.

IV. ANTIBODY DIVERSITY

A. Allotypic and idiotypic variation. In addition to the isotypic (class) variation already described (see II B 1 b), immunoglobulins also display allotypic and idiotypic variation.

  1. Allotypes are allelic variants of isotypes.
    a. Allotypes exist in different individuals within the same species, and are inherited in a mendelian manner.
    b. Allotypes are identified by **allotypic markers** [i.e., structural (antigenic) differences] found in the constant regions of H and L chains.
    c. Nomenclature for allotypic markers has been established for γ, α, and κ chains.
      (1) Markers on **γ H chains** are designated **Gm** (for γ, referring to IgG).
        (a) There are over 20 antigenically different Gm markers.
        (b) All are not found on all IgG molecules; they seem to be restricted to certain subclasses.
      (2) Markers on **α H chains** are designated **Am** (for α, referring to IgA). There are only two alleles at this locus.
      (3) Markers on **κ L chains** are designated **Km.**
        (a) There are three alleles at this locus, and the markers vary only in amino acid composition at positions 153 and 191.
        (b) Km was originally called **Inv** from the source of the antiserum used to identify one of the allelic gene products (from patient "V").

  2. Idiotypes represent the antigen-binding specificities of immunoglobulins.
    a. Overview. Idiotypes represent unique structural (antigenic) determinants (i.e., amino acid sequences) in the variable region that are associated with the antigen-binding capability of the antibody molecule.
      (1) Idiotypic variability pertains to the generation of the antigen-binding site in the variable region of the H and L chains.

    (2) Variability in amino acid sequence in these regions is concentrated in three to four CDRs surrounded by relatively invariant residues (see II D 4).

    (3) These CDRs are the areas that make contact with the epitope of the antigen (see Figure 3-1 inset).

  b. Idiotopes and idiotypes

    (1) **Idiotopes** are antigenic epitopes that occur in the variable region of the Fab portion of an antibody molecule. They may be a part of the CDRs or they may be associated with framework sequences of the molecule (see II D 4 e).

    (2) The **idiotype** of a particular immunoglobulin is the sum of the individual idiotopes.

  c. Anti-idiotypic antibodies (Figure 3-3)

    (1) If an antibody is used as an immunogen, it is possible to induce the production of anti-idiotypic antibodies that structurally resemble the original epitope (see Figure 3-3).

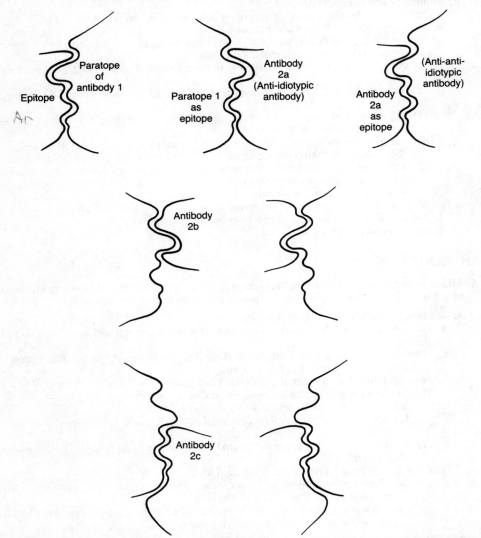

Figure 3-3. The production of anti-idiotypic antibodies. The paratope of an antibody can become immunogenic in an appropriate host and will constitute one of the idiotypes of that antibody. An antibody homologous with the paratope (an anti-idiotypic antibody—e.g., *antibody 2a*) will structurally mimic the original epitope. Similarly, anti-idiotypic antibodies can induce anti-anti-idiotypic antibodies that would structurally mimic the original paratope. Different segments of an antibody's paratope can serve as epitopes, raising antibodies with different specificities (e.g., *antibodies 2a, 2b,* and *2c*).

(2) These second-generation anti-idiotypic antibodies could be used in artificial vaccines, as an immunizing antigen to induce the original antibodies in a "naive" recipient (see Chapter 7 IV B 2 a).

(3) A second potential significance to this anti-antibody circuit is as a mechanism for regulation of the immune response [see Chapter 6 I C 3 and II B 2 d (3)].

B. Genetics of immunoglobulin diversity

1. Overview

a. Similarity

(1) Immunoglobulin gene organization is remarkably similar, whether dealing with H or L chains, or with the different H chain classes.

(2) In fact, the genetics of the T cell receptor also has a pattern of locus clusters that resembles that of immunoglobulins very closely, although different genes are involved.

b. Diversity

(1) The human immune system is capable of producing a vast number of different antibody molecules, each with its own antigenic specificity (see IV C 1).

    (a) This vast diversity is possible because immunoglobulin genes undergo an unusual type of interaction.

        (i) Embryonic DNA contains a great many genes for the variable regions of the H and L chains.

        (ii) A process of **somatic recombination** (DNA rearrangement and deletion), followed by **RNA splicing,** results in a large variety of plasma cell lines that encode different H chains and L chains.

    (b) A fairly high rate of **somatic mutation** in κ, λ, and H chains further adds to the diversity.

(2) A similar process of DNA rearrangement gives the T cell receptor its epitope-binding specificity.

2. Chromosomes, exons and introns, and gene rearrangements

a. Chromosomes. H chains and κ and λ L chains are each encoded on separate chromosomes. In the human these are as follows:

(1) All of the H chain immunoglobulin classes are coded at one site on chromosome 14.

(2) The λ chain gene complex is at one site on chromosome 22.

(3) The κ chain gene complex is at one site on chromosome 2.

b. Variable and constant regions

(1) The H and L chains vary markedly in the amino acid composition of their amino terminal portion (variable region) but are relatively constant in their carboxy terminal portion (constant region).

(2) Analysis of immunoglobulin genes has revealed that the variable and constant regions are separately encoded and located on different fragments of DNA.

c. Exons and introns

(1) As in other genes, **coding sequences (exons)** in the DNA code for the amino acid sequences in immunoglobulin molecules.

(2) The exons are separated by **intervening noncoding nucleotide sequences (introns).**

(3) Both exons and introns are transcribed into RNA, but RNA splicing then removes the introns, leaving the exons joined together.

d. Gene rearrangement

(1) The exons that code for variable domains are split up into smaller segments of DNA along the chromosome.

(2) Making proper exons from these segments requires rearranging and rejoining the segments to form immunoglobulin gene sequences.

3. L chain gene organization

a. Three genes code for each immunoglobulin L chain; the human κ chain (Figure 3-4) is used here as an example.

(1) Two gene segments encode the variable domain.

    (a) The initial gene segment, the variable (V_κ) region, encodes the first 95 amino acids of the variable region protein. Over 200 V_κ region genes exist in this region of human chromosome 2.

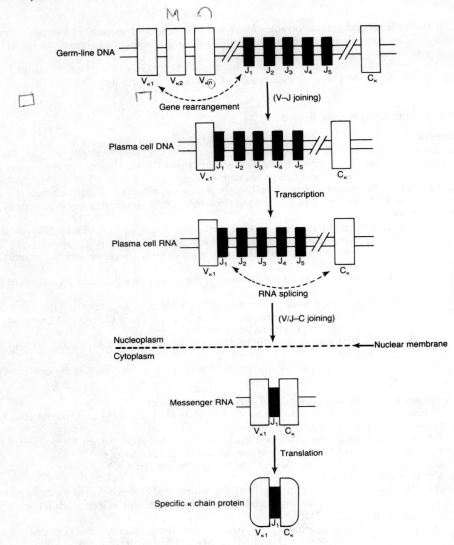

Figure 3-4. Human κ light (L) chain gene organization. The potential for a large variety of κ chains exists due to somatic recombination in the DNA and RNA splicing. As the B cell precursor differentiates into a mature B cell, DNA deletion brings one of the variable (V_κ) genes next to one of the joining (J) genes—in this example, $V_{\kappa 1}$ and J_1. This unit and the remaining J genes are separated from the constant (C_κ) region by an intervening sequence (intron) of DNA. The $V_{\kappa 1}/J_1$ unit codes for one of the numerous possible κ chain variable exons. The plasma cell DNA is transcribed into nuclear RNA, which is spliced to form messenger RNA (mRNA), with $V_{\kappa 1}$, J_1, and C_κ messages joined and ready for translation into the κ chain.

          (b) A second gene, the **joining (J_κ) segment,** encodes the remaining 13 amino acids (96 to 108) of the V exon (this J is unrelated to the J chain found in IgM and IgA). There are five genes at this locus.

      (2) A third gene dictates the amino acid sequence of the constant region. There is only one C_κ **region** on this final segment, which codes for amino acids 109 to 214.

   b. The **λ L chains** arise from a similar gene complex on chromosome 22.

      (1) However, there are six to nine slightly different copies of the C_λ region gene, which correspond to the various subtypes of λ protein. Each λ gene is accompanied by an adjacent J gene segment.

      (2) A V gene segment may fuse with any of these alternative gene combinations, resulting in a **V/J exon** that can be transcribed, in the B cell, with the adjacent **C exon**.

4. H chain gene organization. The **H chain of IgM** (Figure 3-5) is used as an example.
   a. Although similar to that of L chain genes, H chain gene organization is more complex.
      (1) Whereas a L chain gene region encodes only one constant domain, the H chain gene region must code for three or four constant domains (see II E 1 a).
      (2) Also, the H chain C gene region must code for each of the five immunoglobulin classes—and for four IgG and two IgA subclasses as well.
      (3) Furthermore, the exon coding for the variable portion of the H chain is composed of three, not two, segments of DNA.
   b. **Assembly of the V/D/J exon**
      (1) The additional variable region DNA segment is designated the **diversity (D_H) gene region.**
      (2) The D_H gene region accounts for the third CDR of the H chain (see II D 4 c); it comprises only two or three amino acids.
      (3) Gene rearrangements link a D_H to a J_H segment, and then join these to a V_H, to produce the **V/D/J exon.**
   c. There are over 200 V_H genes, at least 20 D_H genes, and 6 J_H genes. This enormous gene pool, with its large potential of combinations, underlies the great diversity of the H chain variable region.

5. The 12/23 spacer rule—a mechanism for joining immunoglobulin gene segments
   a. Each gene segment (H, λ, or κ) is flanked by noncoding **recombination signal sequences (RSSs)** that specify the direction of joining the segments.
      (1) Each RSS consists of a highly conserved sequence containing three parts:
         (a) A **heptamer** (seven DNA base pairs)
         (b) A **spacer** containing either 12 nucleotides (equalling one turn of the DNA helix) or 23 nucleotides (two turns)
         (c) A **nonamer** (nine DNA base pairs)
      (2) Joining of the gene segments occurs only when the spacer nucleotide units are of different lengths.
   b. **Joining of L chain genes**
      (1) For **κ chain** genes, the RSS on the downstream side of each V_κ segment has a 12-nucleotide spacer, while the signal on the upstream side of the J_κ segment is composed of 23 nucleotides, a combination which permits joining.
      (2) For **λ chain** genes, the rule is preserved, but the order is reversed.
   c. **Joining of H chain genes.** This is more complex because three segments are involved.
      (1) The spacers for V_H and J_H genes all have 23 nucleotides and hence cannot be joined.
      (2) However, the spacers that flank the D gene are 13 nucleotides in length, and thus the 12/23 spacer rule is followed once again.

6. VJ and VDJ recombinases
   a. The cleavage and rejoining of the DNA strands are presumed to be carried out by endonucleases and ligases, respectively. These enzymes recognize the heptamer and nonamer RSSs when they are separated by one or two turns of the DNA helix.
   b. Recently, two genes that function in immunoglobulin gene recombination have been identified in mouse pre-B cells. It is not known whether these **recombination-activating genes 1 and 2 (*RAG-1* and *RAG-2*)** code for enzymes or for other regulatory proteins.
   c. These enzymatic processes are active only in the early stages of B and T lymphocyte maturation, during the development of immunologic commitment. The gene products are not functional in mature cells, and thus the immunologic specificity of the B or T cell is maintained.

7. T cell receptor gene organization
   a. The T cell receptor for antigen (see Chapter 5 III B 2 b) is similar to the immunoglobulin molecule in gene organization as well as in molecular structure.
   b. During T cell development in the thymus, the genes for the T cell receptor undergo DNA rearrangements much like those for the immunoglobulin molecule.
      (1) The variable region of the T cell receptor's α chain involves rearrangements of V and J gene segments.
      (2) The variable region of the receptor's β chain involves rearrangements of V, J, and D gene segments.

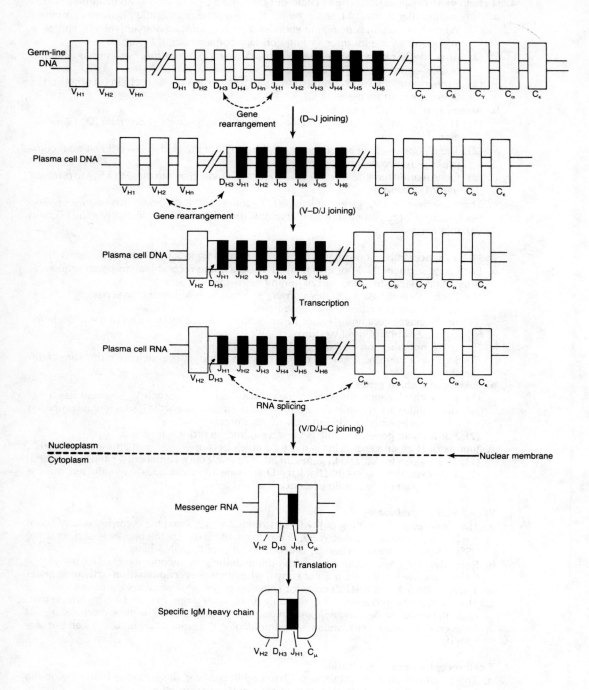

Figure 3-5. Human μ heavy (H) chain gene organization. The potential for variety in H chains, as in κ chains, is due to somatic recombination in the DNA and to RNA splicing. As the B cell precursor differentiates into a mature B cell, DNA deletion brings one of the variable (V_H) genes, one of the diversity (D_H) genes, and one of the joining (J_H) genes together—in this example, V_{H2}, D_{H3}, and J_{H1}. This unit and the remaining J genes are separated from the constant (C) region by an intervening sequence of DNA. The plasma cell DNA is transcribed into nuclear RNA, which is spliced to form messenger RNA (mRNA). In this process, the C_μ gene is selected and joined to the $V_{H2}/D_{H3}/J_{H1}$ complex, and the entire unit is ready for translation into a μ chain.

C. Mechanisms contributing to antibody diversity

1. **Chance recombination** creates a large amount of antibody diversity.
   a. If all events occurred randomly, somatic recombination in the DNA followed by RNA splicing (see Figures 3-4 and 3-5) could produce:
      (1) More than 1000 varieties of κ L chains
      (2) A similar number of λ L chains
      (3) Perhaps as many as 20,000 varieties of H chains
   b. The random combining of H and L chains greatly expands the immunologic repertoire.

2. **Imprecision in the joining of the V, D, and J genes** can also be a source of immunoglobulin diversity. (Wherever genes join, imprecision in joining can occur.)

3. **N region additions** can produce changes in the specificity and reactivity of the immunoglobulin molecule.
   a. **N regions** are very short peptides of variable sequence, often found near the third CDR of the H chain (see II D 4).
      (1) This region, the **most variable region** of the immunoglobulin molecule, contains amino acids encoded by the D_H gene region.
      (2) Furthermore, because the D_H segment is very small, the N region contains two joining boundaries, where exons V and J join D at opposing ends.
   b. Immature lymphoid cells contain an enzyme, **terminal deoxynucleotidyl transferase,** which catalyzes the generation of N regions by the addition of nucleotides at the 3' end of the DNA strands.

4. **Extensive mutation involving variable region genes produces** even further diversity.
   a. Mutations can occur by several mechanisms.
      (1) **Point mutations.** These single-nucleotide substitutions can occur in the variable region of a functional immunoglobulin gene.
         (a) Most mechanisms that generate diversity are active **before** any exposure to antigen.
         (b) The **somatic mutation theory** of antibody diversity suggests that a small number of genes diversify during lymphocyte differentiation—that is, in the pre-B cell or B cell stage—either by point mutation or by recombination events.
            (i) These mutations occur **after** the cells have encountered antigen, especially during intensive immunization.
            (ii) The nucleotide substitutions are found only in variable domains of either H or L chains, predominantly in the CDRs.
      (2) **Gene conversion.** In some immunoglobulin gene families (e.g., chicken λ chain genes), it appears that stretches of nucleotides are translocated from one V gene segment to another in the same V locus. This process may also contribute to the diversity of mammalian variable domains.
   b. The antibodies produced by mutations in variable domain genes may confer a **selective advantage** to the lymphocyte if they possess a **higher affinity** for the antigen.
      (1) Cells coated with high-affinity antibody are better able to interact with antigen and perpetuate the immune response.
      (2) A characteristic of prolonged immunization is the increase in antibody affinity for the antigen as the duration of exposure to that antigen increases, because the longer time increases the chance that a "good" mutation will occur.

D. Immunoglobulin class switching (isotype switching)

1. During the immune response, plasma cells switch from producing IgM to IgG or to another immunoglobulin class (see Chapter 5 V A 2).

2. There is no alteration in the L chain or in the variable portion of the H chain; thus, there is **no change** in antigen-binding specificity.

3. The switch involves a change in the **H chain constant domains (C_H).**
   a. Chromosome 14 contains C_H gene sequences for each of the nine H chain isotypes; these are designated $C_{\mu 1}$, $C_{\delta 1}$, $C_{\gamma 2}$, $C_{\gamma 1}$, and so forth.
   b. When the H chain gene is assembled, all but one of the C_H gene sequences are deleted, thereby producing the desired isotype.

    c. In the process, DNA rearrangement and RNA splicing place the remaining C_H gene sequence adjacent to the V/D/J exon (see IV B 4 c and Figure 3-5).

  4. Repetitive sequences in H chain genes permit immunoglobulin class switching.
    a. The switch is accomplished by recombination between special repetitive switching sequences in the intron upstream from the constant region exons.
    b. The transcriptional enhancer in the intron between the J_H cluster and C_μ exon is upstream of the switching sequence. Therefore every switch carries the enhancer with it, and active transcription is ensured regardless of the H chain class expressed.

  5. Plasma cells can switch successively from C_μ to $C_{\gamma 1}$ to $C_{\alpha 2}$, and so forth.
    a. Regulatory proteins secreted by **T cells** stimulate plasma cells to undergo particular switch recombinations.
    b. For example, **interleukin-4 (IL-4)** promotes switching to the ϵ gene with the resultant production of IgE.

E. Nonproductive rearrangements

  1. The H and L chains are formed during the pre-B cell phase of immunologic maturation.
    a. In the formation of a functional gene, DNA segments must be joined properly to ensure that the correct reading frame is maintained.
      (1) If the joining is erroneous (off by one or two nucleotides), the downstream sequences are out of frame, preventing translation into a functional polypeptide.
      (2) Such erroneous rearrangements occur frequently, and in this case the cell continues to rearrange and join its immunoglobulin gene segments until a functional immunoglobulin is made; then rearrangement ceases.
    b. The appearance of an intact H chain in the cytoplasm seems to be the signal for the end of H chain gene shuffling.
    c. It is also the signal for commencement of L chain gene rearrangement.
    d. The trial-and-error process is repeated until a functional L chain, either κ or λ, is produced.

  2. The pre-B cell then enters the B lymphocyte stage of development, in which the H and L chains are joined by disulfide bonds and are expressed in the B cell membrane.

  3. It is likely that many lymphocytes have nonproductive rearrangements and are of no value to the immune system. This appears to be the price that must be paid to preserve the generation of immunologic diversity by so elaborate a system.

F. Allelic exclusion and clonal restriction. These phenomena are peculiar to antibody-producing cells.

  1. Allelic exclusion is the expression, in a single cell, of **only one allele** at a particular locus.
    a. Two or more alleles frequently exist at the genetic loci for the various components of H and L chains.
    b. Because of allelic exclusion, only one H chain and one L chain gene can be expressed in any given B lymphocyte.
      (1) In individuals who are heterozygous for allotypic forms of H or L chains, individual B cells will express one or the other allele, but not both.
      (2) When a single H or L chain gene is successfully assembled and expressed, this prevents all other genes of that type from undergoing rearrangement in the same cell.

  2. Clonal restriction
    a. When a B cell divides, the chromosomes in its progeny cells bear the selected allelic genes, and these genes do not undergo any further V/J or V/D/J rearrangements.
    b. This is why all the immunoglobulin molecules produced by a given clone (a B lymphocyte and its progeny) are identical in epitope specificity and in κ or λ L chain isotype.

G. Development of malignancy. Errors in immunoglobulin gene rearrangement are thought to contribute to the genesis of several B cell malignancies.

  1. Follicular lymphoma
    a. In many patients with follicular lymphoma, the most common B cell cancer, a putative proto-oncogene (called *bcl-2*) on chromosome 18 is translocated into the H chain gene region on chromosome 14.

    b. It is thought that the close proximity of *bcl-2* to the active H chain gene region enhances the expression of the proto-oncogene and thus contributes to malignant transformation.

2. Burkitt's lymphoma

    a. Similarly, in the malignant cells of this B cell cancer, a portion of chromosome 8 containing the cellular proto-oncogene *c-myc* is translocated into chromosome 14 so that *c-myc* lies right next to the H chain gene region.

    b. The *c-myc* proto-oncogene is thought to be activated as a result of this proximity to the genetically active H gene region.

STUDY QUESTIONS

Directions: Each of the numbered items or incomplete statements in this section is followed by answers or by completions of the statement. Select the **one** lettered answer or completion that is **best** in each case.

1. In comparison to the other classes of immunoglobulins, IgM is predominant in all of the following ways EXCEPT

(A) complement activation
(B) primary immune response to most antigens
(C) enhancing phagocytosis
(D) production by the fetus
(E) heat-sensitivity

2. Components of a Fab fragment include all of the following EXCEPT

(A) an entire light (L) chain
(B) the V_H and C_H1 domains of the heavy (H) chain
(C) the Fd fragment
(D) the carboxy terminal portion of the H chain
(E) the paratope

3. Idiotypic variability pertains to the generation of the antigen-binding site in the

(A) constant region of the heavy (H) chain
(B) constant region of the light (L) chain
(C) variable region of the H chain
(D) C_H1 domain of the H chain
(E) epitope of the molecule

4. All of the following DNA segments contribute to the variable portion of the IgM heavy (H) chain EXCEPT

(A) V_H genes
(B) J_H genes
(C) D_H genes
(D) C_μ genes
(E) N-region additions

5. J chain is a glycopeptide associated with which of the following immunoglobulins?

(A) IgA
(B) IgG1
(C) IgG3
(D) IgD
(E) IgE

6. Structural characteristics of serum IgM molecules include

(A) identical κ or λ light (L) chains
(B) one constant and three variable regions
(C) two identical heavy (H) and two identical L chains
(D) 13 domains
(E) secretory piece

7. Characteristics of IgE, the immunoglobulin involved in atopic allergy, include

(A) the J chain as part of the molecule
(B) the ability to cross the placenta
(C) the ability to activate the classic complement pathway
(D) affinity for cells of the host
(E) opsonic activity

1-E	4-D	7-D
2-D	5-A	
3-C	6-A	

Directions: Each group of items in this section consists of lettered options followed by a set of numbered items. For each item, select the **one** lettered option that is most closely associated with it. Each lettered option may be selected once, more than once, or not at all.

Questions 8–13

For each characteristic listed below, select the immunoglobulin it most appropriately describes.

(A) IgE
(B) IgA
(C) IgG
(D) IgM
(E) IgD
(F) sIgA
(G) sIgM
(H) sIgG

8. Has a half-life of approximately 21 days

9. An elevated level in cord blood may indicate a fetal infection

10. Associated with atopic disease

11. Predominant immunoglobulin in various secretions

12. Predominant antibody in the early (primary) immune response

13. Crosses the placenta in humans

Questions 14–18

Match the descriptions below with the labeled areas in the accompanying diagram.

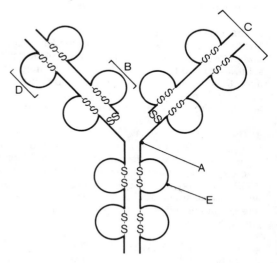

14. Site where papain cleaves the IgG molecule

15. Point of attachment of carbohydrate on heavy (H) chain

16. Area of immunoglobulin molecule where antigen attaches

17. Constant region of light (L) chain

18. Variable region of H chain

ANSWERS AND EXPLANATIONS

1. The answer is E *[III C].*
IgM is not heat-sensitive, as are IgD and IgE. IgM is a cyclic pentamer consisting of five basic units linked at the Fc fragments by the J chain. Because of its relatively high valence (theoretically 10), IgM is the most efficient immunoglobulin at activating complement. IgM antibodies form a major proportion of the primary immune response, whereas the secondary response consists almost entirely of IgG. IgM is synthesized before birth and represents the predominant antibody produced by the fetus. IgM enhances phagocytosis by causing the deposition of complement component C3b opsonin onto target surfaces.

2. The answer is D *[II G 1].*
The Fc (crystallizable) fragment, not the Fab (antigen-binding) fragment, contains the carboxy terminal portion of the heavy (H) chain. Treatment of the basic immunoglobulin monomer with the enzyme papain splits it into two Fab fragments and one Fc fragment. Each monovalent Fab fragment contains an entire light (L) chain and the variable (V_H) and constant (C_H1) domains of the H chain, referred to as the Fd fragment. The epitope-binding region of the molecule (the paratope) is formed by the folding of the variable domains of the H and L chains; therefore, the paratope is part of a Fab fragment.

3. The answer is C *[IV A 2 a (1)].*
Idiotypes represent unique amino acid sequences in the variable regions of the heavy (H) and light (L) chains associated with the antigen-binding site on the immunoglobulin molecule. Variability in amino acid sequence in these regions is concentrated in hypervariable (complementarity-determining) regions (CDRs; "hot spots"). The constant regions of the L and H chains, including the C_H1 domain, demonstrate an unvarying amino acid sequence except for isotypic and allotypic variations. The epitope is the structure on an antigen molecule that is bound by the antigen-binding site (the paratope) on the immunoglobulin molecule.

4. The answer is D *[IV B 4, C 3, D 3].*
In IgM heavy (H) chain gene organization, three segments of DNA [the variable (V_H), diversity (D_H), and joining (J_H) gene regions] join together to generate the variable portion of the H chain (V_H). The D_H gene segment accounts for the third hypervariable (complementarity-determining) region (CDR) of the H chain; this area includes the N region. The C_μ segment of DNA codes for the constant region of the IgM H chain.

5. The answer is A *[II J].*
The J chain is a glycopeptide associated with polymeric forms of immunoglobulins (IgM and some IgA), which contain two or more basic units. The J chain is linked to heavy (H) chains at the carboxy terminal portion of α and μ chains. IgG and IgE exist as monomeric forms and hence contain no J chain.

6. The answer is A *[II B 2 b, D 1, E 1, K; III C 1].*
The structural unit of serum IgM molecules consists of five monomers, each with four polypeptide chains. Thus it has 10 identical heavy (H) chains and 10 identical light (L) chains. All the L chains are of either the κ or λ type, because a given immunoglobulin molecule always contains identical κ or λ chains, never a mixture of the two. Each of the four chains of the monomer has a variable (amino terminal) portion and a constant (carboxy terminal) portion, and the L chains each have two domains, while the H chains of the IgM molecule have five domains. Secretory piece is a component of the secretory IgA molecule.

7. The answer is D *[III E 1, 2].*
IgE is described as homocytotropic because it has an affinity for cells of the host species that produced it. Because of its ability to attach to mast cells, IgE is associated with atopic diseases; that is, immediate hypersensitivity reactions (anaphylaxis, asthma, hay fever). IgE is a monomer and therefore does not contain a J chain as part of the molecule. Unlike IgG, IgE does not cross the placenta; however, IgE production begins in the fetus early in the gestational process. IgE is unable to activate complement via the classic pathway.

8–13. The answers are: 8-C *[III A 2 e; Table 3-1],* **9-D** *[III C 2 a (3)],* **10-A** *[III E 2 d],* **11-F** *[III B 2],* **12-D** *[III C 2 a (2)],* **13-C** *[III A 2 c].*
IgG, the major immunoglobulin in normal human serum (approximately 75% of the total), has a half-life of approximately 21 days, the longest of any of the immunoglobulins. It is the only immunoglobulin that can cross the placenta in humans, thus protecting the newborn during the first months of life. IgE is as-

sociated with immediate types of hypersensitivity reactions (e.g., atopy and anaphylaxis) and also, apparently, with immunity to certain helminthic parasites. Secretory IgA (sIgA) is the predominant immunoglobulin in various secretions (e.g., saliva, tears, colostrum); it consists of two basic units plus the J chain and secretory component. IgM is the predominant antibody in the early (primary) immune response and the predominant antibody produced by the fetus. An elevated IgM level in the cord serum (normal level, 10 mg/dl) of a newborn may indicate a prenatal infection in the fetus.

14–18. The answers are: 14-A *[II G 1, H 2 a],* **15-E** *[II I 1; Figure 3-1],* **16-C** *[II F 2],* **17-B** *[II D 1 b],* **18-D** *[II D 1 a].*
Papain cleaves the IgG molecule at the hinge region into three fragments of approximately equal size. The Fc (crystallizable) fragment is the carboxy, or C, terminal portion of the heavy (H) chain; it contains carbohydrate that is usually bound to the C_H2 or C_H3 domains.. The Fab (antigen-binding) fragments each contain an entire light (L) chain and the variable and constant domains of the H chain (V_H and C_H1, respectively); these fragments hold the antigen-binding site. The variable region of both H and L chains is at the amino, or N, terminal portion of the molecule; the constant region of a L chain is at the carboxy, or C, terminal portion.

6,5

I. INTRODUCTION

A. Overview. The complement system plays a major role in host defense and the inflammatory process.

1. Complement consists of a complex series of at least 15 plasma proteins that normally are functionally inactive.

2. Complement is activated sequentially in a cascading manner, each protein activating the protein that directly follows it in the sequence.

3. Activation of the complement cascade has widespread physiologic and pathophysiologic effects.

B. Metabolism

1. **Synthesis**
   a. The liver is the major site of synthesis of complement proteins, although macrophages and fibroblasts can synthesize some.
   b. Complement proteins first appear in the fetus during the second month of pregnancy.
   c. The concentration of most components at birth is about 50% of adult levels.
   d. Inflammation increases the synthesis of complement components, presumably through the action of interleukin-1 (IL-1) and gamma interferon.

2. **Catabolism.** The catabolic rate of complement proteins is high, 1% to 3% per hour.

C. Nomenclature of complement proteins

1. The nine major **complement components** (Table 4-1) are designated by C followed by an identifying numeral from 1 to 9 (e.g., C1, C2).
   a. The numerals indicate the order in which components are activated, except that component C4 is activated out of numerical order.
   b. This is because components were assigned numbers in the order in which they were discovered, and that did not initially match the sequential order.

2. **Peptide chains** of each component are designated by Greek letters (e.g., C3α, C4β).

3. **Cleaved peptides** from fragmented peptide chains are denoted by lowercase letters (e.g., C3a).

4. If further proteolysis results in loss of fragment activity, an i is added to indicate **inactivation** (e.g., iC3b).

5. A horizontal bar over the numeral of a component (e.g., $\overline{C1}$) indicates that the complement protein has acquired **enzymatic activity;** a horizontal bar over numerals of component complexes (e.g., $\overline{C5b67}$) indicates an **activated state**.

6. Components of the **alternative pathway** are designated by a capital letter (e.g., factor B, factor H).

D. Genetics

1. Most complement proteins have been found to have polymorphic genetic variants. Most variants are specified by autosomal codominant genes.

Table 4-1. Properties of Complement Components

Component	Serum Concentration (µg/ml)	Activation Products	Molecular Weight (kDa)
Classic Pathway			
C1q	70		410
C1r	50	C$\overline{1}$r	85
C1s	50	C$\overline{1}$s	85
C4	500	C4a, C4b	206
C2	25	C2a, C2$\overline{b}$	115
C3	1200	C3a, C3b	195
Alternative pathway			
Factor B	200	Ba, $\overline{B}$b	100
Factor D	1–5	$\overline{D}$	25
Properdin	25		50
Membrane attack (common) pathway			
C5	75	C5a, C5b	200
C6	60		128
C7	55		120
C8	55		150
C9	60		79
Regulatory proteins			
C$\overline{1}$ INH	200		105
Factor I	25		100
C4bp	250		560
Factor H	500		150
S protein	500		84
Anaphylatoxin inactivator	30		300

C$\overline{1}$ INH = C1 esterase inhibitor; C4bp = C4 binding protein.

2. Genes for several polymorphic complement proteins (factor B, C2, C4) are located in the major histocompatibility complex (MHC) on human chromosome 6 in a region called class III (see Chapter 12 II D 1 a).

3. Genes for six of the complement receptors and genes for the regulatory proteins are located on chromosome 1.

4. **Congenital deficiencies** of each of the component proteins except factor B (of the alternative pathway) have been observed in humans (see also Chapter 11 VII).
   a. **Heterozygous** individuals will have about half the normal amount of the protein in question, and usually suffer no ill effects.
   b. Many of those with **homozygous** deficiency suffer from systemic lupus erythematosus (SLE; see Chapter 10 II B) or from increased susceptibility to bacterial infections.
      (1) SLE has been observed in almost all persons with defects in C1 or C4. Of the 100 or more patients with known C2 deficiency, over 50% have SLE or a related illness.
      (2) Individuals with homozygous C3 deficiency suffer from recurrent severe infections caused by a variety of bacteria.
      (3) Absence of factor D, factor I, properdin, or the CR3 receptor predisposes to recurrent pyogenic infections caused by staphylococci, pneumococci, and other potent pathogens.
      (4) Excessive infections are seen in fewer than 5% of persons deficient in C5 to C8; most are caused by *Neisseria* organisms.

E. **Major functions.** Activation of the complement system generates a wide range of biological activities (see V); these can be grouped into three major functions.

1. **Opsonic function.** Opsonization occurs as activated complement components coat pathogenic organisms or immune complexes, facilitating the process of phagocytosis.

2. Inflammatory function. Activation of the complement system results in the release of histamine from mast cells and basophils and in stimulation of the inflammatory response.

3. Cytotoxic function. In the final stage of the complement cascade, the membranes of target cells (e.g., bacteria and tumor cells) are attacked, leading to cell death.

F. Interactions with other systems

1. Overview. Complement activation, kinin generation, blood coagulation, and fibrinolysis are all physiologic processes that occur through the sequential activation of enzymes in cascading fashion. These cascades interact with each other, sharing some activators, inhibitors, and cell membrane receptors.

2. Initiating factors
   a. Tissue injury can initiate each of the cascades.
      (1) Lysosomal enzymes from damaged cells cleave precursor molecules to generate phlogistic (inflammatory) compounds.
      (2) For example, neutrophils are attracted to the site of injury by the chemotactically active C3a that is cleaved from C3 by proteases released from lysosomes.
   b. Cascade-initiating factors can be activated by contact with **negatively charged surfaces** such as heparin or lipid A of the lipopolysaccharide from gram-negative bacterial cells.
   c. Hageman factor (HF; coagulation factor XII) is thereby activated, producing HFa.
      (1) HFa has serine protease activity.
      (2) In the kinin cascade, HFa activates prekallikrein, forming kallikrein.
         (a) Kallikrein in turn generates bradykinin from high-molecular-weight kininogen.
         (b) Bradykinin is a potent vasoactive peptide that causes pain, increases vascular permeability, and causes vasodilation.
      (3) Kallikrein is able to activate HF, and HFa has autoactivating capabilities; thus this system, like the complement system, has an efficient amplification loop.
   d. The three proteins, HFa, prekallikrein, and high-molecular-weight kininogen, are also the initiating factors required for the intrinsic blood coagulation and fibrinolytic pathways.
      (1) HFa activates coagulation factor XI to factor XIa, initiating the blood clotting cascade.
      (2) Kallikrein stimulates the plasminogen activator to generate plasmin, which has a variety of effects.
         (a) Plasmin can activate HF and can initiate the complement cascade.
            (i) It activates certain complement components (e.g., C1 and C3).
            (ii) It enzymatically activates C1s.
            (iii) It generates the anaphylatoxin C3a from C3.
         (b) Plasmin also releases chemotactic and vasoactive fibrinopeptides from fibrin.
   e. Adding **immune complexes** (antigen–antibody complexes) to blood or plasma activates the clotting system. This is caused by:
      (1) Clumping of C3b-coated platelets (immune adherence).
      (2) Release of clot-promoting platelet factors.

3. Inhibiting factors
   a. C1 esterase inhibitor (CT INH) of the complement system (see IV B 1) is an important control mechanism in the various cascading processes.
   b. In addition to inhibiting the serine protease activity of C1s, CT INH also inhibits HFa, XIa, plasmin, and kallikrein.

II. PATHWAYS OF COMPLEMENT ACTIVATION

A. Overview

1. The activation of complement components takes place in a cascading sequence, each component activating its successor protein in the cascade.

2. Complement activation may occur via two pathways, designated **classic** and **alternative**.
   a. The classic pathway is a more recently evolved mechanism of specific adaptive immunity, whereas the alternative pathway provides nonspecific innate immunity.
   b. The classic pathway is initiated primarily by antibody, usually bound to antigen, whereas the alternative pathway is initiated primarily by bacteria.

    c. The classic pathway requires the interaction of all nine major complement components, whereas the alternative pathway does not require components C1, C4, and C2.

    d. Both pathways can be divided into three **phases:**

       (1) A **"recognition" event** that initiates the complement cascade

       (2) An **amplification phase,** in which activation of early complement components culminates in activation of C3, a critical component

       (3) A **membrane attack phase,** which culminates in target cell lysis

    e. The two pathways differ in their initiation and amplification phases, and then share a final common pathway for the membrane attack phase.

  3. Several of the components of the complement cascade, when activated, become **serine proteases** (serine esterases) [Table 4-2].

    a. The substrates for these serine proteases are not hydrolyzed by the enzymes until they are bound into the complex by a "positioning" molecule.

    b. Thus, for example, C4b holds C3 so that C$\overline{2b}$ can hydrolyze it; similarly, C3b holds C5 so that C$\overline{2b}$ can act on it.

B. The classic pathway

1. Activation

    a. The classic pathway may be activated via antigen–antibody complexes or by aggregated immunoglobulins.

       (1) IgG (mainly **IgG1** and **IgG3**) and **IgM** are most efficient in reacting with complement.

          (a) Only one molecule of pentameric IgM is required, whereas at least two adjacent molecules of the monomer IgG are needed.

          (b) IgG4, IgA, IgD, and IgE do not activate the classic complement cascade at all in their native configuration; IgG2 binds complement weakly.

       (2) Classically, an **antigen–antibody complex** is designated **EA,** where **E** is the antigen (erythrocyte in the original historical observations) and **A** is the antibody.

          (a) Other antigens can substitute for E, and EA might not represent an antigen–antibody complex but an antibody-coated bacterial cell, a tumor cell, or a lymphocyte.

          (b) Complement components bind to EA in an orderly sequence to form a macromolecular complex, **EAC142356789.** The numerals indicate the order in which components bind to the complex.

    b. Activation follows the binding of complement component C1 to a site on the Fc fragment of the immunoglobulin. The site is the C_H2 domain on IgG or C_H3 on IgM.

2. Components and steps (Figure 4-1)

    a. C1 (the recognition unit). C1 is a trimolecular complex: it contains three polypeptides—**C1q, C1r,** and **C1s**—held together by calcium ions. With the removal of the calcium, C1 breaks down into its three subunits and loses activity.

       (1) **C1q** is the portion of the C1 molecule that attaches first to immunoglobulin and initiates complement activation.

          (a) C1q has six binding sites, globular structures extending on stalks from a central core (see Figure 4-1).

          (b) Because of its multivalency C1q can cross-link multiple immunoglobulin molecules, a requirement for activation.

          (c) To initiate the process of complement activation, two or more of the six globular domains of C1q interact with the C_H domains of at least two immunoglobulin monomers.

          (d) C1q binding breaks a peptide bond and activates C1r proenzyme to an active serine protease.

       (2) **C1r,** when activated, cleaves the proenzyme C1s.

       (3) **C1s,** when activated, becomes another serine protease, referred to as C$\overline{1}$ esterase (C$\overline{1s}$) because of its esterase activity.

          (a) C$\overline{1s}$ mediates the cleavage of native C4, the next component in the complement cascade.

          (b) One molecule of C$\overline{1s}$ can cleave several C4 molecules, thus serving as one of the sites in the amplification process (see II D).

    b. C4. C$\overline{1s}$ cleaves C4 into C4a and C4b.

       (1) **C4a,** one of three anaphylatoxins (see V B 1 a), is released into the surrounding medium (the fluid phase).

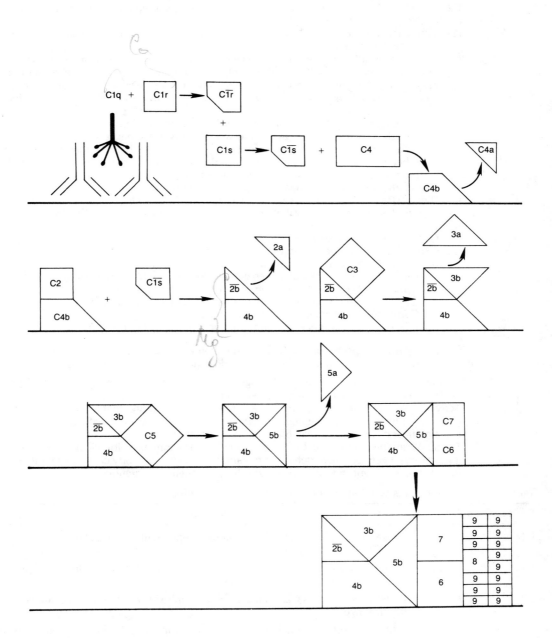

Figure 4-1. The classic pathway of complement activation. A *line* over a component indicates the activated form. See text for details.

(2) C4b can bind to cell membranes. The binding is rather inefficient, but several C4b molecules may cluster about C1s on the membrane surface.

(3) C4b combines with the next component, C2, to provide a substrate for C$\overline{1s}$.

c. C2. Once C2 is bound to the C4b molecule, it becomes susceptible to enzymatic attack by the C$\overline{1s}$ serine protease.

(1) C2b is activated to become the third serine protease in the cascade. Its substrates are C3 and C5 (see Table 4-2).

(2) C$\overline{2b}$ remains linked to the cell-bound C4b, thus forming the enzymatically active bimolecular complex C$\overline{4b2b}$. (Until recently this complex was called C$\overline{4b2a}$, but the International Committee on Complement Nomenclature has decided that this fragment of C2 should be designated C2b, in keeping with the terminology employed for the other complement components).

(a) Formation of the C$\overline{4b2b}$ complex requires magnesium ions.

(b) C$\overline{4b2b}$ is referred to as **classic pathway C3 convertase** because it cleaves C3.

(c) C2b is the enzymatic molecule in the C$\overline{4b2b}$ and C$\overline{4b2b3b}$ complexes, and the other molecules in the complex serve as docking, or attachment, vehicles that hold the substrates in position for enzymatic attack.

(3) The smaller peptide, designated **C2a,** is released into the fluid phase.

d. C3. The substrate for C3 convertase is C3. Circulating C3 binds to the C4b portion of the C$\overline{4b2b}$ complex. It is this binding that renders C3 subject to cleavage by C$\overline{2b}$ into two fragments, C3a and C3b.

(1) C3a is an anaphylatoxin and remains unbound.

(2) C3b is a major component in the complement system, with several key roles:

(a) The C3b bound to the membrane in the vicinity of the C$\overline{4b2b}$ complex (C3 convertase) forms the trimolecular enzymatic complex **C$\overline{4b2b3b}$ (C5 convertase)**. This complex acts on C5, the first component of the membrane attack pathway (see III).

(b) C3b binds the C5 molecule and positions it for cleavage by C$\overline{2b}$.

(c) C3b initiates the alternative complement pathway.

(d) C3b has several other important biological properties (see V B 2).

C. The alternative pathway (properdin pathway). The alternative pathway is considered to be a primitive defense system, a bypass mechanism that does not require C1, C4, and C2.

1. Activation. The alternative pathway can be triggered immunologically (e.g., by aggregated IgA or IgG4) or nonimmunologically (e.g., by certain microbial cell products).

a. Activation by immunoglobulins occurs when antibodies that are unable to interact with C1q in their native state are aggregated, either chemically or by mild heating. The biological significance of this pathway of activation is unclear.

b. The activation of complement by bacterial products has immense biological significance: it represents a very primitive defense mechanism by which the body can activate inflammatory processes and opsonize pathogens for phagocytic destruction.

Table 4-2. Serine Proteases Generated During Complement Activation

Protease	Substrate	Comments
C1r	C1s	These molecules are part of the calcium-dependent trimolecular C1q/C1r$_2$/C1s$_2$ complex
C1s	C4, C2	C4 is the first cleaved; it binds C2 and helps to position it for efficient cleavage into C2a and enzymatically active C$\overline{2b}$
C2	C3	Protease is active as C$\overline{2b}$ in the C$\overline{4b2b}$ complex; C4b binds and positions C3 for cleavage
	C5	Protease is active as C$\overline{2b}$ in the C$\overline{4b2b3b}$ complex; C3b binds and positions C5 for cleavage
D	B	B is bound by C3b on the activator surface and is cleaved by $\overline{D}$ to yield enzymatically active $\overline{Bb}$
B	C3, C5	Needs stabilization by properdin; protease is active as $\overline{Bb}$ in C3bBbP and C3bBb3BP; in the latter complex, first C3b binds and positions B; second C3b positions C5

C designates a component of the classic pathway; D, B, and P (properdin) are proteins of the alternative pathway.

    c. Substances capable of activating complement by the alternative pathway include:
      (1) Polysaccharides of microbial origin
        (a) Lipopolysaccharides of gram-negative bacteria (endotoxins)
        (b) Teichoic acids of gram-positive bacteria (adhesion molecules of some pathogens)
        (c) Zymosan from yeast cell walls
      (2) Surface components of some animal parasites such as *Schistosoma mansoni* larvae
    d. These cell wall components appear to protect C3b from inactivation by the control proteins H and I (see IV A 1 and B 2).

2. Components and steps (Figure 4-2)
    a. C3. The initial recognition event for alternative pathway activation is the presence of C3, specifically **C3b,** which is continuously present in very small amounts in normal serum.
      (1) Initiation by C3b is prevented by interaction with **factors H and I** (see also IV A 1 and B 2).
        (a) If C3b binds to a **nonactivator** (nonprotected) surface, it reacts with factor H and becomes inactivated through the combined actions of factor H and factor I.
        (b) If C3b binds to an **activator** (protected) surface, its ability to bind to factor H is diminished, and it can activate the alternative pathway.
      (2) C3 has two **molecular forms** in the body:
        (a) Native C3, which has an intact thioester bond
        (b) $C3(H_2O)$, in which the thioester bond has been hydrolyzed
    b. Factor B (the C3 proactivator)
      (1) The surface-bound, protected C3b interacts with factor B to form C3bB, a magnesium-dependent complex.
      (2) In the presence of magnesium ions, $C3(H_2O)$, like C3b, can also bind to factor B.
      (3) Factor B is analogous to C2 of the classic pathway.
        (a) The genes for factor B and C2 are adjacent on human chromosome 6.
        (b) C2 probably arises from duplication of the factor B gene.
    c. Factor $\overline{D}$. Factor $\overline{D}$ is a serine protease resembling $C\overline{1s}$.
      (1) Factor B, when bound to C3b [or $C3(H_2O)$], is susceptible to enzymatic cleavage by factor $\overline{D}$.
      (2) Two fragments are formed, Ba and Bb.

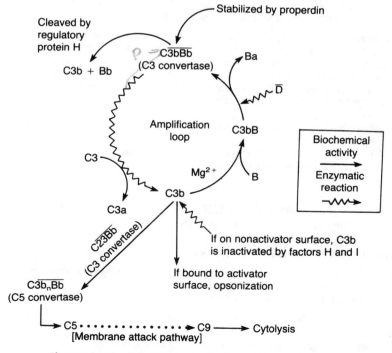

Figure 4-2. The alternative pathway of complement activation.

        (a) The **Ba** fragment is released.

        (b) An active site is exposed in the **Bb** fragment, which remains bound to C3b, forming the enzymatically active $\overline{C3bBb}$ complex.

           (i) $\overline{C3bBb}$ is the **alternative pathway C3 convertase**.

           (ii) The C3b molecule serves to bind substrate, which may be either more C3 molecules or C5 molecules, and hold it for enzymatic action of the activated serine protease, $\overline{Bb}$.

    d. Properdin (P)

        (1) In the presence of properdin, the dissociation of Bb is slowed, stabilizing the $\overline{C3bBb}$ complex.

        (2) When thus stabilized by properdin, the $\overline{C3bBb}$ complex becomes a C3 convertase that cleaves C3 and generates more C3b.

        (3) This creates a positive feedback loop that amplifies the complement cascade (see II D 2).

        (4) As more C3b is generated, the complex expands, with numerous C3b molecules attached to a single Bb ($\overline{C3b_nBb}$, where $n > 1$), and becomes a **C5 convertase** capable of cleaving C5 and thereby initiating the membrane attack pathway.

  3. Cobra venom factor (CVF). A factor contained in cobra venom has the interesting property of activating the alternative complement pathway.

    a. Like C3b, CVF complexes with Bb.

    b. The CVF-Bb thus formed is resistant to factors H and I and is capable of continuously activating the conversion of C3 to C3b, leading to complement depletion.

D. Amplification in the complement cascade. Many of the components of the complement system are enzymes; hence, the potential for self-amplification is tremendous.

  1. In the **classic pathway,** as a consequence of amplification, an enormous number (approximately 1200) of C3b opsonins can be deposited on a membrane near the site of a single IgM molecule.

    a. One IgM molecule is sufficient to bind and activate one C1q; the single C1s molecule is then capable of cleaving approximately one hundred C4 molecules.

    b. Some 20 or so C4b fragments bind to the cell membrane and cleave about 100 C2 molecules.

    c. Although only four to six of the C2b fragments are captured by C4b to form $\overline{C4b2b}$, this enzyme complex can activate thousands of C3 molecules.

  2. The **alternative pathway** represents other options for amplification.

    a. As stated above, approximately 1200 C3b fragments bind the cell membrane in the classic pathway. Each of these can interact with alternative pathway components (factors B and D) to form another molecule of the C3-cleaving enzyme, $\overline{C3bBb}$.

    b. As the C3 convertase of the alternative pathway, $\overline{C3bBb}$, once stabilized by properdin, can cleave thousands of C3 molecules, forming many C3b molecules capable of initiating the alternative pathway.

    c. When these C3b molecules become fixed to an activator surface, more factor B binding sites are exposed.

    d. These C3b molecules can also bind C5 and hold it in a position favorable for $\overline{Bb}$ hydrolysis, thus initiating the membrane attack process.

III. THE PATHWAY OF MEMBRANE ATTACK (THE COMMON PATHWAY). The convergence of the classic and alternative pathways occurs at the point of C5 activation.

A. Activation of the membrane attack pathway

  1. Activation of the membrane attack pathway is initiated by **C5 convertase,** which is

    a. $\overline{C4b2b3b}$ in the classic pathway

    b. $\overline{C3b_nBb}$ in the alternative pathway

  2. These C5 convertases are the only components in the attack pathway that have enzymatic activity.

    a. Thus, cleavage occurs only once in the attack sequence.

    b. Subsequent steps involve spontaneous binding and polymerization of intact proteins.

B. Components and steps

1. **C5.** C5 convertase cleaves C5 into a smaller C5a fragment and a larger C5b fragment.
   a. **C5a,** an anaphylatoxin and chemotactic factor, is released into surrounding fluid medium.
   b. **C5b** is the first component of the membrane attack complex. As such, it is the receptor for C6 and C7 and initiates assembly of the terminal components, C8 and C9.

2. **C6 and C7**
   a. Unstable C5b binds to C6, forming a stable C5b6 complex.
   b. C5b6 then binds to C7, forming the metastable trimolecular C5b67 complex.
   c. The C5b67 complex attaches to the target cell membrane without inflicting any damage.

3. **C8 and C9; formation of the membrane attack complex (MAC)**
   a. **C8** attaches to the membrane-bound C5b67 complex, forming C5b678.
   b. The addition of **C9** to the complex forms C5b6789, the **MAC.**
   c. The MAC is an amphiphilic (loving both lipid and water) molecular complex composed of one molecule each of C5b, C6, C7, and C8 and 12 to 18 molecules of polymerized C9 (see Figure 4-1).
      (1) In plasma, C9 is in soluble, monomeric form.
      (2) When it associates with cell-bound C5b678 complexes, it undergoes a change in shape and polymerizes, a process that requires a divalent cation, either calcium, magnesium, or zinc.
   d. C8 and C9, the final components of the complement cascade, are responsible for the membrane damage that causes cell lysis.

4. **Cell lysis**
   a. Cell lysis can occur when the C5b678 complex forms. In the absence of C9, tiny (3-nm) pores form in the membrane, and the cells become somewhat leaky.
   b. Cell lysis is much enhanced by the addition of C9 molecules to form C5b6789, the MAC. The polymerization of C9 greatly accelerates the process of lysis.
   c. The **C9 polymer** forms a cylindrical transmembrane channel 15 to 16 nm long with an internal diameter of 8 to 12 nm and a wall thickness of 2 nm (see Figure 4-3 inset). Attached to the channel is the C5b678 complex.
      (1) The top of the C9 polymer cylinder is hydrophilic and is capped by a ring which remains outside the cell.
      (2) The other end of the cylinder is lipophilic and forms the transmembrane channel.
   d. The hollow cylindrical channels of the MAC are in the lipid bilayer of the cell membrane.
   e. The channels coalesce into leaky patches, and the surface of the membrane looks like the surface of the moon covered with craters (Figure 4-3).
   f. The channels allow the passage of electrolytes and water across the membrane, leading ultimately to osmotic lysis of the target cells.
      (1) **Target erythrocytes** lose potassium, imbibe sodium and water, swell, and lyse.
      (2) If the target cell is **nucleated,** the cell membrane becomes porous, and low-molecular-weight and then high-molecular-weight substances pass unimpeded; these cells usually do not lyse.
   g. The lysis caused by C5b6789 is restricted to those cells on which the initiating events of the complement cascade have occurred; "innocent bystander" cells in the neighborhood will escape damage. This is because:
      (1) C5b6789 complexes in solution are extremely unstable and quickly lose their cytotoxicity.
      (2) There are inhibitors in plasma (e.g., S protein; see IV B 4) and in cell membranes [e.g., homologous restriction factor (HRF); see IV C 2].
   h. The entire process of cell lysis is nonenzymatic.
      (1) The process is very similar to the membrane damage caused by the perforin molecules secreted by natural killer (NK) cells and cytotoxic T lymphocytes [see Chapter 1 I G 1 c (1) and Chapter 9 V B 4 b (1)].
      (2) Antibodies produced against C9 cross-react with perforin, suggesting structural homology.

IV. REGULATORY MECHANISMS.
Complement activation is associated with potent biological functions that, if left unchecked, would exhaust the complement system and could cause significant damage to the host. Uncontrolled activation of the complement system is prevented by several types of protein–complement interactions.

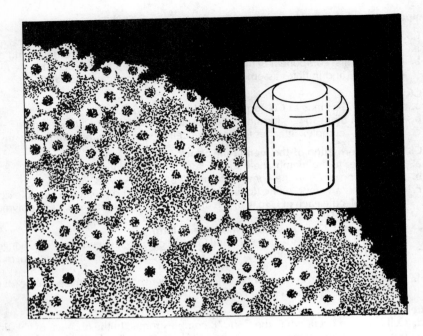

Figure 4-3. Effect of membrane attack complex (MAC; C5b6789) on cell membrane. *Inset* shows a schematic diagram of the transmembrane channel formed by polymerized C9 molecules. Poly C9 channels allow water and ions to cross the cell membrane, leading to cell lysis.

A. **Inactivators.** Some serum proteins enzymatically attack complement components, thereby inactivating them.

   1. **Factor I** (the **C3b inactivator;** hence, formerly called C3b INA)
      a. Factor I is a serine protease that cleaves C3b free in solution or on the surface of cells.
         (1) The degradation products are unable to function in the $\overline{C4b2b3b}$ complex.
         (2) One degradation product, C3c, is converted to C3e (see V B 3 a).
      b. Factor I also degrades C4b, but only in the presence of C4bp.

   2. **Anaphylatoxin inactivator (serum carboxypeptidase N).** This alpha globulin enzymatically destroys the biological activity of C3a, C4a, and C5a by removing the molecules' carboxy terminal arginine.

B. **Inhibitors.** Some serum proteins bind to, and thus inhibit, complement components.

   1. **C1 esterase inhibitor**
      a. $\overline{C1}$ INH is a plasma α_2-globulin that inhibits the enzymatic activity of C1 esterase by dissociating the subunits C1q, C1r, and C1s.
      b. It also inhibits plasmin, kallikrein, activated HF, and coagulation factor XIa.
      c. Deficiency of $\overline{C1}$ INH results in **hereditary angioedema,** an inherited defect characterized by transient but recurrent episodes of local edema due to uncontrolled C1s activity.

   2. **Factor H** (formerly called β1H)
      a. Factor H acts in concert with factor I, binding C3b and allowing factor I to cleave the α chain of C3b.
      b. This leads to formation of cleavage product **iC3b,** which no longer interacts with the alternative pathway components.

   3. **C4 binding protein.** C4bp controls the activity of cell-bound C4b. As with the interaction of factor H and C3b, C4bp binds to C4b and allows cleavage of the α chain and destruction of C4b by factor I.

4. S protein (vitronectin). S protein protects the target cell from lysis by binding to the developing fluid-phase C5b67 complex.
  a. The S protein–C5b67 complex cannot penetrate the target cell membrane.
  b. S protein does not stop the C5b6789 complex from forming, but prevents it from penetrating the lipid layer of the cell membrane.

C. Regulatory proteins in cell membranes

  1. Decay-accelerating factor (DAF) and membrane cofactor protein (MCP)
    a. DAF and MCP have the same functions as factor H and C4bp. However, DAF and MCP inactivate membrane-bound C3b and C4b, whereas factor H and C4bp act on C3b and C4b in solution.
    b. DAF prevents assembly of the two C3 convertases by promoting dissociation of C2b from C4b and Bb from C3b.
      (1) DAF is a membrane glycoprotein found on many cells of the body.
      (2) It is deficient or absent in cells from patients with **paroxysmal nocturnal hemoglobinuria**. The red blood cells of these patients have increased sensitivity to complement-mediated lysis.
    c. MCP is an integral membrane protein that serves as a cofactor for the proteolytic inactivation of C4b and C3b by factor I.

  2. Homologous restriction factor [HRF; also called C8 binding protein (C8bp)]. HRF is found on many cells of the body. HRF binds to C8 and prevents its interaction with cell-bound C5b67.

V. BIOLOGICAL CONSEQUENCES OF COMPLEMENT ACTIVATION (TABLE 4-3)

A. Overview

  1. During complement activation, a number of materials with important biological activities are generated.
    a. The **cleavage products (split products) of C3, C4, and C5** appear to be the most important complement components in terms of biological functions associated with the inflammatory response.
    b. C8 and C9 play a major role in membrane attack and the lytic process.
  2. Cell receptors that have complement fragments for their homologous ligands have significant biological roles (Table 4-4).
    a. Some receptors react with larger fragments such as C3b and promote opsonization and, hence, phagocytosis.
    b. Others are specific for the smaller "a" fragments that play a role in inflammatory processes.

Table 4-3. Principal Inflammatory Activities of Activated Complement Proteins and Their Fragments

Component	Activity
C3a, C4a, C5a	Anaphylatoxin—releases histamine, serotonin, and other vasoactive compounds from mast cells, increasing capillary permeability
C3b, iC3b, C4b	Immune adherence and opsonization—binds antigen–antibody complexes to membranes of macrophages and neutrophils, enhancing phagocytosis; also binds complexes to erythrocytes, facilitating removal by the liver and spleen
C5a	Chemotaxis and chemokinesis—attracts phagocytic cells to sites of inflammation and increases their overall activity
C8, C9	Membrane damage—transmembrane channels form, permitting flux of cytoplasmic constituents. Mammalian cells swell and burst; bacterial cells become leaky and lose vital intracellular metabolites, but usually do not burst
Ba	Neutrophil chemotaxis
Bb	Macrophage activation—causes macrophages to adhere to surfaces and spread on them

Table 4-4. Complement Receptors of Human Cells

Receptor	Ligands	Cell Types	Functions
CR1	C4b, C3b, iC3b	Erythrocytes, phagocytes, B cells, eosinophils	Opsonin: cofactor in factor I cleavage of C3b to C3dg; clearance of antigen–antibody complexes*
CR2	iC3b, C3d, C3dg	B cells, some T cells, NK cells	Immunoregulatory; attachment site for Epstein-Barr virus
CR3	iC3b	Phagocytes	Opsonin; cofactor in C3bi degradation
CR4	C3b, iC3b, C3dg	Phagocytes	Not established; presumably an opsonin
C3aR	C3a	Mast cells, basophils, eosinophils, smooth muscle, phagocytes	Release of histamine and other mediators
C4aR	C4a	Mast cells, basophils	May be same as C3a receptor; same effects as C3a
C5aR	C5a	Mast cells, basophils	Same effects as C3a
C3eR		Neutrophils	Causes PMN release from marrow stores

NK cell = natural killer cells; PMN = polymorphonuclear neutrophil.
*Immune complexes bind rapidly to erythrocytes (by immune adherence) and are transported to the liver and spleen, where macrophages strip the complexes from the cell surface and return the erythrocyte to the circulation.

    c. Complement receptors on human erythrocytes provide an important mechanism for clearing immune complexes from the circulation. They bind the complexes and transport them to the liver and spleen where they are engulfed by phagocytic cells.

B. Cleavage products of C3 and C5

  1. C3a and C5a
    a. C3a and C5a are **anaphylatoxins**. C4a (see V C) is also an anaphylatoxin but is much less active than the other two.
      (1) These molecules react with specific receptors on basophil and mast cell membranes, causing the release of pharmacologic **mediators of inflammation** (e.g., histamine) in a manner that is similar to mediator release by IgE.
      (2) The mediators cause smooth muscle contraction and increased vascular permeability, effects which can be counteracted by antihistamines and anaphylatoxin inactivator.
    b. C3a and C5a also appear to have the ability to contract smooth muscle and increase capillary permeability directly (i.e., without the mediation of mast cells and basophils).
    c. C3a appears to function as an immunoregulatory molecule, demonstrating suppressive activity in immunoglobulin synthesis as well as in T cell functions.
    d. C5a is much more active than C3a on a molar basis and, in addition to anaphylatoxin activity, has a wider **range of biological activity,** including the following:
      (1) C5a seems to be the major complement-derived **chemotactic factor** in serum.
        (a) It causes neutrophils and macrophages to migrate toward the site where it is generated (**chemotaxis**).
        (b) It also increases the overall activity of phagocytic cells (**chemokinesis**).
      (2) C5a causes **neutrophils to adhere** to the endothelium of vessels and to one another, leading to neutropenia.
      (3) It **activates neutrophils,** triggering a bactericidal oxidative burst and degranulation.
      (4) It stimulates the **production of leukotrienes** [e.g., slow-reacting substance of anaphylaxis (SRS-A)], by mast cells.
    e. C5a-des-arg is C5a without the carboxy terminal arginine (removed by anaphylatoxin inactivator). C5a-des-arg lacks the anaphylatoxin activity of C5a but retains chemotactic and neutrophil-activating ability.
  2. C3b. The generation of C3b and the coating of target cells by C3b are perhaps the major biological functions of complement.

    a. The role of C3b in the **activation of the alternative complement pathway** has been described (see II C 2).

    b. C3b is a major **opsonin.**
        (1) Several cell types have surface receptors for C3b and iC3b, including neutrophils, eosinophils, monocytes, macrophages, B cells, basophils, and primate erythrocytes.
        (2) In the case of phagocytic cells, a coating of C3b on particles such as bacteria or antigen–antibody complexes promotes the attachment and ultimate ingestion of the particles.
        (3) The biological significance of the presence of C3b receptors on B cells is not entirely clear, but they may play a role in the induction of certain humoral immune responses.

    c. C3b-coated cells also tend to **aggregate (immune adherence),** a process that also may promote phagocytosis.

    d. Immune adherence of platelets to C3b can also activate the clotting system (see I F 2 e).

  3. Other C3 split products
    a. **C3e** is derived by proteolytic cleavage from **C3c** which, in turn, is derived from C3b by the action of factor H and factor I. C3e provokes a release of neutrophils from bone marrow, causing prompt leukocytosis.

    b. **C3d,** another cleavage product of C3b, can interact with CR2 receptors on B lymphocytes (see Table 4-4) and acts as a growth factor for these cells.

    c. **C3 nephritic factor (C3NeF)** is a **pathologic component** of the alternative pathway.
        (1) C3NeF is found in the circulation of patients with **mesangiocapillary glomerulonephritis.**
        (2) It acts as an antibody against the **C3bBb complex** and leads to a marked hypocomplementemia.

  4. C5b67. The C5b67 complex has been reported to have **chemotactic** activity. However, C5b67 is rapidly inactivated in serum, and hence it is not clear whether the complex plays an important chemotactic role.

C. C4 and its cleavage products

  1. Activated C4 molecules attach to membranes in close proximity to the C1 site. The binding of C1 and C4 by a virus–antibody complex can **neutralize virus activity;** probably, the C4 molecules prevent viral attachment to target cells.

  2. C4a has **anaphylatoxin** activity (see V B 1 a).

  3. C4b receptor sites exist on several cell types (e.g., phagocytic cells, lymphocytes, and primate erythrocytes), suggesting a role for C4b in **opsonization,** as seen with C3b.

D. C2

  1. C2 cleavage has been reported to be linked to the production of a **kinin-like molecule** that increases vascular permeability and contracts smooth muscle.

  2. This molecule is thought to be involved in the symptoms seen in hereditary angioedema (see IV B 1 c).

E. Ba and Bb. These two factors, generated exclusively by the alternative pathway, have important biological functions.

  1. Ba is chemotactic for neutrophils.

  2. Bb activates macrophages and causes them to adhere to and spread on surfaces.

F. C8 and C9. These components are responsible for the membrane damage that causes the lysis of bacteria and other cells (see III B 3, 4).

STUDY QUESTIONS

Directions: Each of the numbered items or incomplete statements in this section is followed by answers or by completions of the statement. Select the **one** lettered answer or completion that is **best** in each case.

1. All of the following complement components are required in the alternative pathway EXCEPT

(A) C1, C2, C4
(B) C5, C6, C7
(C) C3
(D) C8, C9
(E) Properdin

2. Anaphylatoxin inactivator is a serum enzyme that destroys the biological activity of

(A) C1a
(B) C2a
(C) C2b
(D) C3a
(E) C3b

3. Factor I is a serum enzyme that shows which of the following activities? It

(A) enhances opsonization
(B) enhances immune adherence
(C) destroys anaphylatoxin inactivator
(D) cleaves C3b
(E) inactivates anaphylatoxin

4. C3 nephritic factor (C3NeF) has which of the following properties? It is

(A) a pathologic component of the alternative complement pathway
(B) important in neutralizing virus activity
(C) essential for release of neutrophils from bone marrow
(D) an antibody against C3a
(E) an antibody against C3b

5. Magnesium ions are required for the formation of which of the following molecules?

(A) The factor H binding site
(B) C1 esterase
(C) Factor A
(D) The C4b2b complex
(E) C3b

6. C5a stimulates neutrophils to do all of the following EXCEPT

(A) migrate
(B) adhere to the endothelium of vessels
(C) trigger an oxidative burst
(D) produce leukotrienes
(E) release interleukin-1 (IL-1)

7. All of the following are serine proteases EXCEPT

(A) C1r
(B) C1s
(C) C2b
(D) C3b
(E) Bb

8. The binding site for complement on the IgG molecule is in the

(A) V_L domain
(B) C_L domain
(C) V_H domain
(D) C_H1 domain
(E) C_H2 domain

9. Complement regulatory proteins that are active in the cell membrane include

(A) C1q
(B) C1 esterase inhibitor (C1 INH)
(C) C4 binding protein (C4bp)
(D) Decay accelerating factor (DAF)
(E) C3e

1-A   4-A   7-D
2-D   5-D   8-E
3-D   6-E   9-D

Directions: The group of items in this section consists of lettered options followed by a set of numbered items. For each item, select the **one** lettered option that is most closely associated with it. Each lettered option may be selected once, more than once, or not at all.

Questions 10–14

For each characteristic of a complement component listed below, select the component that is most closely associated with it.

(A) C2
(B) C4
(C) C3bBb
(D) C3e
(E) C3b
(F) C5a
(G) C9
(H) C5b6789

10. Neutralizes virus activities

11. Stabilized by properdin

12. Associated with symptoms seen in hereditary angioedema

13. Provokes release of neutrophils from bone marrow

14. Promotes opsonization

10-B   13-D
11-C   14-E
12-A

ANSWERS AND EXPLANATIONS

1. The answer is A *[II C].*
The alternative pathway of complement activation does not require C1, C4, and C2. The alternative pathway, also referred to as the properdin pathway, is considered to be a primitive defense system, a mechanism that bypasses components C1, C4, and C2. The initial requirement for the alternative pathway is the presence of C3, specifically C3b.

2. The answer is D *[IV A 2].*
C3a is destroyed by anaphylatoxin inactivator. C3a, and also C5a and C4a, are referred to as anaphylatoxins. They cause the release of vasoactive amines from mast cells and basophils; the amines, in turn, cause smooth muscle contraction and increased vascular permeability. Anaphylatoxin inactivator (serum carboxypeptidase N) removes the carboxy terminal arginine residue from the anaphylatoxins, destroying their biological activity.

3. The answer is D *[IV A 1].*
Factor I, also known as C3b inactivator (C3b INA), is a serum enzyme that cleaves C3b in solution or on the surface of cells, rendering it unable to function in either the classic or alternative complement pathway. Opsonization and immune adherence, therefore, are inhibited.

4. The answer is A *[V B 3 c].*
C3 nephritic factor (C3NeF) is a pathologic component of the alternative complement pathway that is found in the circulation of patients with mesangiocapillary glomerulonephritis. C3NeF is an antibody against the $\overline{C3bBb}$ complex and leads to a marked hypocomplementemia.

5. The answer is D *[II B 2 c (2) (a) (b), C 2 b (1)].*
In the classic complement pathway, magnesium ions are required for formation of the $\overline{C4b2b}$ complex, the classic pathway C3 convertase. In the alternative pathway, surface-bound, protected C3b interacts with factor B to form C3bB, which is also a magnesium ion–dependent complex. Calcium ions are essential for the activation of C1 esterase in the classic pathway.

6. The answer is E *[V B 1 d].*
C5a does not stimulate neutrophils to release interleukin-1 (IL-1). Besides possessing anaphylatoxin activity, C5a seems to be the major complement-derived chemotactic factor in serum, causing directed migration of neutrophils. It also causes neutrophils to adhere to the endothelial lining of vessels, activates neutrophils towards an oxidative burst, and stimulates mast cells to produce leukotrienes [slow-reacting substance of anaphylaxis (e.g., SRS-A)]. IL-1 is a monokine released by macrophages during antigen presentation to B and T cells. It induces T lymphocytes to release various other interleukins which induce proliferation and differentiation of many different cells of the body.

7. The answer is D *[Table 4-2].*
Five serine proteases become activated in the complement cascade: C1r, C1s, C2b, and factors D and B (as Bb). These serine proteases are proteolytic enzymes that cleave the next components in the cascade. C3b is a potent opsonin that sensitizes bacteria and other foreign particles to phagocytosis. Neutrophils and macrophages have on their membranes a receptor that reacts with C3b and holds the microbe in close proximity to the phagocytic cell, thus enhancing the engulfment process.

8. The answer is E *[II B 1 b].*
In the case of IgG, complement binds to the C_H2 domain on the Fc fragment. With IgM, complement binds to the C_H3 domain. Activation of complement may occur via either the classic or the alternative pathway. The classic pathway may be activated by antigen–antibody complexes involving, primarily, IgG or IgM.

9. The answer is D *[IV C].*
Decay accelerating factor (DAF) is found on the surface of many cells of the body. It prevents the assembly of C3 convertases by promoting dissociation of the enzymatically active fragments C2b and Bb from their membrane-associated ligands, C4b and C3b, respectively. DAF is not an integral membrane protein but is anchored to the membrane by attachment to phosphatidylinositol; the same is true of some cell adhesion molecules, such as lymphocyte functional antigen 3 (LFA-3), found on T cells. These are important biologically because they serve to hold the cells together and enhance intercellular communication. Thus, cytotoxic reactions are enhanced, as are the initial events in cellular collaboration during the induction of immune responses. These molecules are members of a broad group of membrane glycoproteins termed integrins, which are presumed to facilitate cell migration in embryos, wound healing, phagocytosis, and target cell killing.

10–14. The answers are: 10-B *[V C 1]*, **11-C** *[II C 2 c, d]*, **12-A** *[V D]*, **13-D** *[V B 3 a]*, **14-E** *[V B 2 b]*. The binding of C1 and C4 by a virus–antibody complex can neutralize virus activity; it is probable that the C4 prevents viral attachment to target cells. In the alternative pathway, the C3bBb complex is cleaved by factor D̄. The Ba fragment is released, and the C3bBb complex, stabilized by properdin, becomes a C3 convertase. C2 is thought to be involved in the symptoms of hereditary angioedema, a disease caused by uncontrolled C1s activity. C2 cleavage has been reported to be linked to the production of a kinin-like molecule that increases vascular permeability and contracts smooth muscle. C3e provokes a release of neutrophils from the bone marrow, causing prompt leukocytosis. C3e is derived, by proteolytic cleavage, from C3c, which, in turn, is derived from C3b. C3b plays an important role in opsonization.

5
The Immune Response System

I. INTRODUCTION

A. Overview

1. When an individual is exposed to an antigenic substance, either by injection or infection, a complex series of events ensues (Figure 5-1).
   a. An **antigen-presenting cell** (usually a macrophage) processes the antigen and presents it to the lymphoid cells of the immune system.
      (1) For a successful immune response to occur, the **processed antigen** (specifically, its **epitope**) must be **presented to the lymphocytes** in association with a glycoprotein encoded by genes of the major histocompatibility complex (MHC).
      (2) This requirement for effective cell interaction is called **MHC restriction** (see IV D).
   b. The lymphoid cells recognize that particular epitope and acquire the ability to react with it.
   c. The result of this sequence of events is the **activation of antigen-specific B and T cells,** causing them to proliferate and mature.

2. The consequences of the initial interaction between lymphocytes and their homologous epitopes are far-reaching.
   a. A subsequent exposure to antigen will induce some **B lymphocytes** (memory B cells) to proliferate and differentiate into **antibody-secreting plasma cells**.
      (1) These active plasma cells release their specific antibody in large amounts when they contact antigen a second time, a phenomenon known as **anamnesis**.
      (2) The **secreted antibody** reacts specifically with the antigen that originally induced the B cell to proliferate. The potential exists to produce an extremely large (> 100,000) variety of different, specifically reactive, antibodies.
   b. Some **T lymphocytes** (memory T cells) are induced to differentiate and proliferate to form mature progeny that will be triggered to release biologically active metabolites when they contact antigen a second time.

B. Genetic control. The immune response is under highly complex genetic control.

1. Most of the genes that code for chain segments of the immunoglobulin molecule or the T cell receptor are polycistronic (i.e., present in the cell in multiple forms). The process of **DNA rearrangement and deletion,** followed by RNA splicing, selects alleles that code for a particular **immunologic specificity** (see Chapter 3 IV B 1 b).

2. The **ability to respond to antigens** is also under genetic control; the genes that control responsiveness are in the MHC (see Chapter 12 II C 4).

II. THE LYMPHOID SYSTEM

A. Overview. The lymphoid system involves the organs and tissues in which lymphocytic cells originate as lymphocyte precursors and then mature and differentiate; the cells finally lodge in the lymphoid organs or move throughout the body.

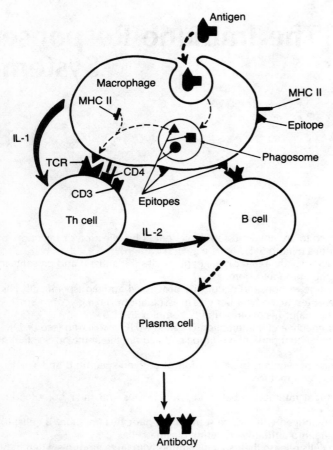

Figure 5-1. Cellular interactions in the humoral immune response. Some antigens do not require participation of helper T (Th) cells. *CD3, CD4* = cluster of differentiation antigens 3 and 4; *IL-1, IL-2* = interleukins 1 and 2; *MHC II* = major histocompatibility complex class II antigen; *TCR* = T cell receptor for antigen.

B. Tissues, organs, and cells of the lymphoid system (Figure 5-2)

1. The lymphoid tissues are divided functionally into primary and secondary organs.
   a. The **central (primary) lymphoid organs** are the **thymus** and the **bursa** or **bone marrow**.
   b. The **peripheral (secondary) lymphoid tissues** are the **lymph nodes, spleen, diffuse lymphoid tissues**, and **lymphoid follicles**.

2. **Precursor cells** of the lymphoid system originate in the yolk sac, the liver, the spleen, or the avian bursa of Fabricius (or its mammalian equivalent, the bone marrow) during fetal development.

3. **Stem cells** from bone marrow or embryonic tissues are deposited in the primary lymphoid organs, where the cells mature into lymphocytes.

4. **Lymphocytes** are precursor cells of immunologic function as well as regulators and effectors of immunity. **T cells** have a long life span of months or years, whereas most **B cells** have a shorter life span of 5 to 7 days.

5. Upon maturation, the lymphocytes seed secondary lymphoid tissue, where the cells undergo further maturation toward immunocompetence and the production of humoral antibodies or specifically sensitized lymphocytes.

C. The two facets of the immune response system

1. The **thymic system** controls the **cell-mediated (cellular) branch** of the immune system.
   a. The immunologic role of the thymus was demonstrated by the following experiment.
      (1) If the thymus of experimental animals is removed (particularly while they are very young), the immune response (primarily cell-mediated immunity) is depressed.
      (2) A thymus graft from another animal restores immunocompetence and cellular immunity. Even if the thymus graft is placed within a bag impervious to cells but not to fluids, the response is restored.

A

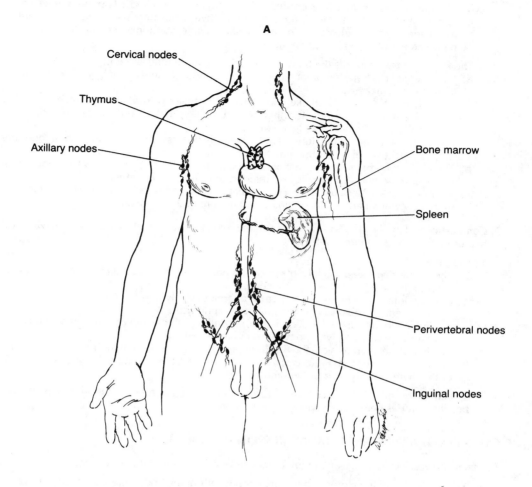

Cervical nodes

Thymus

Axillary nodes

Bone marrow

Spleen

Periervertebral nodes

Inguinal nodes

B

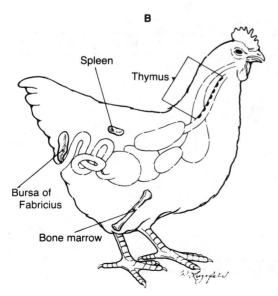

Spleen

Thymus

Bursa of
Fabricius

Bone marrow

Figure 5-2 Tissues, organs, and cells of the lymphoid system (*A*) in humans and (*B*) in birds.

    b. The immunocompetent cells produced in the thymus are called **T lymphocytes (T cells)**.

    c. Epithelial cells of the thymus produce soluble **thymic hormones**—peptides that regulate the differentiation and maturation of T cells. Thymic hormones include thymosin, thymopoietin, and thymic humoral factor.

2. The **bursal system** controls the **humoral branch** of the immune system.

    a. Discovery of the humoral branch of the immune system came about by an accidental observation in chickens.

        (1) A lymphoid organ in chickens known as the **bursa of Fabricius** (see Figure 5-2B) has a role in the development of humoral immunity; that is, in the development of circulating antibodies (e.g., IgG, IgA).

        (2) Removal of the bursa during embryogenesis depresses humoral immunity, but does not affect cellular immune functions.

    b. The immunocompetent cells that arise through this pathway are called **B lymphocytes (B cells)**, and the bursal system is also referred to as the **B cell system**.

    c. Mammals lack a bursa but have a **functional equivalent** that is involved with humoral immunity. Mammalian B cells originate and mature in the **bone marrow**.

D. Compartmentalization. The lymph nodes and the spleen show an anatomic division between the two branches of the immune system.

1. Lymph nodes

    a. The **B cell–dependent regions** of the lymph nodes are called **germinal centers** or **follicles** and are the sites of antibody production.

        (1) The follicles are found in the **cortical area** of the lymph node.

            (a) Primary follicles contain small B lymphocytes.

            (b) Following antigenic stimulation, **secondary follicles** develop which contain many large dividing lymphocytes and plasma cells.

        (2) If the bursa is removed, the B cell–dependent regions of the lymph nodes degenerate.

    b. The **thymus-dependent regions** of the lymph nodes are the **juxtamedullary areas**. Removal of the thymus causes a degeneration of these regions.

2. Spleen. In the spleen, the **B cells** are located in the **white pulp;** the **T cells** ensheathe the **trabecular arteries** before these vessels enter the white pulp.

III. CELLS INVOLVED IN THE IMMUNE RESPONSE (Table 5-1)

A. Macrophages. Macrophages function as **accessory cells** in the immune response.

1. Macrophages are the major **antigen-presenting cells** of the body, interacting with antigen as a primary step in the induction of an immune response. Langerhans cells of the skin, dendritic cells, and B lymphocytes can also present antigen.

Table 5-1. Characteristics of Cells Involved in the Immune Response

Characteristics	T cell	B cell	Macrophage
Antigen-specific	+	+	−
Increased numbers in secondary response	+	+	−
Site of immunoglobulin synthesis	−	+	−
Helper function in antibody response	+	−	−
Effector cell in cell-mediated immunity	+	−	−
Effector cell in humoral immunity	−	+	−
Accessory cell in cell-mediated and humoral immunity	−	−	+
Antigen-binding receptors on surface	+	+	−
Rosette formation with SRBC	+	−	−
Rosette formation with SRBC + antibody + complement	−	+	−
PHA receptors on surface	+	−	−
Con A receptors on surface	+	−	−
Lipopolysaccharide receptors on surface	−	+	−

con A = concanavalin A; PHA = phytohemagglutinin; SRBC = sheep red blood cell.

2. Besides presenting antigen to T and B cells, macrophages release soluble mediators such as the monokine (macrophage-derived mediator with hormone-like effects) interleukin-1 (IL-1), which stimulates T cells to mature and to secrete lymphokines (lymphocyte-derived mediators with hormone-like effects).

B. T lymphocytes

1. **T cell development.** Fetal stem cells that are destined to become T cells enter the thymus and proliferate there. These **immature T cells** (called **thymocytes** while in the thymus) pass through several developmental stages before leaving the thymus for the periphery as mature T cells.
    a. During T cell development in the thymus, several changes occur.
    - **(1)** Some type of selection process occurs which favors the proliferation of thymocytes that are restricted by **self-MHC molecules**. That is, thymocytes are selected for their ability to recognize antigens associated with molecules of the same MHC type (see IV D and Chapter 12 II B 2).
        - **(a)** Precursors of both helper T (Th) cells (MHC class II–restricted) and cytotoxic T (Tc) lymphocytes (MHC class I–restricted) are selected.
        - **(b)** Current evidence suggests that cortical thymic epithelial cells which express both class I and class II MHC glycoproteins are important in this selection event; the mechanism is still unknown.
    - **(2)** **Gene rearrangements** take place that give the mature T cell its **antigenic specificity**.
    - **(3)** There are also changes in certain **antigenic markers** displayed on the T cell surface (see III B 2 a). Ultimately, functional subpopulations of T cells can be differentiated by these identifying surface markers.
    b. In addition, T cells are **suppressed** if they are potentially **reactive against self-antigens** (see Chapter 6 III B 1). This occurs late in their differentiation within the thymus.

2. **General characteristics of T cells**
    a. T cell surface markers
    - **(1)** Monoclonal antibody techniques have identified molecules on the T cell membrane that function chiefly as receptors.
    - **(2)** These surface molecules include:
        - **(a)** Class I and class II **MHC molecules**
        - **(b)** Thy 1, Ly1, Ly2,3, and L3T4 in mice
        - **(c)** **CD (cluster of differentiation) antigens** (e.g., CD3, CD4, and CD8) in humans. (The designation CD replaces various former prefixes, most notably T, for thymus. CD and T numbers do not always correspond; for example, CD2 was formerly T11.)
    - **(3)** As a thymocyte differentiates toward a particular T cell subtype, it acquires certain CD antigens in its membrane and loses others. Thus, the T cell subsets can be distinguished by their CD markers (see Table 5-2).
    - **(4)** **CD3, CD2,** and **CD5** are found on most peripheral blood T cells.
        - **(a)** **CD3** is a heteropolymer with at least five polypeptide chains; it appears late in differentiation when the cells are becoming immunocompetent.
            - **(i)** CD3 is associated with the **T cell receptor for antigen** [see III B 2 b (2) and Figure 5-3]; it is important in intracellular signalling to initiate an immune response once the cell has interacted with a homologous epitope.
            - **(ii)** CD3 is not directly involved in antigen recognition, but antibodies against CD3 will block the antigen-specific activation of T cells.
        - **(b)** **CD2** (the **SRBC receptor**) is responsible for rosetting of sheep red blood cells (SRBCs) in the E-rosette assay for T cell enumeration (see Chapter 8 IV C 1).
        - **(c)** **CD5** is expressed on all T cells and on a subset of B cells that appear to be predisposed to autoantibody production.
    - **(5)** **CD4** and **CD8** are present on different effector T cells (see Table 5-2). These receptors bind the MHC molecule during antigen presentation to the T cell.
    - **(6)** Antiserum against certain of the membrane markers (e.g., against CD3) is immunosuppressive and has been used to prevent rejection of transplanted tissues (see Chapter 12 III G 2 d).
    b. The T cell receptor for antigen
    - **(1)** **Overview.** T cells have an antigen-specific receptor that functions as the **antigen recognition site**. This surface component, the **T cell receptor (TCR),** bears significant structural homology with the Fab portion of an antibody molecule (see Figure 12-3).

(2) Structure and function
  (a) The TCR is a heterodimer.
    (i) It consists of two nonidentical polypeptide chains, an α chain (about 45 kDa) and a β chain (about 40 kDa), linked together by disulfide bonds (see Figure 12-3).
    (ii) Both chains of the heterodimer are variable; there may be more variability in the smaller (β) chain.
  (b) The TCR contains **idiotypic determinants** similar to those of immunoglobulin molecules. **Hypervariability** occurs in particular areas of each polypeptide chain in a manner analogous to the complementarity-determining regions (CDRs) of immunoglobulin molecules (see Chapter 3 II D 4).
  (c) The TCR heterodimer is noncovalently linked in the T cell membrane to the γ, δ, and ε chains of the CD3 molecule (Figure 5-3).
  (d) The TCR–CD3 complex apparently makes contact with both the antigen and a portion of the MHC molecule. Different portions of the hypervariable regions of the α and β chains interact with:
    (i) The helical sides of the epitope-binding cleft of the MHC molecule
    (ii) The epitope lying on the floor of the cleft
  (e) CD4 or CD8 molecules (depending on the T cell subset) also contact a portion of the MHC molecule (see Figure 5-3).
(3) Genetics. Genetically, construction of the TCR is remarkably similar to that of the immunoglobulins (see Chapter 3 II).
  (a) Three gene segments are involved in the synthesis of the α chain: a variable (V), a joining (J), and a constant (C) gene segment.
  (b) In addition, the β chain has a diversity (D) gene segment which is expressed in the intact polypeptide.
  (c) As with immunoglobulins, rearrangements of the V, J, and D gene segments mediate the vast antigenic diversity of the TCR.
    (i) Two of the receptor's hypervariable regions are encoded in the V gene segment.
    (ii) One region is encoded in the VJ (α chain) or VDJ (β chain) segment.

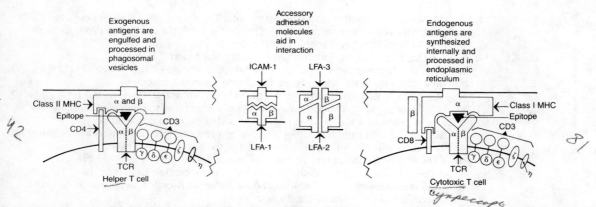

Figure 5-3. Interaction between the T cell receptor (TCR)–CD3–CD4/CD8 complex and the major histocompatibility complex (MHC) restricted antigen-presenting cell. The TCR is a heterodimer with disulfide-linked α and β chains, which functions as the antigen recognition site. The TCR is associated on the T cell surface with cluster of differentiation antigen CD4 or CD8 (depending on the T cell subset), and with five invariant chains (γ, δ, ε, ζ, and η) referred to collectively as the CD3 complex. CD4 or CD8 binds the MHC molecule during antigen presentation to the T cell. CD3 is not directly involved in antigen recognition, but is important in intracellular signalling to initiate an immune response once the T cell has interacted with antigen. The accessory adhesion molecules are important in strengthening the interaction between cells. They come into play after the antigen fragment has interacted with the TCR. The integrin molecules on the T cell interact with specific receptors in the membrane of the antigen-presenting cell. *ICAM* = intercellular adhesion molecule; *LFA* = lymphocyte function–associated antigen [LFA-1 is a dimer of CD11a and CD18; LFA-2 (CD2) and LFA-3 (CD58) are dimeric molecules composed of α and β chains].

    c. Lymphokines. Antigens trigger T cells to release soluble peptide mediators known as **lymphokines** (cytokines produced by lymphocytes), which have various biological activities (see Table 5-3 and Chapter 9 V B 2 d).

  3. Classes of T cells and their functions. Subpopulations of T cells have been defined according to the particular function of the subset and the membrane markers (CD antigens) which they possess (Table 5-2).

    a. Tc lymphocytes [also called **cytolytic thymus-dependent lymphocytes (CTLs)**] cause lysis of antigen-bearing target cells. Tc cells are **CD8$^+$** (i.e., they carry the CD8 surface marker).

      (1) Tc cells rid the body of cells that express foreign or nonself antigens. Tc cells are induced by, and are active against, tumors, viruses, and artificially introduced allogeneic tissue (i.e., tissue transplanted from a genetically different member of the same species).

      (2) Tc cells are usually subject to **MHC restriction** (see IV D and IV E 2).

        (a) In reacting with viral or tumor antigens, the Tc cell recognizes the foreign epitope in association with **class I MHC molecules**. Both the epitopes and the class I molecules must be homologous with the ones that originally induced the Tc function.

        (b) MHC restriction is not involved in graft rejection by Tc cells.

    b. Th lymphocytes are **CD4$^+$** and recognize a specific antigen in association with a homologous **class II MHC molecule**.

      (1) Some Th cells collaborate with B cells and macrophages in the induction of the humoral immune response.

      (2) Similar cells collaborate with other T cells to facilitate the production of Tc cells, primarily via the release of interleukins 2 and 6.

      (3) Subsets of Th cells occur in mice and humans, and probably in other animal species as well. These cells have important regulatory roles in both humoral and cell-mediated immunity.

        (a) Th1 cells mediate functions connected with cytotoxicity and local inflammatory reactions.

          (i) Th1 cells promote the development of Tc cells, the expression of delayed hypersensitivity (via macrophage activation), and the production of IgG2a.

          (ii) Th1 cells secrete gamma interferon predominantly; they also secrete interleukins 2 and 3, tumor necrosis factor α (TNF-α), and lymphotoxin (TNF-β).

Table 5-2. The Functional Heterogeneity of T Cells

T Cell Subtype	Symbol	Identifying Surface Antigen	MHC Restriction	Target Cell	Function
Cytotoxic	Tc	CD8	Class I	Tumors* Virally infected cells Allografts*	Kills foreign cells or cells with new surface antigens
Helper	Th	CD4	Class II	B cells Tc cells	Interleukin secretion
Inducer	Th	CD4	Class II	B cells Tc cell precursors Macrophages	Interleukin secretion
Suppressor	Ts	CD8	Class I	B, Th, Tc cells	Down-regulates cell growth
Delayed-type hypersensitivity	Tdth	CD4	Class II	Langerhans cells Macrophages Tc cells	Releases MAF, MIF, and other lymphokines
Memory	Tm	CD8; CD4†	Both	B cells T cells	Anamnesis

*Not subject to MHC restriction.
†Depends on function.
MAF = macrophage-activating factor; MHC = major histocompatibility complex; MIF = migration inhibiting factor.

(iii) The gamma interferon stimulates the expression of Fc receptors on macrophages, thus enhancing antibody-mediated cellular cytotoxicity. Gamma interferon also regulates Th2 cell function [see II B 3 b (3) (c)].

   (b) Th2 cells direct the immune response toward production of IgE (and hence toward atopic diseases), IgA, and IgG1.

     (i) Th2 cells secrete interleukins 3, 4, 5, 6, and 10.

     (ii) They promote the proliferation of eosinophils (via IL-5) and of mast cells (via IL-3 and IL-4 acting synergistically).

     (iii) Interleukins 4, 5, and 6 stimulate antibody production. IL-4 also enhances class switching to IgE.

   (c) The Th subsets **down-regulate one another**.

     (i) Gamma interferon secreted from Th1 cells suppresses the maturation of Th2 cells and suppresses the enhancing effect of IL-4 (produced by Th2 cells) on IgE and IgG1 synthesis.

     (ii) IL-10 secreted from Th2 cells suppresses the production of Th1 cells.

     (iii) IL-10 has recently been assigned a further cross-regulatory role of inhibiting cytokine synthesis by Th1 cells.

  c. Inducer T lymphocytes are also **CD4$^+$** and recognize antigens associated with **class II MHC molecules**. They activate Th cells, suppressor T (Ts) cells, Tc cells, and macrophages, in contrast to CD4$^+$ Th cells, which act primarily on B cells.

  d. Ts lymphocytes are **CD8$^+$**.

   (1) These cells are induced from precursors by contact with antigens usually independent of MHC association.

     (a) Native (self) antigens may stimulate the development of **autoregulatory Ts cells**.

     (b) Foreign antigens, when present in non-immunogenic forms or in very high concentrations, may also induce specific suppressor cell activity.

   (2) On recognizing the antigen, mature Ts cells interfere with the development of an immune response, by acting either directly on the cell or by releasing **suppressor factors**. Some of the suppressor factors have epitope specificity, suggesting that they may be T cell receptors released from the Ts cell membrane.

   (3) Ts cells may be involved in the prevention of autoimmunity.

   (4) Various lymphocyte populations may have suppressor functions. Two examples follow:

     (a) Tc cells may be able to kill antigen-presenting cells bearing homologous epitopes on their membranes.

     (b) The two **subsets of Th cells** [see III B 3 b (3)] have suppressive activities as well.

  e. Delayed-type hypersensitivity effector cells (Tdth, or TD, cells) are **CD4$^+$** lymphocytic cells and are subject to **class II MHC restriction**. They are responsible for Gell and Coombs type IV (delayed hypersensitivity) reactions (see Chapter 9 V B).

  f. Memory T (Tm) lymphocytes are induced during the primary immune response; they recognize the specific antigen and participate in the anamnestic response (see V A 1 c). Most Tm cells have Th functions and hence are **CD4$^+$** and **class II–restricted**.

C. B cells

  1. B cell development (Figure 5-4)

   a. In mammals, B cells originate from stem cells in the bone marrow.

   b. During maturation, which also occurs in the bone marrow, the B cell undergoes several **gene rearrangements** (see Chapter 3 IV E). These establish the B cell's **antigenic specificity** before it travels to secondary lymphoid organs. Later somatic gene recombinations allow the cell line to **switch** from one **immunoglobulin class** to another (see V A 2) without a change in antigenic specificity.

   c. When the B cell moves to the blood and peripheral lymphoid tissues, it carries immunoglobulin in its surface membrane and is ready to interact with antigen.

     (1) Contact between the antigen's **epitope** and the **immunoglobulin in the B cell membrane** triggers cell division.

     (2) This process is greatly enhanced by interleukins secreted by Th cells.

   d. The B cell **matures** into one of two types of cells.

     (1) The **plasma cell** has abundant rough endoplasmic reticulum and actively secretes large amounts of the antibody that had been anchored in the parent B cell's membrane.

     (2) The **memory B cell** is a long-lived cell that is the progenitor responsible for rapid plasma cell proliferation in the anamnestic response.

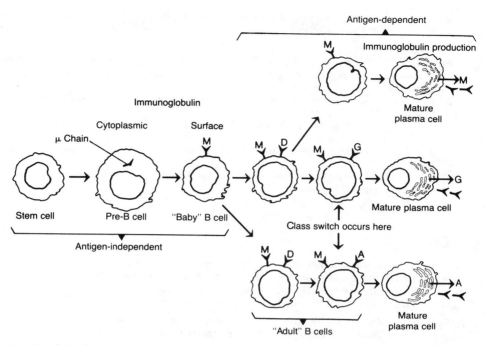

Figure 5-4. B cell development. Gene rearrangements and RNA splicing occur during maturation, which result in the production of a functional μ heavy (H) chain mRNA. The cell is now a pre–pre-B cell. The presence of the μ chain in the cytoplasm identifies the cell as a pre-B cell. Light (L) chain synthesis commences, and soon monomeric IgM appears in the B cell membrane. It has now completed the "antigen-independent" phase of its development; further maturation will be triggered by contact with specific antigen. Subsequent proliferation and differentiation with attendant class switching will be influenced by lymphokines secreted by helper T (Th) cells.

- **2. B cell surface markers**
  - **a. Immunoglobulin** (chiefly **monomeric IgM)** is present as the primary surface marker on the B cell membrane.
    - **(1)** The surface IgM functions as an antigen recognition site and binds specific epitopes.
    - **(2)** This initiates the differentiation of the B cell into plasma cells.
  - **b.** The B cell surface has **other markers** besides immunoglobulins.
    - **(1)** B cells have receptors for the Fc portion of immunoglobulin molecules (e.g., **FcγRII**).
    - **(2) CD antigens** are also found in B cell membranes.
      - **(a) CD10** is found primarily on immature B cells. It is also expressed on the malignant cells from a small percentage of patients with common acute lymphocytic leukemia and hence is called the **CALLA antigen**.
      - **(b) CDs 19, 20, 21, 22, and 23** are also found in B cell membranes; their function is unclear but is likely to be involved in cell activation.
    - **(3)** B cells also have receptors for **complement components** C3b and C3d.
    - **(4)** The B cell surface also carries class I and class II **MHC molecules**.
- **3. Classes of B cells and their functions.** B cells are divided into subpopulations according to the immunoglobulin class they synthesize (see Chapter 3 III).

IV. EVENTS IN THE INDUCTION OF THE IMMUNE RESPONSE

A. Fate of antigen

- **1. Site of deposition.** When an antigen is injected into an animal, it migrates through the circulatory system and is eventually deposited in lymphoid tissue.
  - **a.** If the antigen is injected subcutaneously or intracutaneously, the first deposition of antigen is in the regional **lymph node**. This is followed by hyperplasia of the node; it increases in size due to cellular proliferation.

    b. If the antigen is administered intravenously or intraperitoneally, it locates primarily in the **spleen;** the spleen enlarges and becomes hyperplastic due to cellular infiltration and proliferation.

  2. Antigen processing and presentation. Regardless of the route of injection, the **macrophage** (or other **antigen-presenting cell**—see III A 1) plays a pivotal role in the **preparation of the antigen for presentation** to the lymphoid cells.

    a. Antigen is first bound by the macrophage surface membrane, then is **ingested and processed** within the macrophage.

    b. The antigen is phagocytized or pinocytosed and is partially digested into smaller, more readily handled fragments.

    c. The **display of MHC determinants** by macrophages is a prerequisite for antigen presentation.

      (1) The processed epitopes are coupled to class II MHC glycoprotein molecules within the macrophage cytoplasm.

      (2) The epitope–MHC complex is then transported to the macrophage membrane where it is displayed, or ''presented,'' to B and T cells.

B. Collaboration between cells

  1. In the **humoral immune response,** when processed antigen is presented to the lymphocytes on the macrophage membrane, antigen-specific Th cells recognize the antigen, as do B lymphocytes. The three cells—**Th cell, B cell,** and **macrophage**—interact, perhaps in a tricellular complex, and the B cell undergoes blastogenesis and differentiation (see Figure 5-1).

  2. Cell-mediated immunity is produced in a similar manner, except that the three interacting cells are the **Th cell, Tc cell precursor,** and **macrophage**.

C. Epitope recognition

  1. Two recognition events must occur.

    a. The **epitope** is recognized by a component of the lymphocyte cell membrane which is specifically reactive with that particular epitope.

      (1) For **B cells,** the specifically reactive membrane component is a **monomeric IgM** molecule.

      (2) For **T cells,** the analogous membrane component is the **TCR** [see III B 2 b (2)].

        (a) The TCR also has immunologic specificity.

        (b) The α chain–β chain heterodimer TCR recognizes and binds the processed foreign epitope complexed with the variable-region segment of the self MHC molecule (either class I or class II).

    b. The **MHC molecule** on the antigen-presenting cell must be recognized by the appropriate CD membrane component on the T cell: either **CD4** of the Th cell or **CD8** of the Tc cell. (This phenomenon is referred to as **MHC restriction;** see IV D.)

  2. This stringent requirement for a dual signal prevents the induction of immune responses by autologous (self) cells or proteins that have not been ''processed'' and ''presented'' appropriately.

D. MHC restriction. The requirement for MHC recognition in epitope presentation is the **major control mechanism** for immune responses.

  1. Activation of T cells requires that the epitopes of processed antigen be presented to the cells in close association with MHC- encoded cell membrane glycoproteins (see Chapter 12 II C 4).

    a. The **induction of Tc cells** from immunologically committed precursors requires that the epitope must be presented to the precursor in association with a **class I MHC molecule**. The **participation of Th cells** can only occur if the epitope is presented to the Th cells in association with a **class II MHC molecule**. Thus, there is dual restriction in the **induction of Tc cells.**

    b. Mature Tc cells (CD8$^+$) must recognize antigen in conjunction with **class I MHC molecules**. The epitopes (e.g., viral or tumor antigens) are synthesized within antigen-presenting cells and are coupled to the MHC carriers prior to their appearance in the cell membrane.

    c. Th cells (CD4$^+$) must recognize antigen in conjunction with **class II MHC molecules**. The epitopes are attached to the MHC molecules intracytoplasmically after partial degradation.

2. Similarly, **B cell activation** requires that the epitope be presented in conjunction with **class II** molecules, which are recognized by **Th cells**.

E. T cell activation

1. Activation of Th and Tdth cells

  a. Activation of Th and Tdth cells by antigen requires **two signals,** each of which is mediated by **macrophages** (see Figure 5-1).

    (1) The **first signal** requires the **presentation of antigen** in a manner suitable for recognition by T cells, namely, in conjunction with class II MHC molecules.

    (2) The **second signal** involves the synthesis and release of **IL-1**.

  b. The synthesis of IL-1 induces the synthesis of a second distinct interleukin, **IL-2,** by the T cells. It is the action of IL-2, in concert with other interleukins (see Table 5-3), that allows full T cell activation to proceed.

  c. The responding T lymphocytes synthesize more IL-2 receptors (CD25 molecules), thus forming an **autocatalytic (autocrine) cycle**.

  d. The complex network of interleukin immunoregulatory activity is shown in Figure 5-5; the many functions of interleukins are given in Table 5-3.

2. Activation of Tc cells

  a. To be induced to the killer function, the $CD8^+$ Tc precursor cells must be stimulated by antigen that is associated with class I MHC molecules in the membranes of antigen-presenting cells.

  b. **Two activating signals** are required:

    (1) One signal involves interaction between two complexes:

      (a) The **TCR–CD8 complex** on the Tc cell

      (b) The **specific epitope–class I MHC complex** on the antigen-presenting cell

    (2) The second signal is the **release of interleukins** by macrophages and Th cells in the vicinity.

  c. The **Th cell** is pivotal in the activation of Tc cells: it supplies essential cytokines that enhance the proliferation of Tc cells and their maturation to functional cytotoxic cells.

  d. Thus Tc cell activation has **two levels of MHC restriction**:

    (1) **Class I restriction** in epitope presentation to the **Tc cell precursor**

    (2) **Class II restriction** in epitope presentation to the **Th cell**

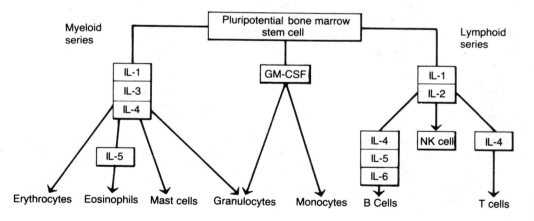

Figure 5-5. Cytokine regulation of the immune system. Shown are the major interleukins and their target cells. Note the redundancy of stimuli and the multiplicity of targets for each lymphokine. Note also that more than one interleukin may have a similar effect. The interleukins (*IL-1* to *IL-6*) are lymphokines; granulocyte–monocyte colony-stimulating factor (*GM-CSF*) has multiple sources, including monocytes. *NK cell* = natural killer cell.

Table 5-3. Cytokines of Importance in Immune Response Induction[*][†]

Cytokine	Sources	Targets	Effects
IL-1	Macrophages B cells NK cells	T cells B cells Macrophages	Lymphocyte activation Macrophage stimulation Pyrexia Acute-phase reaction[‡] Increased cell adhesion
IL-2	T cells	B cells T cells NK cells Macrophages	Lymphocyte activation Macrophage activation Stimulation of lymphokine secretion
IL-3	T cells	Stem cells	Proliferation
IL-4	T cells	B cells Macrophages	Lymphocyte proliferation Macrophage activation Influence on class switching: 　　Promotes IgG1 and IgE production 　　Decreases IgG2 and IgG3 　　　production
IL-5	T cells	B cells Stem cells	Proliferation Differentiation Promotion of switch to IgA Eosinophilia
IL-6	Numerous	B cells Macrophages	Proliferation Stimulation of immunoglobulin 　secretion Acute-phase reaction[‡]
IL-7	Stromal cells	Pre-B cells T cells	Proliferation
IL-8	Vascular 　endothelium	Neutrophils	Inhibition of leukocyte adhesion
IL-9	T cells	Th cells Mast cells	Proliferation
IL-10	T cells	T cells	Proliferation
GM-CSF	T cells Monocytes	Stem cells Monocytes Granulocytes	Proliferation Differentiation
TNF-α	Macrophages T cells NK cells	B cells	Growth and differentiation[§]
IFN-γ	T cells	B cells	Differentiation[§]

GM-CSF = granulocyte–monocyte colony-stimulating factor; IFN = interferon; IL = interleukin; NK cells = natural killer cells; Th cells = helper T cells; TNF = tumor necrosis factor.
[*]Lymphokines that are important in the expression of immunity are discussed in Chapter 9 V B 3 e.
[†]Cytokines are soluble mediators with hormone-like actions. Cytokines produced by macrophages and other mononuclear phagocytes are called monokines; those produced by lymphocytes are called lymphokines.
[‡]Acute-phase reaction = increased concentration of certain serum proteins (C-reactive protein, amyloid A, haptoglobin, ceruloplasmin, and many complement components) in response to acute inflammation.
[§]Other major effects are given in Table 9-3.

    e. Mature, activated Tc cells recognize epitopes bound to class I molecules on the surface of the target cell.

      (1) It is the **CD8 molecule** in the Tc cell membrane that is important in this recognition event, since cells bearing this membrane marker will release cytotoxins, and so forth.

      (2) **Specificity** of the response is assured by the **TCR,** which will only interact with its homologous epitope.

      (3) The **killing of virus-infected cells** is the most common example of Tc cell function and its MHC restriction.

        (a) During viral replication, viral peptides bind to class I MHC molecules in the infected cell's cytoplasm.

        (b) The peptide–MHC complex is transported to the cell surface where it is recognized by Tc cells.

        (c) Expression of cell-mediated immunity and killing of virus-modified target cells can only occur if the target cell and the Tc cell have the **same class I MHC molecule** in their membranes.

          (i) The response mounted by the host is restricted to the elimination of cells bearing a complex consisting of the same virus antigen that the Tc cell originally recognized and the same class I molecule that the Tc cell carries.

          (ii) The Tc cells do not kill cells bearing the same viral antigen and a different class I molecule, nor do they kill cells bearing a different viral antigen and the same class I molecule.

        (d) MHC restriction in viral diseases is important to the host in that it prevents the premature release of lymphokines from Tc cells that encounter extracellular virus or viral antigens at sites removed from infected cells.

      (4) A similar event probably occurs in the **recognition and destruction of some tumor cells,** where tumor antigens, synthesized in the cytoplasm, complex to class I MHC molecules and are transported to the cell membrane.

      (5) In **graft rejection,** allogeneic MHC antigens are targets recognized directly by Tc cells; the process of MHC restriction is **not** involved in **rejection,** although induction of Tc cells is dually restricted (see IV D 1 a, E 2 d).

  3. Activation of Ts cells. The requirement for macrophages in the activation of Ts cells differs from that noted for the activation of other T cells.

    a. Ts activation does not appear to be under MHC control.

    b. Antigen presentation by the macrophage may not be required. In its absence, antigen appears to be capable of directly activating Ts cells.

    c. Whether or not activation of Ts cells requires the liberation of a soluble substance by accessory cells is not known. Neither IL-1 nor IL-2 is sufficient to induce Ts cell activation.

F. B cell activation and antibody synthesis

  1. Antibody production takes place in lymphatic tissues, either in specialized organs such as the spleen or lymph nodes, or at sites of inflammation.

  2. Plasma cells are responsible for antibody synthesis. B cells can also produce antibodies, but the major production is by the plasma cell.

  3. Two signals are involved in the differentiation of B cells into antibody-secreting plasma cells.

    a. One signal is provided by interactions between **antigen** and the **IgM immunoglobulin receptor** on the B cell surface.

    b. The second signal is mediated by **Th cells**.

      (1) This signal requires contact between Th cells and B cells and is primarily mediated by soluble materials.

      (2) Also, Th cells can only help B cells bearing identical class II MHC determinants; thus, this response is **MHC-restricted**.

  4. Most humoral immune responses are **thymus-dependent**: they need participation of the Th cell.

  5. A few antigens are **thymus-independent**: they are able to induce antibody synthesis without the aid of Th cells.

  6. Also affecting B cell proliferation and maturation are various **interleukins** formerly referred to broadly as **B cell growth factors**.

    a. IL-1, IL-2, and IL-6 enhance antibody production, acting alone or synergistically.

b. **IL-1** also has a positive effect on pre–B cell maturation, as well as on clonal expansion of B cells following antigen stimulation.

c. **IL-4 and IL-5** influence immunoglobulin class switching.

d. **Gamma interferon** also acts as a stimulant of B cell differentiation.

V. PHASES OF THE HUMORAL IMMUNE RESPONSE

A. The primary and secondary immune responses

1. **Characteristics** (Figure 5-6)

   a. The **primary immune response** occurs following the **first exposure to antigen** and produces a relatively **small amount of antibody**.

   b. If a sufficient length of time elapses after the primary antigenic stimulation, the antibody level will decrease markedly.

   c. However, subsequent exposure to even a small amount of antigen will evoke an **anamnestic response** (also called **booster response, memory response,** or **secondary immune response**).

   (1) The anamnestic response consists of a **rapid proliferation of plasma cells,** with the concomitant production of **large amounts of specific antibody**.

   (2) The anamnestic response occurs because a large population of **memory B and T cells** are recruited into the humoral immune response.

   (a) These memory cells are produced during the initial exposure to the antigen.

   (b) The memory cells are precursors of Th cells and plasma cells, and represent another product of the collaboration between T cells and B cells (see IV B).

2. **Immunoglobulin class switching**

   a. **The IgM–IgG switch**

   (1) In the **primary immune response,** the immunoglobulin produced is mainly **IgM**. **Subsequent exposures** to antigen will cause the response to **shift to IgG** production.

   (2) This changeover occurs within individual plasma cells; it is not the result of recruitment of new IgG-producing cells to replace effete IgM-producing plasma cells.

   (3) The individual plasma cell splices out the μ constant-region gene complex and replaces it with a γ3, γ1, or another constant-region gene (see Chapter 3 IV D).

   (4) The entire light (L) chain gene complex and the variable, diversity, and joining segments of the heavy (H) chain remain intact. Thus, the antigenic specificity of the plasma cell and its immunoglobulins is not changed.

   b. **Class switching to IgA, IgD, or IgE** takes place by similar splicing processes.

B. Ontogeny of the immune response

1. **IgG** is the major fetal antibody, and it is **acquired from the mother** through the placenta.

   a. Transplacental passage of IgG occurs almost exclusively during the last 4 to 6 weeks of gestation.

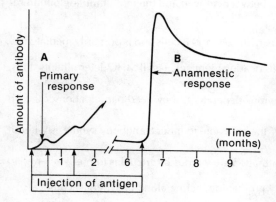

Figure 5-6. Phases of the humoral immune response. The time between initial and subsequent exposure to a specific antigen must be sufficient for an adequate immune response to be mounted. (*A*) A primary immune response occurs upon initial exposure; if the time between initial and subsequent antigen exposure is short, only a low-grade immune response is mounted. (*B*) If sufficient time elapses between exposures, an anamnestic response occurs, in which there is a rapid proliferation of plasma cells and production of a large amount of antibody specific for the antigen.

    b. Serum antibody levels in the newborn are directly related to gestational age.

        (1) Term newborns have adult levels of IgG.

        (2) Infants of less than 32 weeks' gestational age have extremely low levels of immuno-globulins and have heightened susceptibility to infections of all types.

2. **IgM** synthesis begins prior to birth and IgM is the major antibody **produced by a fetus**. If IgM levels are elevated at birth, the infant may have an infection.

3. The **secretory IgA** in maternal **colostrum** provides local immunity for the infant's upper respiratory and intestinal tracts.

4. During the **null period,** several months after birth, the maternal IgG is being rapidly degraded and the infant has not yet begun to synthesize large quantities of IgG. This is the most dangerous time for an infant.

5. The development of **full immunocompetence** takes several years in humans and occurs in an ordered sequence that in many ways parallels the phylogenetic development of immune responses. Adult levels of antibodies are not reached until the teenage years.

STUDY QUESTIONS

Directions: Each of the numbered items or incomplete statements in this section is followed by answers or by completions of the statement. Select the **one** lettered answer or completion that is **best** in each case.

1. The rapid rise, elevated level, and prolonged production of antibody that follows a second exposure to antigen is known as the

(A) delayed hypersensitivity reaction
(B) autoimmune response
(C) anamnestic response
(D) conditioned response
(E) thymus-independent response

2. One of the characteristics of the secondary immune response is that it

(A) is mainly IgM antibody
(B) requires a low dose of immunogen for induction
(C) has low-affinity antibodies
(D) has a short duration of antibody synthesis
(E) has a slow rate of antibody synthesis

3. The thymic lymphocytes that recognize an antigen and interfere with the development of a humoral immune response are called

(A) killer (K) cells
(B) helper T (Th) cells
(C) null cells
(D) contrasuppressor cells
(E) suppressor T (Ts) cells

4. A secondary immune response differs from a primary immune response in each of the following ways EXCEPT the

(A) length of the latent period
(B) amount of antibody produced
(C) duration of antibody production
(D) class of immunoglobulin produced
(E) antibody specificity

5. Most antibody is synthesized within which of the following structures?

(A) Central lymphoid organs
(B) Peripheral lymphoid organs
(C) Thymus
(D) Macrophages
(E) Golgi apparatus

6. The monokine (macrophage-derived hormone) that is intimately involved in the immune response is

(A) interleukin-1 (IL-1)
(B) IL-2
(C) IL-3
(D) macrophage-activating factor (MAF)
(E) migration-inhibiting factor (MIF)

7. The mammalian counterpart of the avian bursa of Fabricius is the

(A) spleen
(B) gut-associated lymphoid tissue (GALT)
(C) thymus
(D) bone marrow
(E) liver

8. The anamnestic response is defined as

(A) a gradual rise in antibody titers
(B) true immunologic paralysis
(C) the prompt production of antibodies after a second exposure to antigen
(D) species-specific antibodies
(E) the lag in antibody production after initial antigen exposure

9. Which of the following characteristics best describes the anamnestic response in comparison with the primary immune response?

(A) Lag period is longer after antigenic stimulus
(B) More antibody is produced
(C) IgM production predominates
(D) More immunogen is required
(E) It characterizes the immune response to carbohydrate antigens

1-C	4-E	7-D
2-B	5-B	8-C
3-E	6-A	9-B

Directions: Each group of items in this section consists of lettered options followed by a set of numbered items. For each item, select the **one** lettered option that is most closely associated with it. Each lettered option may be selected once, more than once, or not at all.

Questions 10–12

For each cell characteristic or function described below, select the cell with which it is most closely associated.

(A) T cell
(B) B cell
(C) Macrophage
(D) Natural killer (NK) cell
(E) Eosinophil
(F) Basophil
(G) Neutrophil
(H) Mast cell

10. Functions as helper in antibody response

11. Functions as suppressor cell

12. Phagocytizes and processes antigen in the immune response

Questions 13–16

For each characteristic of an interleukin listed below, choose the interleukin that it best describes.

(A) Interleukin 1 (IL-1)
(B) IL-2
(C) IL-3
(D) IL-4
(E) IL-6
(F) IL-8
(G) IL-9
(H) IL-10

13. Plays an important role in class switching

14. Is the endogenous pyrogen produced by macrophages

15. Promotes IgE production

16. Is the cytokine synthesis-inhibiting factor

10-A	13-D	16-H
11-A	14-A	
12-C	15-D	

84 *Chapter 5*

ANSWERS AND EXPLANATIONS

1. The answer is C *[V A 1 c].*
Immunologic memory (anamnesis) is an important characteristic of the immune response. It allows booster shots 5 to 7 years after a primary immunization. More importantly, the rapid rise in antibody levels after re-exposure to a particular infectious agent is responsible for long-lasting "convalescent" immunity.

2. The answer is B *[V A 1 c].*
The secondary immune response, also referred to as the booster or anamnestic response, is triggered by relatively low doses of immunogen. The secondary immune response is mainly IgG antibody, and the antibodies produced have a high affinity for the antigen. Another feature of the secondary immune response is a rapid rate of production of antibody, usually accompanied by an antibody level which exceeds the previous, or primary, immune response.

3. The answer is E *[III B 3 d (2)].*
Suppressor T (Ts) cells interfere with the development of humoral immune responses. Helper T (Th) cells, on the other hand, participate in an immune response in a positive manner. Both Ts and Th cells are of thymic origin. The Th cells release soluble hormone-like mediators, known as lymphokines, which enhance the immune response. These interleukin mediators induce the proliferation of other T cells as well as B cells.

4. The answer is E *[V A 1].*
The secondary immune response differs from a primary immune response in that the interval between antigen exposure and antibody production is shorter in the secondary immune response, and more antibody is produced for a longer period of time. Usually the immunoglobulin produced in the primary response is IgM, and it is during the secondary response that IgG begins to appear, due to immunoglobulin class switching. The antibody specificity does not change within a particular plasma cell line, although subtle mutations in B cell immunoglobulin genes may produce a paratope with greater affinity for the epitope.

5. The answer is B *[IV F].*
Antibody synthesis occurs in peripheral (secondary) lymphoid organs such as the tonsils, Peyer's patches, lymph nodes, and spleen. The central (primary) lymphoid organs are the thymus and the bursa of Fabricius or its mammalian counterpart, the bone marrow: these are the sites where lymphocytes receive their immunologic education and become committed to life as T or B cells.

6. The answer is A *[IV E 1 a; Table 5-3].*
Interleukin-1 (IL-1) is a product that the macrophage secretes during antigen processing. IL-1 reacts with the helper T (Th) cell, inducing it to produce IL-2. IL-2 in turn acts on other Th cells and causes them to proliferate and elaborate IL-3 and a host of other interleukins which cause the proliferation of many cells. Among these are B cells, which would be the most important in the context of the humoral immune response. IL-1 is also known as endogenous pyrogen.

7. The answer is D *[II C 2 c].*
In birds, the bursa of Fabricius is the organ responsible for the maturation of the B cell component of the immune system. Although gut-associated lymphoid tissue (GALT) was once considered to be the likeliest mammalian counterpart of this avian organ, the bone marrow is now believed to be the site where mammalian B cells mature. The thymus is the organ (in birds as well as in mammals) that is responsible for the maturation and differentiation of T cells. Splenectomy will decrease the antibody content of serum transiently, but would not cause permanent immunosuppression. This procedure is used in the therapy of idiopathic thrombocytopenic purpura (ITP) and a few other immunologic diseases. Removal of the spleen renders an individual susceptible to bacterial sepsis; *Streptococcus pneumoniae* is a common etiology.

8. The answer is C *[V A 1 c].*
The anamnestic response, or anamnesis, is also called the booster response, memory response, or secondary immune response. It is characterized by the prompt production of high levels of antibody (i.e., a rapid rise in antibody titers) following secondary exposure to antigen. Anamnesis is due to the presence of B and T memory cells that were induced during the primary immune response. Immune paralysis is the inability to mount a response to a normally immunogenic substance.

9. The answer is B *[V A 1].*

A characteristic of the anamnestic (secondary) immune response is the greater amount of antibody produced during this response versus the primary immune response. In addition, there is a more rapid production of antibody during the anamnestic response. IgM is characteristic of a primary immune response; the antibody that predominates during the anamnestic response is IgG. It usually takes less immunogen to induce a secondary response than a primary response.

10–13. The answers are: 10-A *[III B 3 b (1)],* **11-A** *[III B 3 d],* **12-C** *[IV A 2].*

The T cell—specifically the helper T (Th) cell—can help with the B cell proliferation and differentiation to an antibody-secreting plasma cell that occurs in the antibody response. If antigen on an accessory cell (e.g., a macrophage) interacts with its homologous receptor on a T cell surface, this will trigger lymphokine release from the Th cell, as well as proliferation and differentiation of the B cell, if both the cells are identical at the class II major histocompatibility complex (MHC). The Th cells that participate in B cell maturation also show this MHC restriction.

There are several functional subsets of T cells. Cytotoxic T (Tc) cells cause lysis of antigen-bearing target cells (virally infected cells, tumor cells, transplanted allogeneic cells). Besides being important in B cell maturation, Th cells also function in Tc cell development. The suppressor T (Ts) cell has an opposing function; it serves to down-regulate (depress) the immune response. Ts cells suppress directly, or via suppressor factors, the function of other immunologically active cells (e.g., Th cells). Ts cells and Tc cells bear the CD8 membrane antigen but not the CD4; hence they are $CD8^+$, $CD4^-$. Therefore, Ts and Tc cells are easily distinguished from Th cells, which are $CD8^-$, $CD4^+$.

Macrophages and the dendritic cells of the spleen and the Langerhans cells of the skin are responsible for the initial processing of an antigen as it enters the spleen or lymph nodes. The processed antigen is complexed with class II MHC molecules in the cytoplasm and is presented to the lymphocytes on the membrane of the antigen-presenting cell. Peripheral blood neutrophils are phagocytic, as are the macrophages, but do not process antigen effectively.

13–16. The answers are: 13-D *[Table 5-3],* **14-A** *[Table 5-3; Ch 1 II D 7 d],* **15-D** *[III B 3 b (3); Table 5-3],* **16-H** *[III B 3 b (3) (c) (iii)].*

Interleukin 4 (IL-4) plays a significant role in class switching and promotes the synthesis of IgG1 and IgE. IL-4 is produced by helper T (Th) cells of the Th2 subset. Acting synergistically with IL-5, IL-4 enhances the production of IgA; it also can stimulate mast cell proliferation and maturation in synergy with IL-3. One of the actions of the monokine IL-1 is the production of fever; hence the name "endogenous pyrogen." IL-1 reduces the concentration of prostaglandins in the region of the hypothalamus and thus causes an increase in body temperature. IL-10 is a Th2 cell product that tends to down-regulate cytokine production by Th1 cells.

6
Immune Regulation

$\mathcal{U}$

I. INTRODUCTION

A. In clinical medicine, there are special instances when suppression or enhancement of immune responsiveness to selected antigens is desired.

1. **Immunosuppression** may be desirable under the following circumstances.
   a. **Allergic conditions** of all sorts, both immediate and delayed hypersensitivities, can be handled by suppressing the immune response.
   b. **Autoimmune disease** is so-called immunologic suicide where the body destroys its own tissues. If normal tissues are being destroyed by an immune mechanism, suppression of the immune response would be rational treatment.
   c. The rejection of grafted tissues and organs has an immunologic basis. Therefore, **prolongation of graft survival** can be enhanced by suppressing the patient's immune response.

2. **The enhancement of immune responsiveness** would be advantageous in the management of **immunodeficient patients**.

B. Responsiveness is the key to immune regulation.

1. **Unresponsiveness**
   a. Unresponsiveness is the absence of an immune response to a substance that, under ordinary conditions, would be immunogenic: the substance has all the features necessary for antigenicity, but there is no immune response to it.
   b. Unresponsiveness can be divided into two broad categories: immunosuppression and tolerance. The difference between the two is primarily quantitative.
      (1) **Immunosuppression** refers to a reduction in a large portion of the host's immune responsiveness. The reduced responsiveness may be due to:
         (a) A congenital defect
         (b) An acquired immunocompromising condition; examples include infection [e.g., with human immunodeficiency virus (HIV)], malignancy, malnutrition, or medication
      (2) **Tolerance** is more restrictive; it implies the absence of a selected immune response, and thus a state of specific unresponsiveness (i.e., an immunotolerant state).

2. **Enhancement of responsiveness**
   a. Enhancement of responsiveness (**immunopotentiation**) can be specific or nonspecific.
   b. Materials that possess the ability to enhance or augment an immune response are often referred to as **adjuvants** (see IV B 1).

C. Natural processes exist which act to **control the immune response**.

1. **Suppressor T (Ts) cells** are induced during an immune response. Ts cells control the proliferation and maturation of immunocompetent T and B cells.

2. **Major histocompatibility complex (MHC) restriction** (see Chapter 5 IV D) is a self-imposed regulatory mechanism.
   a. Effective collaboration between helper T (Th) cells, B cells, and antigen-presenting cells can only occur if the antigen's epitope is linked to the appropriate class II MHC molecule.
   b. Thus, immune responses to self antigens such as red blood cells will not occur because these antigens will not be linked to the class II MHC molecule in the macrophage membrane.

3. The **idiotypic network** [see II B 2 d (3) and Chapter 3 IV A 2] has been proposed as a negative regulatory system. In this proposed system:
   a. The immune response stimulates the formation of **anti-idiotypic antibodies;** that is, antibodies to the epitope-binding region of the original antibody.
   b. These anti-idiotypic antibodies can **down-regulate the immune response**.
      (1) They do so by mimicking the original epitope and binding with epitope-specific immunoglobulins or T cell receptors on immunocommitted lymphocytes.
      (2) Because this binding takes place in the absence of class II MHC molecules that are present on antigen-processing cells, it interferes with effective epitope triggering of the cell to proliferate and mature.

4. **Neuroendocrine control** of the immune system is suggested by considerable evidence.
   a. The **sympathetic nervous system** interacts with the immune system.
      (1) Lymphocytes and macrophages have membrane receptors for:
         (a) Neurotransmitters (acetylcholine and norepinephrine)
         (b) Endorphins
         (c) Enkephalins
      (2) Neurons in the brain, particularly in the hypothalamus, have membrane receptors for:
         (a) Interleukins
         (b) Interferons
         (c) Histamine, serotonin, and other mediators of inflammation
         (d) Prostaglandins, which are mediators of inflammation and also act like cytokines
      (3) Lymphocytes secrete endorphinlike compounds.
      (4) **Stress** usually produces immunosuppressive effects in the body.
   b. The **endocrine glands** appear to be involved in these regulatory networks as well.
      (1) Lymphocytes and macrophages have receptors for adrenocorticotropic hormone (ACTH), corticosteroids, insulin, growth hormone, prolactin, estradiol, and testosterone.
      (2) Lymphocytes secrete ACTH.

D. This chapter approaches the topic of immune regulation as a pyramid, dealing first with the broadest type of immunosuppression (the base of the pyramid) and progressing from here through stages of greater specificity to epitope-specific immunologic tolerance.

II. IMMUNOSUPPRESSION

A. **Physical means of immunosuppression**

1. **Surgical manipulation** can have a major impact on immune responsiveness.
   a. **Removal of central (primary) lymphoid organs** has effects that vary depending on the time of removal.
      (1) Lymphoid cells require programming in a central lymphoid organ if the cells are to differentiate appropriately in response to antigen in peripheral lymphoid tissues, but once that programming has been achieved, cells react as mature cells in peripheral tissues for months or years.
      (2) Surgical removal of central lymphoid organs demonstrates this clearly.
         (a) If the **bursa of Fabricius,** the **thymus,** or both are surgically removed **in the neonatal period,** immunologic competence will not develop in the corresponding lymphoid cell line.
            (i) It is necessary for future antibody-producing cells to receive some influence from the bursa before they can become responsive in peripheral lymphoid tissues.
            (ii) Similarly, it is necessary for small lymphocytes to differentiate in the thymus before they can function in peripheral tissue.
         (b) However, if these tissues are surgically removed **after immunologic development,** immune competence is affected very little, at least for a considerable period.
   b. **Removal of peripheral lymphoid tissue** has effects that vary depending on the tissues removed.
      (1) Surgical removal of the **lymph nodes** and **lymphoid cells** in connective tissue has little effect, because these tissues are too diffuse to be removed completely by surgical procedures.

(a) If they all could be removed, the animal would be immunologically completely unresponsive.

(b) While this cannot be done surgically, total removal can be approximated through the use of antilymphocyte antibodies [see II B 2 d (1)] or whole body irradiation (see II A 2).

(2) Removal of the **spleen,** or its ablation due to diseases such as sickle cell anemia, does not grossly impair antibody production but it does render the individual susceptible to bacterial infections, particularly septicemias, owing to the loss of this organ's blood-filtering ability.

2. Ionizing radiation damages the lymphoid organs and bone marrow.

a. Radiation damages DNA; thus, cells that are in the process of division or that need to divide in order to express their immunologic role will be most affected by this exposure.

(1) Therefore, irradiation produces various immunosuppressive effects on the **inductive** phase of the primary immune response.

(2) The secondary immune response is affected less by irradiation because the cells involved are not as dependent on DNA synthesis (i.e., they do not need to divide; many are in the maturational phase of the immune response, such as class switching).

b. Shielding the lymphoid organs from whole body irradiation protects against diminished immune capacity.

B. Chemical and biological means of immunosuppression

1. General considerations

a. Chemical and biological immunosuppressive agents are used **clinically** for several purposes:

(1) In **transplantation procedures** to suppress graft rejection reactions

(2) As therapeutic agents for **autoimmune disease**

(3) As **cancer chemotherapeutic agents**. Most anticancer agents have some degree of immunosuppressive activity because they inhibit DNA synthesis and thus are most effective against rapidly dividing cells.

b. All chemical and biological immunosuppressive agents are more effective in **preventing a primary immune response** than they are in preventing a secondary immune response or in interrupting an ongoing response. Therefore, in order to block responsiveness, it is important that the immunosuppressive agent be given before the antigen.

(1) For example, kidney transplant patients are started on immunosuppressive therapy before the transplant operation. Once the patient has started to respond immunologically to the transplant, the injection of immunosuppressive agents is less effective.

(2) Immunosuppressive drugs are more effective in preventing homograft rejection than they are in treating allergies or autoimmune diseases. In the latter two cases, the disorder is diagnosed by the presence of antibody or sensitized lymphoid cells in the patient's tissues; hence, the immune response has already been induced.

c. Since a role of the immune response is to protect against infectious diseases, the result of immunosuppression is an **increased incidence and chronicity of infection**.

d. When immunosuppressive agents are used, the patient is also more likely to develop **malignancy**.

2. Types of immunosuppressive agents and their actions

a. Lympholytic agents

(1) Lympholytic agents can block the expression of the immune response (through cell lysis) but still are more effective in blocking the initiation of the immune response.

(2) The two major **types** of lympholytic immunosuppressants are **ionizing radiation** (see II A 2) and **antibodies** (i.e., antilymphocyte serum or antithymocyte serum; see II B 2 d).

(a) Both types are effective against cell-mediated immunity and block both the induction of an immune response and the expression of one already induced.

(b) These agents are used in situations such as renal and cardiac transplantation.

b. Lymphocytotoxic agents

(1) Lymphocytotoxic agents are most efficient at interrupting the induction of an immune response.

(a) These agents interfere with cellular metabolic processes (usually DNA synthesis).

(b) The effect is to block cell division or otherwise interrupt vital cell functions such as RNA or protein synthesis.

(2) There are several major **types** of lymphocytotoxic agents.
  (a) Antimetabolites, such as purine and pyrimidine analogs and folic acid antagonists (e.g., methotrexate), interfere with DNA synthesis.
  (b) Alkylating agents (e.g., cyclophosphamide) interfere with cell division by altering guanine so that DNA base-pairing errors occur. They also can cross-link the two DNA strands, thus blocking replication.
  (c) The **antibiotic** cyclosporine inhibits interleukin action, thus blocking the expansion of the helper/inducer T cell population.
(3) Cyclosporine is particularly effective in suppressing graft rejection reactions. The **immunologic effects** of cyclosporine include:
  (a) Blocking transcription of the genes for interleukins 2, 3, and 4 and for gamma interferon
  (b) Inhibiting antigen processing by dendritic cells
  (c) Enhancing the production of Ts cells
c. Corticosteroids
  (1) Corticosteroids (e.g., cortisone) are both immunosuppressive and anti-inflammatory.
  (2) Corticosteroids are **lympholytic** in laboratory animals but not in humans, where they seem to **alter cell migration,** causing:
    (a) Neutrophilia
    (b) Lymphopenia, especially of Th cells
    (c) Monocytopenia
    (d) Depressed macrophage chemotaxis
  (3) Other immunologic effects of corticosteroids include:
    (a) Decreasing the binding of immune complexes to Fc and C3b receptors of phagocytic cells
    (b) Depressing bactericidal activity, antigen-processing activity, and interleukin-1 (IL-1) production by macrophages
    (c) Increasing the influx of calcium into cells, with concomitant activation of a cellular endonuclease, resulting in DNA fragmentation
    (d) Depressing the release or the effect of various lymphokines, namely IL-2, tumor necrosis factor (TNF), macrophage migration inhibition factor (MIF), and macrophage-activating factor (MAF)
    (e) Blocking the cleavage of membrane phospholipids, thus lowering prostaglandin and leukotriene levels by inhibiting arachidonic acid release from the membrane
d. Antibodies. Antibodies can be used to inhibit immune responses in three ways.
  (1) Antibodies that react with lymphoid cells (i.e., **antilymphocyte globulins** or **antilymphocyte serum**) can be produced that will react more or less specifically with T cells or with B cells.
    (a) If injected into the body, antibodies against T cells can find all the T lymphocytes in the blood and lymph nodes. This is the means of attacking peripheral lymphoid tissue to produce wanted immunosuppression.
    (b) Antilymphocyte serum, particularly **antithymocyte serum,** is most useful in inducing immune deficiency in transplant patients by suppression of cell-mediated immune responses (see Chapter 12 III G 2 d).
  (2) If a preformed antibody is injected, followed by injection of specific antigen, the injected antibody binds the antigen and prevents its access to lymphoid tissue. The immune response in the host will thereby be blocked.
    (a) This is the principle through which **Rh$_o$(D) immunoglobulin (RhoGAM)** was developed to combat Rh incompatibility (**erythroblastosis fetalis;** see Chapter 9 III C 1 b).
    (b) Antiserum against the immunogen (Rh antigen) will opsonize the Rh-positive erythrocytes and facilitate their clearance from the body by the liver; thus, an immune response is aborted.
  (3) Antibodies can be produced that are specific for the antigen-combining site (the idiotype) of an antibody. If these **anti-idiotypic antibodies** (see I C 3) are injected, they can specifically abort the immune response between the original antibody and its homologous epitope.
    (a) The anti-idiotype mimics the original epitope structurally (see Figure 3-3); hence, it can react with IgM bound to the surface of a B cell. This will block B cell activation by the original epitope when it is present on an antigen-presenting cell in association with class II MHC molecules.
    (b) An anti-idiotype can react similarly with a T cell receptor and thus block T cell activity.

C. Immunosuppression associated with diseases. A reduction of immune competence may accompany various disease states (see Chapter 11). This is usually due to a direct effect on the immune apparatus itself, but it may also occur as a side effect of the primary disease.

   1. Congenital immunodeficiencies
   a. In **Bruton's hypogammaglobulinemia** (see Chapter 11 III A), **B cell (humoral) immunity** fails to develop. Patients form antibodies very poorly and suffer from repeated bacterial infections.
   b. In **DiGeorge syndrome** (see Chapter 11 IV A), **T cell immunity** is deficient because the third and fourth pharyngeal pouches fail to develop during embryogenesis. Patients have a great deal of trouble with recurrent viral diseases.
   c. In **chronic granulomatous disease** (CGD; see Chapter 11 II B 1), **phagocytes** are unable to kill ingested microorganisms. Patients have recurrent bacterial infections.

   2. Malignancies. These are potentially immunosuppressive, particularly if they involve lymphoid tissues. **Lymphomas** (e.g., **Hodgkin's disease** and **sarcoidosis**) may disrupt normal lymphocyte functions directly or may "crowd out" normal lymphocytes from bone marrow and peripheral lymphoid tissues.

   3. Infections
   a. **Measles** and certain **other viral diseases** cause a transient depression in cell-mediated immune responses.
   b. Viral infections can also have an adverse effect on various macrophage functions (Table 6-1).
   c. **HIV** infection (see Chapter 11 VI C) causes a profound immunosuppression which renders patients susceptible to fatal opportunistic infections. Recrudescence of latent viral infections [e.g., herpes zoster (shingles)] is also common, as are certain types of tumors, particularly Kaposi's sarcoma.
   d. **Specific anergy** is seen in **lepromatous leprosy** and the terminal stages of **tuberculosis**; in these conditions, delayed hypersensitivity is impaired.

   4. Malnutrition
   a. Adequate nutrition is essential for proper functioning of the immune system.
   b. Cell-mediated immunity appears to be the most sensitive to nutritional deprivation, but humoral immunity, complement, and phagocytic functions are also affected.
   c. **Nutrient deficiencies that adversely affect immune functions** include:
      (1) Protein deficiency
      (2) Vitamin deficiencies, particularly those involved in DNA and protein synthesis (e.g., vitamins A, B_6, B_{12}, and folic acid)
      (3) Mineral deficiencies, particularly of zinc or iron, which can cause decreases in T cell functions and in microbicidal activity of phagocytes

III. TOLERANCE

A. Overview

   1. Tolerance is the absence of specific immune responses in an otherwise fully immunocompetent person.

   2. This type of unresponsiveness can be either naturally acquired (**autotolerance**) or specifically induced (**acquired or immune tolerance**).

   3. Tolerance is of importance in **clinical medicine** in several ways.
   a. Escape from autotolerance may result in **autoimmune diseases**.
   b. Specifically induced tolerance could represent an avenue for the **therapy** of autoimmune diseases, allergic conditions, and allograft rejection.

Table 6-1. Macrophage Functions Adversely Affected by Viral Infections

Phagocytosis	Presentation of antigens
Degranulation	Cytokine secretion
Microbicidal activity	Cytocidal activity
Processing of antigens	Suppressor activity

B. Autotolerance and acquired tolerance

1. Autotolerance (neonatal, natural, or self tolerance)
  a. Autotolerance is tolerance to one's own antigens.
  b. Autotolerance is acquired early in life, probably in utero.
  (1) During fetal development, the ability to recognize one's own tissues is acquired.
  (2) From that point, individuals do not ordinarily produce antibodies against their own normal (self) tissue antigens.
  c. There are many theories as to how autotolerance comes about, but the most favored is the **clonal deletion theory:**
  (1) It is probable that clones of cells capable of responding to an individual's own tissues arise throughout life.
  (2) These clones, called **forbidden clones,** are immediately deleted by encountering an overwhelming amount of self antigens or by the activity of antigen-specific suppressor cells.
  (a) The cell that is most susceptible to deletion is the Th cell.
  (b) In probability, functional B cells exist that are potentially reactive against self antigens.
  d. Very often the suppression of forbidden clones (i.e., autotolerance) works less effectively than it should, the result being autoimmune disease.

2. Acquired (immune) tolerance
  a. Autotolerance can be simulated by a simple experiment. However, because the procedure is contrived and the unresponsive state is not natural, the phenomenon is called **acquired or immune tolerance**.
  (1) Unresponsiveness can be induced in a fetal animal by the injection of a foreign substance (this mimics the autoantigen exposure that induces autotolerance).
  (2) The animal will assume that the substance is self and will not produce an antibody response to that substance later in life.
  (3) However, the only way to perpetuate this unresponsiveness is by continually maintaining a low level of that substance in the animal.
  b. Immune tolerance is usually induced by excessive amounts of antigen.
  (1) The antigen that induces tolerance is known as the **tolerogen,** and the large dose of antigen that will induce tolerance is referred to as the **tolerogenic dose**.
  (2) The mechanism whereby immune tolerance is induced is probably quite similar to that of autotolerance:
  (a) The antibody-producing B cells or the T cells capable of mounting a response are overwhelmed and deleted.
  (b) Tolerance is not simply in vivo neutralization or absorption of the antibody—it is the specific absence of antibody formation induced by tolerogen.

C. Characteristics of immune tolerance

1. Tolerance is a **specific cellular defect** that is probably due to the absence of an immunologically reactive lymphocyte.
  a. This may involve two of the three cells in the immune response.
  (1) The macrophage does not have immunologic specificity, so it cannot be directly involved in tolerance.
  (2) The T cells and B cells have specificity, so they can be involved.
  b. The **roles of the T cell and the B cell** have been extensively investigated in mice. In this experimental system, it is the Th cell which is most susceptible to tolerance induction, an event which seems also to occur in nature.
  (1) In mice, Th cell tolerance occurs 1 day after the tolerogen is given and lasts 120 to 150 days.
  (2) In contrast, it takes 5 to 7 days for the B cell to become tolerant, and this tolerance lasts for only about 50 days.
  (3) Further, inducing Th cell tolerance requires one thousand times less the amount of antigen required for B cell tolerance.

2. Gradations of tolerance are possible.
  a. In **partial tolerance,** the individual is unable to respond to some of the epitopes on the antigen but can respond to others.

    b. In **immune deviation (split tolerance),** one of the immune responses can be interfered with but not another. For example:

      (1) The **IgG** response may be blocked, but **not the IgM** response.

      (2) The **cell-mediated** response may be blocked, but **not the humoral** response.

3. Tolerance is **antigen-specific:** the unresponsiveness is to all or only some of the epitopes of one particular antigen.

    a. Cross-reacting antigens can break tolerance to some epitopes if two conditions are met.

      (1) The immunogen (i.e., the cross-reacting antigen) must contain one or more new epitopes plus a common (shared) one to which the animal is unresponsive.

      (2) The unresponsiveness must affect the T cell compartment only: epitope-specific responsive B cells must be available to be "triggered" to differentiate into plasma cells.

    b. When the immunogen is injected, it will recruit Th cells that are reactive with the new epitope, and cooperation of these cells with the responsive B cells will ensue.

4. Several **factors influence the induction of tolerance.**

    a. Immune tolerance (in either the T cell or B cell) is easier to induce in the **prenatal animal** or the **neonate,** because the ease of induction is greatest when immunologic maturity is least. It then follows that **immunosuppression** will also enhance tolerance induction.

    b. The **simpler the antigen,** the better tolerogen it will be. The more complex it is, the less effective it will be in inducing tolerance.

      (1) Thus, bacterial and mammalian cells are extremely poor tolerogens.

      (2) This is probably related to two factors:

        (a) These cells have a high density of different epitopes.

        (b) They also have a propensity for phagocyte interaction, an event that seems to drive the immune response forward in a positive direction.

    c. A **threshold amount of antigen** is required to induce tolerance.

      (1) An increase over this threshold amount will not hasten the onset of tolerance.

      (2) However, an increase over the threshold amount may increase the **duration of tolerance.** Also, the longer a tolerogen can persist in an animal above the threshold, the longer the duration of tolerance will be.

D. The induction of immune tolerance

1. Methods of inducing immune tolerance in adult animals

    a. Adult animals are often immunosuppressed by the injection of cyclosporine or another suitable immunosuppressant before they receive antigen.

    b. Alternatively, they can be injected with a tolerogenic form of antigen.

      (1) For example, a saline solution of human gamma globulin would normally be immunogenic in a non-human species.

      (2) However, if the aggregated forms of the antigen are removed by ultracentrifugation, the gamma globulin solution becomes tolerogenic.

    c. The antigen can be **complexed with a toxic compound** such as ricin or daunorubicin, or **labeled with a radioactive isotope** such as iodine-125 (^{125}I). The B cells and T cells bearing membrane receptors for the antigen can thereby be destroyed, eliminating that specific immune reactivity.

    d. Anti-idiotypic cytotoxic antibody can be injected to eliminate a specific clone of B cells.

    e. Similarly, an animal can be treated with an antiserum specific for the epitope-reactive portion of the T cell antigen receptor (a **clonotypic antibody**), thus blocking cell-mediated immune responses.

2. Theories of how immune tolerance is induced. Two mechanisms of tolerance induction have been postulated; both are probably operative in nature.

    a. One theory states that the B cell is rendered tolerant by an **antigen blockade** at the membrane. Tolerance in the T cell may have a similar mechanism.

      (1) The cell has a specific membrane receptor for antigen (and tolerogen).

      (2) When the receptor reacts with its homologous epitope, the receptor is fixed, or frozen, so that no messages for antibody production can get into the cell. The cells may, in fact, be killed by interaction with tolerogen.

    b. An alternative theory states that tolerogen induces the generation of **specific suppressor cells.**

      (1) These cells interact directly with Th cells or plasma cell precursors to block their maturation.

      (2) In addition, both antigen-specific and nonspecific soluble factors that suppress the immune response have been isolated from T cells.

IV. IMMUNOPOTENTIATION

A. Overview

1. The immune response can be **enhanced** by increasing the rate at which the response occurs, elevating its magnitude, or increasing the duration of the response. In some instances, one particular response can be enhanced with no change in other responses; for example, the presence of certain mycobacterial cell wall components will favor the development of cell-mediated immunity.

2. Substances capable of these actions may be specific or nonspecific potentiators.

B. Adjuvants (nonspecific potentiators of the immune response)

1. **Mechanisms of potentiation**
   a. **Adjuvants** are substances that enhance the immunogenicity of molecules without altering their chemical composition.
   b. Adjuvants enhance immune responses by several **mechanisms**:
      (1) Increasing the efficiency of macrophage processing of antigen
      (2) Prolonging the period of exposure to the antigen
      (3) Amplifying the proliferation of immunologically committed lymphocytes by enhancing lymphokine activity

2. **Freund's adjuvant** is a classic adjuvant used in experimental animals. It is an emulsion of paraffin or mineral oil (usually Bayol F) and water. Lanolin or Arlacel A is used as an emulsifying agent.
   a. **Incomplete Freund's adjuvant (IFA)** is a water-in-oil emulsion with antigen in the water phase. IFA increases the **humoral immune response** about 100-fold, greatly reduces the amount of antigen required, and prolongs the phase of active immunoglobulin synthesis by months.
   b. If **mycobacteria** or their cell wall components are added, the product is called **complete Freund's adjuvant (CFA)**.
      (1) The addition of the bacteria does not markedly enhance the antibody response, but the response of the host will now include **cell-mediated immunity** as well as antibody synthesis.
      (2) Thus, if an antigen like ovalbumin is injected with CFA, the animal will develop both high levels of circulating antibody and a strong T cell response to ovalbumin.

3. Another example of a **directional influence** of an adjuvant is the elevated IgE response seen when heat-killed *Bordetella pertussis* organisms are present in a vaccine.

4. **Aluminum hydroxide, alum,** and other **precipitants** or **adsorbents** used in humans have a mechanism of action similar to Freund's adjuvant.
   a. These substances retard the absorption of the antigen and thus prolong the exposure to antibody-forming tissues.
   b. They also will cause local inflammation, thus increasing mononuclear cell exposure.

5. **Lymphokines,** such as **interleukins 1, 2,** and **3** and **gamma interferon,** enhance lymphocyte proliferation and differentiation and activate phagocytic cells (see Table 5-3).

6. **Mitogenic substances,** such as **endotoxin** and plant lectins like **phytohemagglutinin (PHA),** produce an immunostimulatory effect by increasing the clonal expansion of B cells and T cells.

7. **Bacille Calmette-Guérin (BCG)** is a well-studied immune potentiator.
   a. BCG is an attenuated tubercle bacillus that is used as a vaccine against tuberculosis. It causes macrophage activation and also enhances natural killer (NK) cell activity. The **adjuvant activity** resides in a glycolipid.
   b. A synthetic muramyl dipeptide, **N-acetyl-muramyl-ʟ-alanyl-ᴅ-isoglutamine,** has similar properties.

8. **Synthetic polynucleotides** stimulate antigen processing and Th cell activity and may induce interferon production as well.

C. Specific potentiators. Some factors have immunologic specificity.

1. **Helper factors** are secreted by T cells following interaction of their antigen-specific receptor with its homologous epitope.

2. **Transfer factor** is an antigen-specific dialyzable extract of immune T cells that is capable of transferring cell-mediated immunity.

3. An **immunogenic RNA** has been extracted from lymphoid tissues of experimental animals following antigen injection. This appears to be an antigen epitope complexed with cellular RNA which greatly increases the immunogenicity of the molecule.

STUDY QUESTIONS

Directions: Each of the numbered items or incomplete statements in this section is followed by answers or by completions of the statement. Select the **one** lettered answer or completion that is **best** in each case.

1. The injection of large doses of protein results in immune tolerance that is due to

(A) removal of antibody by excess antigen
(B) catabolism of antibody as rapidly as it is formed
(C) production of a nonreacting antibody
(D) suppression of B cells, T cells, or both
(E) induction of cytotoxic anti-idiotype antibodies

2. The immunosuppressive effect of cortisone is attributed to its ability to

(A) produce lymphopenia
(B) destroy immunoglobulins
(C) block DNA synthesis
(D) stabilize lysosomal membranes
(E) cross-link DNA strands

3. Erythroblastosis fetalis can be prevented if the mother is injected, at parturition, with an antibody called

(A) blocking antibody
(B) $Rho_o(D)$ immunoglobulin (RhoGAM)
(C) antilymphocyte globulin
(D) antithymocyte serum
(E) univalent antiserum

4. Which of the following adjuvants will induce an increase in the IgE response?

(A) Incomplete Freund's adjuvant (IFA)
(B) Complete Freund's adjuvant (CFA)
(C) *Bordetella pertussis*
(D) Mycobacteria
(E) Alum

5. A serious complication of the use of immuno-suppressive agents is the

(A) increased incidence of autoimmune diseases
(B) increased susceptibility to opportunistic infections
(C) loss of tuberculin sensitivity in tuberculosis patients
(D) loss of hair
(E) decrease in complement levels

6. An immunosuppressive agent that is lympholytic in humans is

(A) cortisone
(B) actinomycin D
(C) x-irradiation
(D) cyclosporine
(E) methotrexate

7. If the emergence of forbidden clones is not continuously suppressed throughout life, a person may develop

(A) hypergammaglobulinemia
(B) allergic conditions
(C) autotolerance
(D) autoimmune disease
(E) serum sickness

8. Immunosuppressive measures are most effective when administered

(A) just prior to antigen exposure
(B) 1 week before antigen exposure
(C) 1 week after antigen exposure
(D) 1 month before antigen exposure
(E) 1 month after antigen exposure

1-D	4-C	7-D
2-A	5-B	8-A
3-B	6-C	

ANSWERS AND EXPLANATIONS

1. The answer is D *[III B 2 b].*
Large doses of antigen induce immune tolerance by eliminating helper T (Th) cells and specifically re-active B cells. In most experimental systems, circulating antibody would not be present prior to tolerogen administration. In fact, free antibody can interfere with induction of tolerance. Cytotoxic anti-idiotype antibodies can induce immune tolerance, but their production would not be induced by the injection of antigen.

2. The answer is A *[II B 2 c (2)].*
Cortisone produces lymphopenia, either by direct lympholytic action, as seen in rodents, or by altering the tissue distribution of these cells, as seen in humans. T cells are more sensitive than B cells to this effect of corticosteroids. These drugs also have an anti-inflammatory action and interfere with the formation of phagolysosomes.

3. The answer is B *[II B 2 d (2) (a)].*
Rh_o(D) immunoglobulin (RhoGAM) reacts with Rh-positive fetal erythrocytes in the Rh-negative mother's circulation and opsonizes them, so that they are phagocytized by the mother's reticuloendothelial system and destroyed before they can induce an immune response. RhoGAM cannot interfere with a secondary response to the D (Rh) antigen; therefore, it must be used in the first pregnancy. It is a blocking agent, not a means of inducing immune tolerance to the D antigen; hence, it should be administered at the end of each subsequent pregnancy.

4. The answer is C *[IV B 3].*
Bordetella pertussis has an adjuvant action that induces the production of IgE antibodies in experimental animals. Freund's adjuvants (either complete or incomplete) are water and oil emulsions in which the antigen is emulsified in the oil phase. Complete Freund's adjuvant has mycobacteria or mycobacterial cell products incorporated into the emulsion. Both of these adjuvants are used in experimental situations, but are not used in humans because they cause granuloma formation. They function, as does alum, by being irritants, causing an inflammatory response at the site of adjuvant deposition, and by serving as depots from which antigen is slowly released to the antibody-forming system of the body.

5. The answer is B *[II B 1 c].*
Drug-induced immunodeficiency commonly increases the incidence of infections, particularly by op-portunistic pathogens. The frequency of cancer also is higher in individuals receiving immunosuppressive therapy. Tuberculin sensitivity would probably not be affected as immunosuppression is not very effective against established responses. Hair loss is a common complication of cancer chemotherapy, but the dos-ages of immunosuppressive drugs used in the control of autoimmune diseases, graft rejection episodes, and so forth usually are not high enough to manifest this unpleasant side effect.

6. The answer is C *[II A 2, B 2 a, c (2)].*
In humans, lysis of lymphoid cells can be caused by ionizing radiation and by specific antibodies to ap-propriate cell membrane markers. Cortisone causes lympholysis in some animal species but not in humans. Here its action is more directed to changing the traffic patterns of the cells. Actinomycin D, cy-closporine, and methotrexate interfere with DNA replication or function and hence cause immunosup-pression.

7. The answer is D *[III B 1 d].*
One theory concerning the origin of autoimmune diseases hypothesizes that these diseases are due to the emergence of clones of cells that are autoreactive. These "forbidden" clones are triggered to proliferate and mature into immunologically competent effector cells that attack self antigen by contact with anti-gens or altered native molecules. Another theory suggests that B cells reactive with self antigen are present naturally and their development into plasma cells secreting autoantibodies occurs because a helper T (Th) cell has been recruited by a second epitope on the immunogen.

8. The answer is A *[II B 1 b].*
Immunosuppressive therapy is usually directed at cells in the process of proliferation and hence is most effective if given just before, or at the time of, antigen administration. It is far more difficult to block on-going responses and booster responses because the need for cell proliferation is not as marked. If the suppression occurs too far in advance of the immunization, the drug effect will have worn off.

I. INTRODUCTION

A. History

1. The practice of immunization began in antiquity with the realization that individuals who recovered from certain diseases were often protected against recurrence of the same illness.

2. In 1798, Edward Jenner introduced the use of vaccination with cowpox to protect individuals against smallpox.

3. Some years later Louis Pasteur observed that attenuated rabies virus would protect individuals against rabies.

4. The contributions of Jenner and Pasteur ushered in a modern era devoted to the search for immunizing agents that would, with a minimum of risk to the host, provide long-term protection against infectious diseases.

B. Types of immunization. Agents used for immunization can be divided into two categories based on the **type of immunity** that they induce.

1. **Vaccines** are used for **active** artificially acquired immunization.
   a. Vaccines are able to induce an immune response without producing disease.
   b. Vaccines consist of either intact **microorganisms** (killed or attenuated) or their immunogenic **components** (e.g., hepatitis B surface antigen; HBsAg) or **products** (e.g., bacterial toxoids).

2. **Serum preparations** are used for **passive** artificially acquired immunization.
   a. Passive immunization provides protective antibodies for a particular disease, but does not stimulate an immune response.
   b. Thus, passive immunity is effective and acts immediately, but is only temporary in its effect.
   c. Three basic **types of serum preparations** are used:
      (1) Antitoxin
      (2) Immune globulin (gamma globulin)
      (3) Specific immune globulins

C. Routes of administration. Agents used for immunization can be administered by several routes.

1. **Injection** is the most common method used for immunization. Several injection routes are available.
   a. **Intramuscular** and **subcutaneous injections** are the methods used most often.
   b. **Intradermal (intracutaneous) injection** is often used for revaccination of previously inoculated individuals.
   c. **Intravenous injection** is sometimes used for administration of immune globulin.

2. **Oral administration** came into widespread use with the introduction of the oral polio vaccine (OPV; Sabin vaccine).
   a. The Sabin vaccine contains a live attenuated virus that multiplies, infects, and immunizes the recipient.
   b. In the process, the vaccine virus is disseminated in the community and induces immunity in those it infects—for example, family members of the recipient.

3. **Intranasal administration** has gained interest in recent years.
    a. In upper respiratory disease, natural infection results in the production of specific antibodies both in serum and in secretions at the local site of infection.
    b. Intranasal immunization should stimulate an immune response that mimics the response induced by natural infection. The procedure is currently being evaluated with influenza vaccination.

II. ACTIVE IMMUNIZATION

A. Bacterial vaccines

1. **Intact bacteria** used for immunization may be either dead or living.
    a. For the preparation of **dead bacterial vaccines,** the organisms are cultured, harvested after suitable incubation, and then killed with heat or chemicals (e.g., acetone, formalin, thimerosal, phenol). Killing must be designed to preserve the immunogenicity of the preparation.
    b. **Live attenuated (weakened) bacterial vaccines** can be prepared by frequent subculture on artificial media.
    c. Live attenuated agents are generally preferable because they provide a superior and longer-lived immunity. However, they do have some risks (see V A).

2. **Bacterial products** used for immunization are usually either **structural components** or **detoxified products (toxoids).**
    a. **Structural components**
        (1) The **capsule** of certain bacteria (e.g., *Streptococcus pneumoniae*) is an example of a structural component that has proved to be valuable in vaccination. It induces the production of anticapsular antibodies that neutralize the antiphagocytic effect of the capsule.
        (2) Viral envelope proteins (HBsAg) and **pili** (*Neisseria gonorrhoeae*) are other examples of structural components of value in immunization.
    b. **Toxoids.** Toxoids are nontoxic but still immunogenic preparations produced from toxins.
        (1) Heat or formalin can be used in their preparation to inactivate the toxic portion of the molecule. The resulting immunogen induces the production of antitoxic antibodies.
        (2) **Adjuvants** (see Chapter 6 IV B) are sometimes used to prolong the antigenic stimulus and enhance its immunogenicity.
            (a) **Alum-precipitated toxoid** is toxoid that has been precipitated by the addition of potassium aluminum sulfate, then washed and suspended in saline.
            (b) **Adsorbed toxoid** is toxoid that has been adsorbed onto particles of aluminum hydroxide or aluminum phosphate.

3. **Representative currently used vaccines**
    a. **Diphtheria toxoid** is available as a fluid toxoid of *Corynebacterium diphtheriae,* but is more immunogenic when precipitated with potassium alum or adsorbed onto aluminum hydroxide or aluminum phosphate. It is commonly combined with tetanus toxoid and pertussis vaccine as **DPT vaccine.**
    b. **Pertussis (whooping cough) vaccine** consists of a thimerosal-killed or heat-killed preparation of *Bordetella pertussis* organisms.
        (1) Only bacteria in a capsular form can be used for this vaccine, since the presence of a capsule correlates with virulence.
        (2) The killed, whole-bacterial vaccine can cause complications such as high fever and convulsions, which require discontinuing the vaccination series. An **acellular pertussis vaccine** producing fewer side effects is in use in Japan and is currently being evaluated in the United States.
    c. **Tetanus toxoid** is a preparation of inactivated *Clostridium tetani* toxin. It is available as fluid toxoid but the adsorbed form is most immunogenic.
    d. **Bacille Calmette-Guérin (BCG)** vaccine is a live attenuated strain of *Mycobacterium bovis* used as a vaccination against tuberculosis, primarily in developing countries.
    e. **Typhoid vaccine** is a suspension of heat-killed or acetone-killed *Salmonella typhi.*
    f. **Pneumococcal polysaccharide vaccine** provides immunity against bacteremic pneumococcal disease.
        (1) The vaccine was originally prepared from the polysaccharide capsule of 14 antigenically different strains of *S. pneumoniae.*
        (2) Capsular material from 23 antigenic types of organisms is currently pooled.

g. *Neisseria meningitidis* **vaccine,** for prevention of meningococcal meningitis, is available for use in epidemic situations, for military recruits, and for patients with asplenia or with congenital absence of the terminal components of the complement cascade.

h. *Haemophilus influenzae* **vaccine** is prepared from the polysaccharide capsule of *H. influenzae* type b to provide immunity against *H. influenzae* meningitis, which occurs in preschool-age children. Low immunogenicity in those under 18 months old has prompted a search for an effective carrier molecule (see IV B 1 h).

B. Viral and rickettsial vaccines

1. Live attenuated viral vaccines
a. These vaccines have the advantage of mimicking natural infection. They multiply in the vaccinated host and stimulate long-lasting antibody production.
b. However, they carry the risk of reversion to virulence.
c. Attenuation can be accomplished by repeated subculture in tissue culture or by serial passage in various animal hosts.

2. Killed (inactivated) vaccines
a. These preparations are safer than live attenuated vaccines, in general.
b. However, the immunity conferred is often brief and must be boosted.
c. Inactivation can be accomplished with formalin or ultraviolet light.

3. Representative currently used vaccines
a. Viral vaccines
  (1) Rubella (German measles) vaccine contains live attenuated virus grown in tissue culture, which may be either rabbit kidney, duck embryo, or, preferably, human diploid cells.
  (2) Influenza virus vaccine
    (a) This vaccine consists of whole virus or disrupted (split) virus products grown in chick embryo and inactivated by formalin or ultraviolet light.
    (b) The composition of the vaccine varies depending on epidemiologic circumstances.
      (i) Of the three serotypes of influenza virus, only types A and B are involved in human influenza vaccine. However, new antigenic subtypes continually evolve.
      (ii) To compensate for the frequent antigenic drift of the influenza virus, new vaccines that will be effective against new strains must be developed each year.
  (3) Measles and **mumps vaccines** are live attenuated viruses grown in chick embryo.
  (4) Poliomyelitis vaccine is currently available in two forms.
    (a) Inactivated polio vaccine (IPV; Salk vaccine) is made from virus that is grown in tissue culture (e.g., monkey kidney) and inactivated with formalin or ultraviolet light.
      (i) This form of the vaccine is administered intramuscularly.
      (ii) It protects against paralytic or systemic disease but not against poliovirus infection.
    (b) Oral polio vaccine (Sabin vaccine) is made from a **live attenuated virus** grown in tissue culture (monkey kidney or human diploid cells).
      (i) This form of the vaccine is given orally.
      (ii) It provides more complete protection by stimulating not only systemic humoral immunity but also intestinal (mucosal) immunity, thereby protecting against viral implantation.
  (5) Rabies vaccine
    (a) Vaccine for use in humans is currently available in two forms.
      (i) One vaccine uses virus grown in duck embryo and inactivated with β-propiolactone. This form can cause neurologic complications.
      (ii) The preferred vaccine uses virus grown in human lung fibroblasts (i.e., in human diploid cells free of nerve tissue) and inactivated with tributyl phosphate.
    (b) Live attenuated virus vaccines have also been developed for use in immunizing dogs, cats, and domestic livestock.
  (6) Hepatitis B vaccine. HBsAg produced by a genetically engineered strain of *Saccharomyces cerevisiae* is available for use as vaccine.

   b. Rickettsial vaccines
      (1) Typhus vaccine is prepared from formalin-killed *Rickettsia prowazekii* grown in the yolk sac of chick embryos.
      (2) Rocky Mountain spotted fever vaccine is prepared from formalin-killed *Rickettsia rickettsii* grown in chick embryos.

III. PASSIVE IMMUNIZATION

A. Antitoxins

1. Antitoxins consist of toxin-neutralizing antibodies (**antiserum**) specific for a given toxin. Antitoxins have no effect on the microorganism that produced the toxin.

2. Most commercial preparations are produced from horses or cows immunized with toxin or toxoid.
   a. The serum or plasma is harvested and processed to concentrate the antitoxin and eliminate as much equine or bovine serum protein as possible. The preparations are then sterilized by filtration, treated with a chemical preservative, and standardized.
   b. Such animal-derived antitoxins are used only when a specific human immune globulin is not available because, being foreign proteins, they can cause adverse effects such as anaphylactic shock or serum sickness.

3. **Representative currently used preparations**
   a. **Botulism antitoxin** is prepared in horses. It contains polyvalent antitoxin to three types of toxin (types A, B, and E) produced by *Clostridium botulinum*.
   b. **Diphtheria antitoxin** is prepared by injecting horses with the toxoid of *C. diphtheriae*. The antitoxin is used in the treatment of diphtheria. (For prevention of diphtheria, see section II A 3 a.)
   c. **Tetanus antitoxins** derived from animals are no longer recommended, since tetanus immune globulin (see III C 2 c), derived from humans, is now available.

B. Immune globulin (gamma globulin)

1. Immune globulin is prepared from pooled normal adult human plasma or serum by cold ethanol fractionation.

2. It contains antibodies (mainly IgG) to a variety of different microorganisms and is used for passive immunization against those diseases or for maintenance of immunodeficient individuals.
   a. **Hepatitis A** and **measles** are two diseases for which immune globulin may be given.
   b. **Measles immune globulin** is immune globulin that has been specifically tested for its measles antibody content.

C. Specific immune globulin

1. A specific immune globulin is a gamma globulin that is derived from human plasma obtained either from volunteers who have been hyperimmunized against a specific infectious disease or from people who have recently recovered from the disease.

2. **Representative currently used preparations**
   a. **Hepatitis B immune globulin** is derived from human plasma that demonstrates a high titer of antibody to HBsAg.
   b. **Rabies immune globulin** is prepared from humans who have been hyperimmunized against rabies (usually veterinary students or veterinarians). It is used, in conjunction with rabies vaccine, to treat individuals exposed to rabid animals.
   c. **Tetanus immune globulin** is derived from humans hyperimmunized with tetanus toxoid; it is specific for the tetanospasmin toxin of *C. tetani*.
   d. **Varicella–zoster immune globulin** is prepared from human-derived serum selected for high titers of antibody to varicella–zoster. It will modify or prevent varicella (chickenpox) in immunodeficient children but is of no benefit to people with active varicella or herpes zoster (shingles).
   e. **$Rh_o(D)$ immunoglobulin** (Rh_oGAM) is a human-derived preparation used in Rh-negative women within 72 hours of delivery, miscarriage, or abortion of an Rh-positive baby or fetus to prevent sensitization of the mother to possible Rh-positive fetal red blood cells in future pregnancies (see Chapter 9 III C 1).

IV. EXPERIMENTAL IMMUNIZATION PROCEDURES. Concern over the safety and efficacy of currently used immunization techniques has led to the development of various means to augment the immune response (immunopotentiation), either specifically or nonspecifically, and to the development of a number of newer vaccines. Some examples are presented here.

A. Nonspecific immunopotentiation

1. **BCG** (see II A 3 d) has been used with varying degrees of success to immunize against tuberculosis. Through its ability to stimulate the immune response nonspecifically, administration of BCG can also inhibit the development of certain malignant tumors or induce their regression. It can be given by intradermal injection or by the scarification method, either alone or in conjunction with chemotherapy.
   a. BCG appears to activate T cells and macrophages and stimulate natural killer (NK) cells. Further, it cross-reacts antigenically with certain tumor cells, suggesting the possibility that it might also stimulate a specific antitumor immune response.
   b. Intralesional injection of BCG in cutaneous melanoma causes regression of both the injected and distant tumors.
   c. Intravesical treatment of superficial bladder carcinoma with BCG is now widely accepted in the management of such patients.
   d. Its sometimes severe side effects (e.g., chills, fever, anaphylaxis, and, in immunosuppressed individuals, occasional BCG infection) have led to attempts to prepare purified subfractions of the organism designed to reduce such complications.
      (1) A methanol-extractable residue of phenol-treated BCG appears to have some promise.
      (2) **Muramyl dipeptide,** a synthetic product that can mimic the adjuvant activity of mycobacterial cell wall preparations, is also under investigation.

2. *Corynebacterium parvum,* a gram-positive bacterium, is used as a heat-killed, formaldehyde-treated suspension.
   a. Given orally or injected intralesionally, it is reported to cause regression of certain tumors (e.g., malignant melanoma), probably by activating macrophages.
   b. Undesirable side effects include fever and vomiting.

3. **Levamisole** is a potent anthelmintic drug that is also an interesting immunostimulant.
   a. It appears to inhibit suppressor T (Ts) cell activity and enhances delayed hypersensitivity.
   b. Clinical studies have shown levamisole to be of limited value in such conditions as herpesvirus and staphylococcal infections, melanoma, and colorectal cancers.
   c. Complications include nausea, rash, and neutropenia.

4. **Interferons** (see Chapter 1 II F 2 c) were originally of interest because of their antiviral effects. However, interferons are now recognized as having important immunoregulatory properties.
   a. Their major regulatory effect seems to be enhancement of NK cells and macrophages.
   b. All three classes of interferon (alpha, beta, and gamma) are currently produced by recombinant DNA techniques, which will greatly facilitate investigation of these promising immunomodulators.
   c. Interferons have been found to be of value in the treatment of hairy cell leukemia, some lymphomas and other tumors, herpesvirus infection, hepatitis B, and the common cold.
   d. Complications from their use include reversible granulocytopenia. Most patients develop fever, chills, headache, and myalgia while receiving an interferon drug; some develop significant fatigue and anorexia.

5. **Interleukin-2 (IL-2)** is a T cell lymphokine that is now produced in large amounts by recombinant DNA techniques.
   a. IL-2 stimulates the growth of activated T cells and converts quiescent lymphocytes into active cytotoxic cells known as lymphokine-activated killer (LAK) cells (see Chapter 1 II G 3).
   b. IL-2 also appears to augment the cytotoxicity of NK cells.
   c. IL-2 also stimulates the development of **tumor-infiltrating lymphocytes (TILs).**
      (1) Certain cytotoxic lymphocytes, when extracted from a tumor and cultured in the presence of tumor cells and IL-2, expand in number. These cells are TILs, which show enhanced tumoricidal activity when infused back into the donor of the lymphocytes and tumor cells.
      (2) Clinical trials are in progress to investigate the effectiveness of TILs in the management of certain types of cancer.

B. Specific immunization. Numerous attempts to develop both new and improved vaccines, as well as to develop techniques for antigen specific immune modulation, are currently in progress.

1. Vaccines for specific agents

a. Pneumococci. Mutants of *S. pneumoniae* that are able to colonize the upper respiratory tract are under investigation, as are attempts to improve the immunogenicity of the polysaccharide capsule by coupling it to a protein carrier molecule.

b. Group A streptococci
   (1) Group A organisms and their products are associated with sore throat, endocarditis, rheumatic fever, glomerulonephritis, and other diseases.
   (2) Type-specific **M protein** (an antiphagocytic virulence factor), freed of toxic and tissue cross-reactive materials by salt fractionation and ion-exchange chromatography, is being evaluated as a vaccine.

c. Group B streptococci
   (1) Group B organisms, particularly serotype III, are a major cause of neonatal meningitis.
   (2) Purified capsular polysaccharide prepared from type III organisms has been found to be a well-tolerated immunogen; it is being investigated as an immunizing agent for the mother to provide the newborn with protective antibody levels.

d. Gonococci
   (1) Despite extensive control efforts, *N. gonorrhoeae* infection rates remain high, emphasizing the need for a vaccine.
   (2) It is possible that gonococcal **pili** can be used as an immunogen to protect against gonococcal infection.
      (a) The attachment of gonococci to host tissue is an important part of the disease process. Only types 1 and 2 appear to be virulent and possess pili that facilitate attachment.
      (b) Antibody against pili not only blocks attachment but also enhances the phagocytosis of gonococci.
      (c) The existence of multiple antigenic types of pili may pose a problem.

e. Meningococci
   (1) *N. meningitidis* is an important cause of bacterial meningitis in both children and adults.
   (2) Immunity to *N. meningitidis* infection is associated with complement-dependent bactericidal antibodies. The antibodies are group-specific.
      (a) The protection-inducing antigen for groups A, C, Y, and W135 meningococci is capsular polysaccharide. Though a vaccine is available (see II A 3 g), group A and group C polysaccharides are relatively poor immunogens in young infants.
      (b) The protection-inducing antigen for group B appears to be a type-specific protein. Group B polysaccharide is poorly immunogenic.
      (c) Studies are in progress aimed at enhancing the immunogenicity of capsular material by coupling it to protein (e.g., tetanus toxoid).

f. *S. typhi.* The current vaccine for typhoid fever, whole killed *S. typhi,* affords only partial resistance and is relatively toxic. Oral administration of a live attenuated mutant strain has been studied in controlled field trials and found to be extremely effective.

g. Enterotoxicogenic *Escherichia coli* (ETEC)
   (1) This agent appears to be a major cause of traveler's diarrhea ("turista") precipitated by an enterotoxin-induced hypersecretion in the small intestine.
   (2) The plasmids carrying genes for enterotoxins may also carry genes for colonization factors that aid in the attachment of organisms to the intestinal epithelium.
   (3) Both toxin and colonization factor antigens (CFAs) are being examined for use as vaccine.

h. *H. influenzae*
   (1) The currently used vaccine for *H. influenzae* meningitis is made from the polysaccharide capsule of *H. influenzae* type B.
   (2) Unfortunately, this vaccine is not effective in infants younger than age 18 months, the age group that suffers the highest attack rate.
   (3) The immunogenicity of the capsular material can be increased by conjugating it to a **protein carrier**.
      (a) Diphtheria toxoid as a carrier was licensed in the United States in 1988.
      (b) Tetanus toxoid and meningococcal outer membrane proteins are under investigation as other possible carriers.

   i. ***Vibrio cholerae***
      (1) Only limited protection against cholera is conferred by the conventional vaccine (killed *V. cholerae*). This has led to the development of experimental vaccines.
      (2) New approaches include the use of combined antigens, consisting of toxoid or a sub-unit of toxin together with conventional vaccine or vibrial lipopolysaccharide.
      (3) Avirulent mutants of *V. cholerae* are also under investigation for use as live oral vaccine.
   j. ***Pseudomonas aeruginosa.*** This important pathogen can cause serious wound and burn infections, meningitis, and infections of the urinary tract, ears, and other sites. Detoxified lipopolysaccharide, lipopolysaccharide–protein conjugates, and toxoid are being evaluated as vaccines.

2. **Vaccines using anti-idiotypic antibodies or monoclonal antibodies**
   a. **Anti-idiotypic antibody vaccines**
      (1) Immunoglobulin idiotypes represent unique amino acid sequences in the variable region associated with the antigen-binding capacity of the molecule.
      (2) Idiotypic sites are capable of inducing the production of anti-idiotypic antibodies (see Figure 3-3).
      (3) Anti-idiotypic antibodies that are directed at the hypervariable region of antimicrobial antibodies can be used as vaccines, since the anti-idiotypic preparation contains an internal image component that mimics the epitope of the microbial antigen.
      (4) Anti-idiotypic antibodies have been used experimentally in animals to induce an immune response to a variety of infections, including trypanosomiasis and a number of viral infections (reovirus, Sendai virus, and rabies, polio, herpes, and hepatitis B viruses).
   b. **Immunotoxins** can be produced by linking **toxins** to highly specific **monoclonal antibodies**. These have shown promise in recent experimental studies.
      (1) A popular toxin used is **ricin,** extracted from castor oil plants.
         (a) Ricin can inhibit protein synthesis and cause cell death.
         (b) An immunotoxin that could be of potential value in **cancer therapy** would be one consisting of ricin coupled to monoclonal antibody specific for tumor cell antigens. Such a preparation should have no effect on normal tissue.
      (2) Another potential use for immunotoxins is in the management of **autoimmune disease**.
         (a) In the disease myasthenia gravis, neuromuscular transmission is impaired because the patient makes antibodies to the acetylcholine receptor.
         (b) Studies are in progress to construct an immunotoxin that would eliminate the set of lymphocytes that make anti–acetylcholine-receptor antibody.

3. **Transfer factor for cell-mediated immunity**
   a. **Transfer factor** is a dialyzable, low-molecular-weight nucleopeptide derived from activated T cells. It is capable of transferring antigen-specific cell-mediated immunity (delayed skin test reactivity) from specifically sensitized donors to nonsensitized recipients.
   b. To date, transfer factor has been reported to be of some clinical value in the management of several types of diseases:
      (1) Certain viral diseases (e.g., measles, herpes, and chickenpox in children with leukemia)
      (2) Fungal infections (e.g., mucocutaneous candidiasis and histoplasmosis)
      (3) Bacterial diseases (e.g., tuberculosis)
      (4) Parasitic infections (e.g., leishmaniasis)
      (5) Cancers (e.g., osteosarcoma and malignant melanoma)

V. ADVERSE REACTIONS FROM VACCINES.
Federal law requires that all vaccines licensed in the United States be safe, effective, and essentially free of side effects. However, each has been shown to cause adverse reactions in a small number of recipients.

A. Adverse effects specific to live vaccines

1. Live vaccines such as those used to prevent many viral diseases have the potential to "revert" to a virulent state.

2. Live vaccines can also cause disease in particularly vulnerable individuals.
   a. Because of possible fetal infection, live vaccine should not be given to a **pregnant woman** unless there is an imminent risk such as an epidemic or unless the woman is planning to travel in an area endemic for a particularly serious disease.

    b. Live vaccines can cause serious and even fatal infections in **immunologically incompetent individuals**.

        (1) Such persons include those with:

            (a) Congenital defects in cell-mediated immunity, such as DiGeorge syndrome or severe combined immunodeficiency

            (b) Acquired defects in cell-mediated immunity due to leukemia, lymphoma, or acquired immunodeficiency syndrome (AIDS)

            (c) Bruton's agammaglobulinemia

                (i) These individuals have a 10,000-fold increased risk of paralytic complications from the Sabin polio vaccine.

                (ii) Because the Sabin virus is shed in the feces of vaccinees, family members of Bruton's patients also should not be vaccinated.

        (2) Live vaccines should also generally not be given to patients receiving corticosteroids, alkylating agents, radiation, or other **immunosuppressant therapy**.

B. Other adverse effects

1. Allergic reactions to vaccine components such as egg proteins, antibiotics, or mercurial preservatives can occur.

2. Serum sickness may result from the injection of large quantities of foreign proteins such as diphtheria antitoxin.

C. Assessing the risk:benefit ratio. All vaccines can have side effects that are undesirable. The potential benefits must be evaluated with the possibility of these unwanted effects in mind.

1. For example, rubella is a relatively benign disease, but can be devastating in the fetus; it would definitely be contraindicated to give this vaccine to a woman during pregnancy.

2. However, the same pregnant woman traveling in an area endemic for yellow fever should be immunized against yellow fever because the risk of infection exceeds the small theoretical hazard to fetus and mother.

STUDY QUESTIONS

Directions: Each of the numbered items or incomplete statements in this section is followed by answers or by completions of the statement. Select the **one** lettered answer or completion that is **best** in each case.

1. The preferred vaccine for diphtheria consists of

(A) heat-killed *Corynebacterium diphtheriae*
(B) attenuated *C. diphtheriae*
(C) precipitated or adsorbed toxoid
(D) capsular polysaccharide
(E) capsule plus carrier protein

2. Bacille Calmette-Guérin (BCG) is sometimes used for

(A) passive immunization for tuberculosis
(B) inducing the production of neutralizing antibody
(C) nonspecific suppression of the immune response
(D) inducing the production of antipili antibody
(E) nonspecific potentiation of the immune response

3. The major immunoregulatory effect of interferon seems to be

(A) differentiation of plasma cells
(B) enhancement of natural killer (NK) cells and macrophages
(C) suppression of cell-mediated immunity
(D) enhancement of antibody production
(E) provision of passive immunity

4. An immune response that mimics the response induced by natural infection is believed to be stimulated by administering agents via the

(A) subcutaneous route
(B) percutaneous route
(C) intradermal route
(D) intramuscular route
(E) intranasal route

5. Purified polysaccharide capsule is used to vaccinate against infection caused by

(A) *Bordetella pertussis*
(B) *Corynebacterium diphtheriae*
(C) *Salmonella typhi*
(D) *Streptococcus pneumoniae*
(E) *Clostridium tetani*

6. Active artificial immunization is induced by the administration of all of the following EXCEPT

(A) bacterial products
(B) toxoids
(C) vaccines
(D) antitoxins
(E) attenuated pathogens

7. Specific immune globulin is preferred for passive immunization against all of the following EXCEPT

(A) tetanus
(B) rabies
(C) chickenpox (varicella)
(D) botulism
(E) hepatitis B

8. A component of a virus synthesized by a genetically engineered yeast comprises the vaccine used for

(A) rubella
(B) measles
(C) poliomyelitis
(D) hepatitis B
(E) mumps

9. Examples of specific immune globulins include all of the following EXCEPT

(A) rabies immune globulin
(B) measles immune globulin
(C) hepatitis B immune globulin
(D) varicella–zoster immune globulin
(E) Rh_o (D) immune globulin

1-C	4-E	7-D
2-E	5-D	8-D
3-B	6-D	9-B

Directions: The group of items in this section consists of lettered options followed by a set of numbered items. For each item, select the **one** lettered option that is most closely associated with it. Each lettered option may be selected once, more than once, or not at all.

Questions 10–12

Match each description below to the type of immunizing agent that it best characterizes.

(A) Bacterial vaccine
(B) Rickettsial vaccine
(C) Antitoxin
(D) Immune globulin
(E) Specific immune globulin
(F) Viral vaccine
(G) Protozoan vaccine
(H) Antivenom

10. Contains products that are detoxified

11. Prepared from hyperimmunized human volunteers

12. Prepared from pooled normal adult human plasma

10-A
11-E
12-D

ANSWERS AND EXPLANATIONS

1. The answer is C *[II A 3 a]*.
The preferred vaccine for diphtheria is fluid toxoid precipitated with potassium alum or adsorbed onto aluminum hydroxide or phosphate. Since diphtheria results primarily from the action of the toxin formed by *Corynebacterium diphtheriae* rather than from invasion by the organism, resistance to the disease depends on specific neutralizing antitoxin such as that induced by vaccination.

2. The answer is E *[IV A 1]*.
Bacille Calmette-Guérin (BCG) is a live attenuated strain of *Mycobacterium bovis*. It has been used with varying degrees of success for active immunization against tuberculosis. Administration of BCG can also nonspecifically stimulate the immune response. It appears to activate T cells and macrophages and to stimulate natural killer (NK) cells. Its primary effect is on cell-mediated immunity, not humoral antibody–mediated immunity.

3. The answer is B *[IV A 4]*.
Interferon, while it was originally associated with antiviral effects, is now recognized as having important immunoregulatory properties, mainly enhancement of natural killer (NK) cells and macrophages. Interferon would thus be expected to enhance cell-mediated immunity but to have little effect on humoral antibody–mediated immunity.

4. The answer is E *[I C 3]*.
Administering an immunizing agent intranasally appears to stimulate an immune response that mimics the response induced by a natural infection, particularly in upper respiratory tract disease. That is, this route results in the production of specific antibodies both in serum and in secretions at the local site of infection. Evaluation of the intranasal route for administering influenza vaccine is currently under way.

5. The answer is D *[II A 3 f]*.
Polysaccharide capsular material is used to vaccinate against pneumococcal pneumonia and against bacterial meningitis caused by meningococci and *Haemophilus influenzae* type B. Vaccines for typhoid fever (*Salmonella typhi*) and pertussis (*Bordetella pertussis*) consist of intact killed organisms. Vaccines for diphtheria (*Corynebacterium diphtheriae*) and tetanus (*Clostridium tetani*) are made from toxoid.

6. The answer is D *[I B 2 c; III A]*.
Antitoxins are used to induce passive, not active, immunity. Active immunity is artificially induced by the use of vaccines containing either intact microorganisms (killed or attenuated), their component parts (e.g., capsule), or their products (e.g., toxoid). These immunogens are treated so as to be unable to produce disease, but they are still antigenic and able to induce an immune response.

7. The answer is D *[III C 2]*.
Antitoxin prepared in horses is used to provide passive immunization against botulism. Equine antisera are also used in botulism and in some victims of snake and spider bites. A specific immune globulin is gamma globulin obtained from people who have recently recovered from a specific infectious disease or from hyperimmunized human volunteers. Specific immune globulins are available for passive immunization against tetanus, rabies, hepatitis, and chickenpox (varicella).

8. The answer is D *[II B 3 a]*.
Hepatitis B vaccine consists of chemically inactivated, adsorbed surface antigen particles purified from plasma of human carriers. Surface antigen produced by genetically engineered *Saccharomyces cerevisiae* is the vaccine of choice for hepatitis B. A surface antigen preparation purified from chemically inactivated virus is also available. For the vaccines against rubella (German measles), measles (rubeola), and mumps, and for the Sabin poliomyelitis vaccine, a live attenuated virus grown in tissue culture is used. An inactivated virus preparation (Salk vaccine) is also available for poliomyelitis.

9. The answer is B *[III B 2 b, C 2]*.
Measles immune globulin is immune globulin derived from pooled normal human plasma or serum that has been specifically tested for its measles antibody content. It is not a specific immune globulin: since immune globulin is derived from pooled plasma, it contains antibodies (mainly IgG) to a variety of different microorganisms and can be used for passive immunization against several diseases. Immune globulin is also used for maintenance of immunodeficient people. Specific immune globulin is an immune

globulin obtained from hyperimmunized human volunteers or from people who have recently recovered from a specific infectious disease. Examples of specific immune globulins are rabies immune globulin and varicella–zoster immune globulin. Rh_o (D) immune globulin is a hyperimmune preparation used in Rh-negative women within 72 hours after delivery, miscarriage, or abortion of an Rh-positive baby or fetus to prevent sensitization of the mother to possible Rh-positive red blood cells in future pregnancies.

10–12. The answers are: 10-A *[II A 2],* **11-E** *[III C 1],* **12-D** *[III B 1].*
Bacterial products used for immunization are usually structural components or detoxified products known as toxoids. Toxoids are toxins that are converted (via heat or formaldehyde treatment) into a non-toxic but immunogenic material, which induces the production of antitoxic antibodies. Specific immune globulin is a gamma globulin obtained from people who have recently recovered from a specific infectious disease or from human volunteers who have been hyperimmunized against that disease; examples include hepatitis B immune globulin and rabies immune globulin. Specific immune globulin is used to provide specific passive immunity. Immune globulin (gamma globulin) is prepared from pooled normal adult human plasma or serum by cold ethanol fractionation. Immune globulin contains antibodies to many common infectious agents that affect humans (e.g., measles, hepatitis A), and is used for passive immunization in people at risk of developing measles or hepatitis A, or for maintenance of passive immunity in immunodeficient people.

8
Laboratory Methods

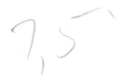

I. GENERAL CONSIDERATIONS. Serologic reactions—that is, in vitro antigen–antibody reactions—provide methods for the diagnosis of disease and for the identification and quantitation of antigens and antibodies.

A. The antibody titer, or level of antibody in serum, can be measured by using known antigens.

1. Antibody titers can be of diagnostic and prognostic importance.

2. For example, a rise in the antibody titer between serum taken during the acute phase of an illness and during the convalescent phase (acute and convalescent serums) can be diagnostic for that illness.

B. Environmental factors can profoundly affect the forces involved in antigen–antibody interactions. For example:

1. Physiologic **pH** and **salt concentration** promote optimal union. Forces of attraction tend to be weaker in conditions that are acid (below pH 4.0) or alkaline (above pH 10.0).

2. **Temperature** can be important: the higher the temperature (up to a maximum of 50° to 55° C), the greater the kinetic motion of the reactants and therefore the more rapid the rate of reaction.

C. The serologic identification of antibody types and types of antigen–antibody reactions are based on the physical state of the antigen:

1. **Agglutinins** are antibodies that aggregate cellular antigens.

2. **Lysins** are antibodies that cause dissolution of cell membranes.

3. **Precipitins** are antibodies that form precipitates with soluble antigens.

4. **Antitoxins** are antibodies that neutralize toxins.

D. The relative sensitivity of the various tests for antigens and antibodies are presented in Table 8-1.

II. PROCEDURES INVOLVING DIRECT DEMONSTRATION AND OBSERVATION OF REACTIONS

A. Procedures involving cellular antigens

1. **Agglutination reactions**
   a. Agglutination reactions serve to detect and quantitate agglutinins and to identify **cellular antigens** such as bacterial cells, white blood cells, and red blood cells.
      (1) When cells interact in vitro with the appropriate antibody, they clump together and eventually form masses that become large enough to be seen. (When antibody agglutinates bacteria in the body, opsonization occurs; see Chapter 1 II E.)
         (a) Agglutination occurs because antibodies are at least bivalent (i.e., they have at least two combining sites).
         (b) Two sites on the antibody and multiple sites on the antigen result in antigen–antibody lattice formation that can build up into increasingly larger complexes (Figure 8-1).

Table 8-1. Relative Sensitivity of Tests Measuring Antibody and Antigen

Test	Approximate Detectable Amount (μg/ml)	
	Antibody	**Antigen**
Precipitation	20.0	1.0
Immunoelectrophoresis	20.0	...
Double diffusion in agar gel	1.0	...
Complement fixation	0.5	...
Radial immunodiffusion	0.05	0.5
Bacterial agglutination	0.01	...
Hemolysis	0.01	...
Passive hemagglutination	0.01	...
Hemagglutination inhibition	...	0.001
Antitoxin neutralization	0.01	...
Radioimmunoassay (RIA)	0.0005	0.000005
Enzyme-linked immunosorbent assay (ELISA)	0.0005	0.000005
Virus neutralization	0.000005	...

      (2) The aggregates may be seen in the test tube or under the microscope.
      (3) If red blood cells are employed as the agglutinogen, the process is **hemagglutination**.
  b. The classic application of the agglutination reaction is the **Widal test** for the diagnosis of typhoid fever.
      (1) In this test, the antibody content of the patient's serum is measured by adding a **constant amount of antigen** (e.g., *Salmonella typhi*) to **serially diluted serum**—that is, to progressively more dilute serum samples.
      (2) After appropriate incubation, the serum samples are examined for visible agglutination. The highest dilution of serum that shows agglutination is referred to as the **titer**.

  2. Lysis
    a. Principle
      (1) In the presence of complement, an antigen–antibody reaction on a cell membrane may damage the membrane, leading to cell lysis (**cytolysis**).
      (2) The damage is presumed to be due to the enzymatic activity of activated complement components and the membrane-altering properties of complement components C8 and C9 (see Chapter 4 III B 3).
      (3) The phenomenon is probably of importance in the host's defense against microbial infections, cancer, and so forth.
      (4) Cytolysis in vivo can be a major cause of tissue damage.
    b. Types of cytolysis
      (1) In **hemolysis,** hemoglobin is released from the red blood cell; this is a requisite phenomenon for the complement fixation test.

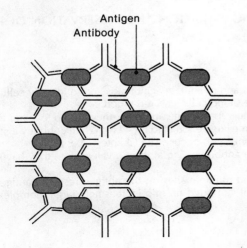

Antigen
Antibody

Figure 8-1. Lattice structure composed of antigen and antibody.

(2) In **bacteriolysis,** cells of gram-negative bacteria undergo immune lysis.

(3) Cytolysis can also involve the destruction of other cell types (e.g., tumor cells) under appropriate conditions in the presence of specific antibody and complement.

B. Procedures involving soluble antigen

1. Precipitation

a. When **soluble antigens** come in contact with specific antibody, they aggregate (i.e., precipitate).

(1) Because the antigen is soluble instead of cellular, a large number of molecules are required for lattice formation.

(2) Moreover, a large lattice must be formed in order for the aggregate to be visible.

b. Changing the amount of antigen affects precipitation (Figure 8-2).

(1) When the antigen concentration is very low and the antibody relatively superabundant (**zone of antibody excess**), formation of small complexes occurs.

(a) However, residual antibody will remain in the supernatant after the mixture has been centrifuged.

(b) This area containing excess antibody is known as the **prozone.**

(2) As more antigen is added, large aggregates form. In the **zone of equivalence,** there is neither antigen nor antibody in the supernatant.

(3) With increasing amounts of antigen (**zone of antigen excess**), the lattice size becomes too small to precipitate. Hence, instead of reaching a plateau, the curve (see Figure 8-2) comes back down to zero.

(a) The area containing excess antigen is known as the **postzone.**

(b) In extreme antigen excess, the complex will be **trimolecular** (i.e., one antibody molecule for every two antigen molecules).

2. In vivo consequences of soluble complexes

a. When soluble complexes form in vivo, they may cause serum sickness (see Chapter 9 IV C 2).

(1) An example of this is the administration of **diphtheria antitoxin** made from horse serum, which is a foreign protein to humans.

(2) People given too much antitoxin (i.e., antigen) may develop serum sickness.

b. The soluble complexes are not handled well by the reticuloendothelial system (RES).

3. Immunodiffusion. This laboratory technique is based on the phenomenon of precipitation.

a. If an antigen–antibody reaction takes place in a **semisolid medium** (e.g., agar), bands of precipitate will form.

b. The **Ouchterlony technique,** a **double immunodiffusion** method, is a useful example.

(1) The technique is called **double diffusion** because the two components diffuse toward each other. (In **single diffusion,** one component is fixed in place.)

(2) In the Ouchterlony procedure, antigen and antibody preparations are placed in separate wells that are cut into a thin layer of agar in a Petri dish.

(a) The reactants diffuse toward each other through the agar until they meet.

(b) At optimal antigen–antibody proportions, bands of precipitate form (Figure 8-3).

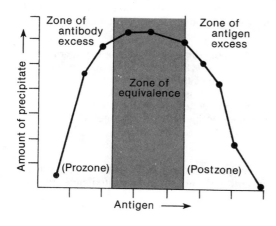

Figure 8-2. Effect of increasing amounts of antigen on the total immune precipitate obtained in a mixture of soluble antigen and its homologous antibody.

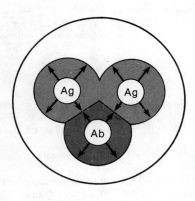

Figure 8-3. Diffusion of reactants in double immunodiffusion. *Ag* = antigen; *Ab* = antibody.

   c. One advantage of immunodiffusion procedures is that **antigenic relationships** can be detected from **precipitation patterns** (Figure 8-4).
   (1) In **reactions of identity,** two identical antigens will diffuse at the same rate, and their two precipitin bands will merge into a solid **chevron**.
   (2) In **reactions of nonidentity,** the two antigens are completely different, and the lines of precipitate will **cross**.
   (3) In **reactions of partial identity,** a **spur** will form, indicating that the two antigens are cross-reactive but not identical.
      (a) The spur occurs because one of the antibodies does not react with the cross-reacting antigen but migrates past that antigen until it reaches an antigen with the epitope for which it has specificity.
      (b) The spur in Figure 8-4 contains antibody b only; antibody a reacted with epitope a on antigen ac.

4. Quantitative radial immunodiffusion is a variation that allows the quantitation of antigens. It is used routinely to determine human serum immunoglobulin levels—in this case, the **immunoglobulin** is the **antigen**.
   a. For this purpose, an agar-coated slide is used, the agar being impregnated with antiserum (e.g., antibody to human IgG). Serum samples are then placed in wells in the agar.
   b. As each sample diffuses through the agar and encounters the antibody, the IgG will form a concentric ring, or halo, of precipitate. The **diameter of the halo** directly correlates with the **concentration of IgG** in the sample.
   c. The level of IgG in the sample can be determined by reference to a standard curve based on halo diameters of known concentrations of IgG.

5. Immunoelectrophoresis. The double-diffusion technique could not always resolve highly complex mixtures of antigens; therefore, this more sophisticated technique was developed.
   a. In immunoelectrophoresis, antigen is placed in wells in agar on a glass slide and is then subjected to electrophoresis via application of an electric current. Under these conditions, the individual antigenic components will migrate through the agar at variable rates.
   b. If antibody is then placed in a well running the length of the slide and parallel to the path of migration, the reactants will diffuse toward one another and form separate arcs of precipitation for each antigenic component.

6. Counterimmunoelectrophoresis. This variant of double diffusion adds an electric current as the migratory force, which greatly speeds up the reaction (18 to 24 hours by double diffusion; 30 to 90 minutes with electric propulsion) and intensifies the precipitin bands.
   a. Antigen and antibody are placed in wells and current is applied.
   b. In suitable buffer, the negatively charged antigen migrates toward the anode, whereas the antibody (with no significant net charge) migrates in the opposite (counter) direction as a result of endosmosis. Precipitation occurs where the reactants meet.

C. Toxin–antitoxin reactions. If a serum contains an antitoxin (i.e., an antibody to a toxin), the antibody will neutralize the toxin. The **presence of antitoxin** can be demonstrated either directly or indirectly.

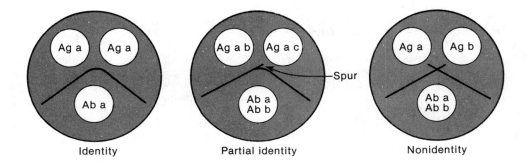

Figure 8-4. Types of patterns seen in immunodiffusion. *Ag* = antigen; *Ab* = antibody.

1. **Direct testing.** The presence or absence of antitoxin in an individual's serum can be shown by intradermally injecting a small amount of the toxin. An example is the **Schick test,** which is used to test for immunity to diphtheria by testing for antibody to diphtheria toxin.
   a. A **positive test** (inflammation that develops at the injection site within a few days) indicates the **absence of antibody**.
   b. A **negative test** (no reaction) indicates that there was **sufficient antitoxin** to neutralize the toxin injected, and the individual is immune.

2. **Indirect testing.** Antitoxin can also be detected via neutralization in vitro.
   a. An individual's serum is mixed with toxin in vitro, and then, after a few minutes, a small amount of the mixture is injected into an experimental animal.
   b. If the serum contains antitoxin, the animal will be protected against the deleterious effects of the toxin.

D. **Procedures involving insoluble particulates. Flocculation** is an antigen–antibody reaction that occurs if the antigen is neither cellular nor soluble, but is an **insoluble particulate**.

   1. The **Venereal Disease Research Laboratory (VDRL) test** and the **rapid plasma reagin (RPR) test** are flocculation tests used for the diagnosis of syphilis.

   2. These tests make use of **cardiolipin,** a hapten from normal beef heart that cross-reacts with a heterophile (heterogenetic) antigen of the spirochete of syphilis.

   3. Cholesterol particles with water-insoluble cardiolipin on their surface are used in the test. Visible aggregates form in the presence of an antibody (**reagin**) in the serum of patients with syphilis.

III. COMPLEX SEROLOGIC PROCEDURES. In some antigen–antibody reactions, the visible manifestation requires the participation of accessory factors, indicator systems, or specialized equipment.

A. **Complement fixation**

   1. **General considerations**
      a. **Complement,** a protein constituent of normal serum, is **consumed (fixed)** during the interaction of antigens and antibodies.
         (1) This interaction between complement and antigen–antibody complexes is called **complement fixation** when it occurs in vitro.
         (2) When the same interaction occurs in vivo it is known as **complement activation**.
      b. This phenomenon forms the basis for the **complement fixation test,** a sensitive in vitro procedure that is widely used to detect or quantitate antigens or antibodies.

   2. The primary reacting ingredients are antigen, antibody, and complement.
      a. Normal guinea pig serum is often used as a source of complement because the animal has high levels of complement with efficient lytic properties.

    b. Different sources of complement are used in other tests; rabbit complement, for example, is used in cytotoxicity tests performed for transplantation antigen detection.

  3. Complement fixation is often used to determine whether a patient's serum contains antibody to a particular antigen. Both a **test system** and an **indicator system** are required, because the reaction cannot be seen without an indicator system.

    a. Test system

      (1) The serum to be tested is heated to 56° C to inactivate native complement, and measured amounts of the antigen and complement (guinea pig serum) are then added.

      (2) If antibody specific for that antigen is present in the serum, antigen–antibody complexes will be formed that will fix all the complement.

    b. Indicator system

      (1) **Sheep red blood cells (SRBCs)** plus **hemolysin,** an antibody specific for SRBCs, are added to test for the presence of free (active) complement.

      (2) Interpretation of the test is based on the presence of **hemolysis.**

        (a) If all the complement has been fixed, none will be free to lyse the SRBCs; this constitutes a **positive** complement fixation test.

        (b) If no antibody is present in the patient's serum, then the complement is not fixed and is free to interact in the indicator system, lysing the SRBCs; this constitutes a **negative** complement fixation test.

  4. Complement fixation tests require appropriate controls to ensure that no **anticomplementary (AC) factors** are present to affect the results adversely.

    a. The antigen or the serum itself may have anticomplementary properties (e.g., they may contain denatured or aggregated immunoglobulin, heparin, chelating agents, or microbial contaminants).

    b. The AC factors may fix all the complement in the system.

    c. They may remove calcium or magnesium ions, both of which are essential for complement-mediated lysis.

B. Immunofluorescence. If a fluorescent dye (e.g., fluorescein isocyanate) is conjugated to antibody molecules, the molecules will be visible via ultraviolet light in a fluorescence microscope. Such labeled antibody can be used to identify antigens. Both direct and indirect techniques are available.

  1. Direct immunofluorescence. This is a rapid, useful test for the identification of antigens in tissues or other specimens.

    a. Antibody specific for a particular antigen (e.g., a microorganism) is labeled (tagged) with a fluorescent dye, usually fluorescein, and is allowed to react with the tissue or organism in question.

    b. If the antibody reacts, it will be visualized as a green stain on the specimen when it is examined under ultraviolet light.

    c. For the **identification of *Treponema pallidum*** in an exudate from a patient suspected of having syphilis, the following procedure would be used.

      (1) A slide of exudate is prepared and flooded with tagged antibody specific for *T. pallidum*. If these organisms are present in the exudate, they will bind the tagged antibody.

      (2) Excess, unbound antibody is then washed from the slide, and the slide is examined under ultraviolet light with a fluorescence microscope; *T. pallidum* will fluoresce and appear green against the black background.

  2. Indirect immunofluorescence

    a. Indirect immunofluorescence procedures employ antibody against antibody (e.g., rabbit antiserum against human gamma globulin), with a fluorescent compound covalently coupled to it.

    b. The "sandwich" technique allows for detection of antibody.

      (1) This technique is used in the **fluorescent treponemal antibody absorption (FTA–ABS) test** for the serodiagnosis of **syphilis.**

        (a) *T. pallidum* is fixed to a slide, and the slide is flooded with the patient's serum to be tested for antibody. If antibodies to the spirochete are present in the patient's serum, they will bind to the organisms on the slide.

        (b) Excess antibody is removed by washing, and the preparation is then overlaid with fluorescein-tagged antibody to human gamma globulin.

> > **(c)** If the patient's s rum contains antibodies to *T. pallidum,* the tagged antibody will bind to the patient's antibodies, and fluorescing organisms will be seen when the slide is examined with the fluorescence microscope.
> **(2)** The sandwich technique is also used in detecting **antinuclear antibodies** (antibodies to components of the cell nucleus, such as DNA, RNA, or histone).
> > **(a)** Antinuclear antibodies are present in systemic lupus erythematosus (SLE) and sometimes in rheumatoid arthritis and other autoimmune collagen vascular diseases (see Chapter 10 II B 2 b).
> > **(b)** For serodiagnosis of **SLE,** the procedure is essentially identical to that described above for *T. pallidum* except that the antigen is DNA in animal or human buffy coat cells, rat kidney sections, or beef thymus sections.

C. Virus neutralization. These assays are based on the ability of specific antibodies to interfere with some biological function of the virus, usually its attachment to host cells.

> **1.** When certain viruses (e.g., herpesviruses) are added to appropriate target cells growing in tissue culture (e.g., rabbit kidney cells), the viruses will produce observable cytopathic effects (CPE).
> **2.** The phenomenon of CPE is useful in the search for **virus-neutralizing antibodies** in a serum sample. The serum suspected of containing antibody is added to a virus suspension and then a culture of susceptible (target) cells is inoculated with the mixture.
> > **a.** If CPE develops in the cell culture, no neutralizing antibodies were present:
> >
> > $$\text{Virus + target cell} \rightarrow \text{CPE}$$
> >
> > **b.** If CPE fails to develop, then neutralizing antibodies were present in the serum sample:
> >
> > $$\text{Serum antibody + virus + target cell} \rightarrow \text{no CPE}$$

D. Procedures involving agglutination

> **1. Hemagglutination inhibition**
> > **a. General considerations**
> > > **(1)** Hemagglutination involves the agglutination of red blood cells by antibodies (hemagglutins) or by certain particles (e.g., influenza or mumps viruses) or other substances.
> > > **(2)** The inhibition of hemagglutination can be used for virus identification and to test for the presence of various antigens.
> > **b. Virus identification.** A valuable viral diagnostic test demonstrates the presence of serum antibody to hemagglutinating viruses.
> > > **(1)** Although hemagglutination by a virus is not an immunologic phenomenon, its inhibition by specific antibody is. Indeed, the inhibition of viral hemagglutination is a form of virus neutralization.
> > > **(2)** The serum of a patient suspected of having **influenza,** for example, can be examined for influenza antibody by mixing the patient's serum with known influenza virus and red blood cells.
> > > > **(a)** If no anti-influenza antibody is present, hemagglutination will occur:
> > > >
> > > > $$\text{Virus + red blood cells} \rightarrow \text{hemagglutination}$$
> > > >
> > > > **(b)** If antibody is present, hemagglutination will be inhibited because the antibody will bind to the virus and block its ability to hemagglutinate:
> > > >
> > > > $$\text{Serum antibody + virus + red blood cells} \rightarrow \text{no hemagglutination}$$
> **2. Passive (indirect) agglutination.** In tests based on passive, or indirect, agglutination, a reaction system is converted from one that precipitates to one that agglutinates, thus yielding a more sensitive indication of antibody.
> > **a. Tests for rheumatoid factor.** People with rheumatoid arthritis produce an antibody (mainly IgM) to their own IgG; this anti-IgG autoantibody is known as **rheumatoid factor.** Several passive agglutination tests for rheumatoid factor are useful in the diagnosis of **rheumatoid arthritis.**
> > > **(1)** The **latex agglutination test** consists of coating latex particles with IgG and reacting them with the patient's serum. Agglutination indicates the presence of anti-IgG antibodies, or a positive test.

      (2) In the **Rose-Waaler test,** tannic acid–treated SRBCs are coated with rabbit IgG antibodies specific for the SRBCs, and the patient's serum is added. Again, agglutination indicates the presence of rheumatoid factor.

    b. **Bis-diazotized benzidine** is a coupling reagent that can be used to conjugate proteins or haptens to red blood cells, thus allowing the detection of specific antibodies to the antigenic materials by passive hemagglutination procedures.

    c. **Test for soluble antigens.** A two-step test can be employed to detect soluble antigens that react with and neutralize a hemagglutinating antibody.

      (1) Antibodies to a soluble antigen such as IgG will cause the agglutination of red blood cells that have IgG coupled to their membranes.

      (2) However, if soluble IgG is added to the antiserum before the IgG-coated red blood cells are admixed, the anti-IgG antibody will react with the soluble IgG and hemagglutination will be inhibited.

  3. **Coombs (antiglobulin) tests.** The **direct and indirect Coombs tests** are modified agglutination procedures.

    a. **General considerations**

      (1) In certain cases, antibodies directed against antigenic determinants are unable to form visible aggregates when subjected to precipitation or agglutination procedures. In order to demonstrate the presence of antibody (gamma globulin) in such cases, Coombs (antiglobulin) testing may be employed.

      (2) The Coombs tests involve adding an anti–gamma globulin antibody from a different species (e.g., from the rabbit). This induces the lattice formation necessary for agglutination by providing a bridge between two antibody-coated cells or particles.

    b. **Direct Coombs test**

      (1) The direct Coombs test is used to detect **cell-bound antibody**. It is of value in the detection of antibodies attached to red blood cells in syndromes such as **hemolytic disease of the newborn (erythroblastosis fetalis)** and **autoimmune hemolytic disease**.

      (2) In the direct procedure, red blood cells are washed free of serum and unbound antibody, and the antiglobulin reagent is added directly to the cell suspension. If the red blood cells had antibody adsorbed to their surfaces, they will now be agglutinated.

    c. **Indirect Coombs test**

      (1) The indirect Coombs test is used to detect the presence of **circulating nonagglutinating antibody**. It is of value in detecting IgG-associated Rh antibody in the serum of a woman who is thought to be sensitized to the Rh antigen and at risk for carrying an erythroblastotic fetus.

      (2) In the indirect procedure, a serum sample is incubated with appropriate red blood cells, the cells are washed, and the antiglobulin reagent is added. If antibody from the serum sample has adsorbed to the red blood cells, they will now be agglutinated.

E. Radioimmunoassay (RIA)

  1. **General considerations**

    a. RIA procedures can be used for the quantitation of any immunogen or hapten that can be labeled with a radioactive isotope such as iodine-125 (^{125}I). These extremely sensitive methods are capable of measuring picogram quantities or less, depending on the substance being assayed.

    b. **Serum levels** of a wide range of substances can be measured, including:

      (1) Hormones (e.g., insulin, growth hormone, adrenocorticotropic hormone, triiodothyronine, thyroxine, estrogen)

      (2) Serum proteins [e.g., carcinoembryonic antigen (CEA), IgE]

      (3) Metabolites [e.g., cyclic adenosine 3,5-monophosphate (cyclic AMP), folic acid]

      (4) Drugs (e.g., digoxin, digitoxin, morphine)

      (5) Microbial agents and antibodies [e.g., hepatitis B surface antigen (HBsAg)]

    c. RIA procedures are based on the competition between labeled (known) and unlabeled (unknown) antigen for the same antibody.

  2. **Liquid-phase RIA**

    a. A known amount of labeled antigen, a known amount of specific antibody, and an unknown amount of unlabeled antigen are allowed to react together.

    b. The antigen–antibody complexes that form are then separated out by either physicochemical or immunologic means (e.g., by precipitation using either ammonium sulfate or a second antibody, respectively).

c. The radioactivity remaining in the supernatant (representing unbound, labeled antigen) is measured, and the percentage of labeled antigen bound to the antibody is calculated from this.

d. The concentration of the unknown (unlabeled) antigen can be determined by reference to a standard curve constructed from data obtained by allowing known amounts of unlabeled antigen to compete.

3. Solid-phase RIA

a. Solid-phase RIA involves adsorption or covalent linkage of antibody to a solid matrix. Unlabeled antigen is then added, followed by labeled antigen.

b. Determination of bound versus free labeled antigen is made, and the amount of antigen in the unknown sample is calculated again by reference to a standard curve.

F. Enzyme-linked immunosorbent assay (ELISA)

1. ELISA can be used to assay both antigens and antibodies. It has virtually the same sensitivity as RIA.

a. The principles are as follows:

(1) Antigen or antibody can be adsorbed to a solid-phase support (e.g., a plastic surface or paper disk) and still retain its immunologic activity.

(2) If the antigen or antibody is linked to an enzyme (e.g., horseradish peroxidase or alkaline phosphatase), the antigen–enzyme complex retains both immunologic and enzymatic activity.

b. The test is designed so that the enzyme–substrate reaction will produce a color change if the test is positive.

2. One variant of ELISA, the **double antibody sandwich** for the assay of an antigen (e.g., HBsAg), is performed as follows:

a. Antibody specific for the antigen being assayed is coated on a polystyrene plate. The solution being tested for antigen is applied to the surface, and any unreacted material is removed by washing.

b. Enzyme-labeled antibody specific for the captured antigen is then applied, and any excess conjugate is removed by washing.

c. Finally, the substrate of the enzyme is added. A substrate that will give a color change on degradation is chosen, so that spectrophotometry can be used to measure the extent of substrate degradation.

d. The measurement of substrate degradation gives the amount of enzyme-labeled antibody that was bound, and from this value one can determine the amount of antigen in the solution being tested.

IV. ASSAYS OF IMMUNE COMPETENCE: EVALUATING PHAGOCYTIC CELLS, B CELLS, AND T CELLS

A. Analysis of phagocytic cells

1. Assays for metabolism and the generation of toxic molecules

a. General considerations. These assays are used in the diagnosis of **chronic granulomatous disease (CGD)**. They determine whether phagocytic cells are using the hexose monophosphate (HMP) shunt and are going through the oxidative burst, thereby generating toxic materials to kill microorganisms.

b. Chemiluminescence. Singlet oxygen produces a small amount of light when its electron returns to its original orbit. If normal levels of singlet oxygen are being generated, the light produced can be measured as chemiluminescence.

c. Nitroblue tetrazolium (NBT) reduction. The NBT test is usually used to assay the phagocytic function of neutrophils.

(1) NBT, a yellow, water-soluble dye, converts to **formazan,** a purple, water-insoluble intracellular precipitate, when functioning neutrophils produce hydrogen peroxide and superoxide anion during the phagocytic process. Thus, counting the formazan-positive (f+) cells gives an indication of neutrophil function.

(2) The assay has two **parts**:

(a) Resting. Dye is placed on the cells, but nothing is administered to trigger oxidation. Normally, 1% to 2% of resting neutrophils are f+.

(b) Stimulated. Neutrophils are stimulated to phagocytize.

    (i) In normal individuals, 100% of the neutrophils can be stimulated to be f+.

    (ii) Patients with CGD lack certain enzymes associated with the HMP shunt [e.g., nicotinamide-adenine dinucleotide phosphate (NADPH) oxidase] and therefore their neutrophils do not kill intracellularly; no cells are f+ in either the resting or stimulated states.

(3) The NBT test is particularly useful in **genetic counseling** (CGD is usually an X-linked disease). If the mother is a carrier, she may have 1% to 2% f+ in resting neutrophils and an intermediate value (e.g., 50%) when stimulated.

2. Assay for ingestion and killing of microorganisms. In some phagocytic disorders, the cells show a defect in uptake or in killing, with normal NBT values. In these cases, the cells are evaluated for their phagocytic and microbicidal activities.

a. Phagocytosis. Cells can be incubated with bacteria or other engulfable materials (e.g., latex or polystyrene particles) for 1 to 3 hours, then stained and examined for uptake of the foreign bodies.

b. Microbicidal activity. Intracellular killing by phagocytic cells can be measured by direct plate counting of mixtures of microorganisms and cells.

(1) In this test, the **microbicidal or intracellular killing assay,** viable bacteria are added to a tube of neutrophils and incubated for 30 to 60 minutes.

(2) Counting the surviving bacteria by culture of the mixture, and comparing the counts to a control tube with bacteria but no neutrophils, gives the percentage of kill. A normal population of cells will kill 85% to 90% of the bacteria within 30 minutes.

(3) The viability of the engulfed microbes can be determined more easily if acridine orange, a fluorescent dye, is added to the culture medium. When observed with a fluorescence microscope, live bacteria will stain green while dead organisms will appear red.

3. Assays for chemotaxis

a. Two procedures are available for testing the ability of neutrophils to move in a directed migratory pattern toward a chemotactic stimulus such as endotoxin or the complement split product C5a.

(1) The neutrophils and the stimulus can be separated by a nitrocellulose membrane with a pore size of 3 to 5 μ; the cells that migrate through the small pores can be counted by staining and observation of the opposite side of the membrane.

(2) The migration may occur through an agar menstruum, with the cells migrating from a well punched in the agar toward a chemoattractant placed in a second well.

b. The assay must be done in parallel with a normal blood specimen to provide a frame of reference.

B. Analysis of B and pre-B cells. In all evaluations of immunity, it is important to establish both the number of immune cells that are present and whether these cells are functional.

1. Enumeration of B cells

a. Membrane marker assays are used to measure lymphocyte subpopulations.

(1) For B cells, the marker can be a **surface immunoglobulin molecule** or a **cluster of differentiation (CD) molecule** such as CD19 or CD20 (see Chapter 5 III C 2); these molecules are all integral membrane components (not just absorbed by a receptor).

(2) The **procedure employing immunoglobulin** is as follows:

    (a) Since the immunoglobulin is a protein, it can serve as an antigen.

    (b) The B cells are mixed with an antibody to gamma globulin that has been labeled with fluorescein dye.

    (c) The antibody will recognize the antigen, so that after incubation the cell will have fluorescent antibody all around its membrane.

    (d) Under a fluorescence microscope, B cells can be identified by their bright green halo.

    (e) The cells are commonly enumerated by flow cytometric techniques (see IV C 1 b)

b. The **erythrocyte–antibody–complement (EAC) rosette assay** can be performed to quantitate B cells. This assay is similar to the erythrocyte rosette (E-rosette) assay for T cells (see IV C 1 a), but the SRBCs must first be coated with antibody and complement.

2. Enumeration of pre-B cells

a. The pre-B cell has μ heavy (H) chain in its cytoplasm but none on its membrane. Antibody does not normally enter the cell cytoplasm, and can only label the membrane if it contains IgM molecules.

b. Pre-B cells are incubated with fluorescein-labeled anti–human μ chain antiserum.

c. The cells are then washed and fixed on a slide. At this point, the membrane is permeable, and rhodamine (red)-labeled anti–human μ serum is added to label any μ chain in the cytoplasm.

d. Pre-B cells show red fluorescence in the cytoplasm and no fluorescence on the membrane. Mature B cells will have a red cytoplasm and a green membrane.

3. Evaluation of function

a. Serum immunoglobulin levels. The quantitation of serum immunoglobulin levels is accomplished by radial immunodiffusion (see II B 4).

b. Antibody synthesis. Some patients have normal serum immunoglobulin levels but lack specific antibodies. In this case, it must be determined whether the patient can respond to antigens by synthesizing antibodies.

(1) Possible **test antigens** include poliovirus, tetanus toxoid, diphtheria toxoid, pneumococcal polysaccharide, and keyhole-limpet hemocyanin (KLH).

(2) The patient's immunization history and past medical history are examined prior to deciding which antigen to use.

(a) Since most individuals have had immunizations, they should respond to poliovirus, tetanus toxoid, and diphtheria toxoid antigens.

(b) If the patient has not been immunized, vaccination would be necessary. A killed vaccine is used, because attenuated vaccines can cause infection and death in the immunodeficient patient.

(c) If an antibody assay of an immunized patient is negative, a booster injection could be given, again using a killed vaccine.

c. Isohemagglutinin levels. People in blood group A, B, or O should have anti-B, anti-A, or anti-A and anti-B antibodies, respectively, in their serum by the age of 2 years. If these antibodies are absent, it would indicate a defect in B cell function.

d. Lymphocyte proliferation assays

(1) Principle

(a) T cells and B cells have receptors for various plant lectins. When the cells interact with the lectins, the cells are stimulated to undergo mitosis; hence, the stimulating molecules are called **mitogens**.

(b) Some mitogens stimulate the transformation of B cells into plasma cells [this may have implications in the etiology of autoimmune disease; see Chapter 10 I A 3 b (2)].

(2) Procedures

(a) Lipopolysaccharide induces mitosis in B cells. This can be quantitated through the use of a **radioactive DNA precursor** (tritiated thymidine).

(i) The mitogen is mixed with the B cells and the tritiated thymidine.

(ii) B cells have a specific receptor for the mitogen, causing the B cell to undergo rapid proliferation.

(iii) Determining the amount of radioactive tritium that is incorporated into the DNA of the cell will quantitate the degree of mitosis.

(iv) If the count is lower than one for normal blood done on the same day, the patient has deficient B cell proliferation.

(b) The **relative proportions of B cells and T cells** in a population can be estimated by using appropriate mitogens and measuring the uptake of radioactive thymidine.

(i) Phytohemagglutinin (PHA) and concanavalin A (con A) are considered to be **T cell–specific** mitogens.

(ii) Pokeweed mitogen stimulates mitosis in **both T cells and B cells**.

(iii) Bacterial lipopolysaccharide (endotoxin) is mitogenic for **B cells only**.

C. Analysis of T cells and their subsets

1. Enumeration

a. T cells. The **E-rosette assay** is a marker test for enumerating T cells regardless of subtype.

(1) If peripheral blood lymphocytes (both T cells and B cells) are mixed with a suspension of SRBCs, the T cells will bind the SRBCs to their membranes and form **rosettes** (mulberry-shaped cell aggregates); the B cells will not do this.

(2) Since the T cells in rosette form can be distinguished from other lymphocytes, they can be enumerated.

b. T cell subsets. Fluorescent monoclonal antibodies can be used to assay specific T cell subsets, since different monoclonal antibodies interact with different subsets of cells (Table 8-2).
   (1) T cells, once labeled with a fluorescent dye, can be observed via ultraviolet darkfield microscopy or they can be quantitated by sophisticated machines and methodologies.
   (2) One such machine is the **fluorescence-activated cell sorter (FACS;** Figure 8-5), which uses flow cytometric techniques to analyze and separate cells according to their fluorescence and light-scattering properties.
      (a) A cell suspension is stained with a fluorescent dye conjugated to a particular monoclonal antibody.
      (b) The suspension is forced through a narrow aperture so that the cells are lined up single-file.
      (c) The stream passes through a laser beam, and photocells measure fluorescence emission and light scatter, giving an index of cell size and granularity.
      (d) Vibrations in the flow chamber disperse the particles into droplets.
      (e) The falling droplets are next given an electrical charge, the nature of the charge depending on the photocell measurements.
      (f) The droplets then pass between a pair of charged plates, where they are deflected into new paths according to their electrical charge; thus the cells can be separated and sorted.
      (g) The viability of the cells is not affected by this procedure; hence, they can be used in subsequent experiments such as in vivo reconstitution of immunodeficient animals.

2. Evaluation of function
   a. Delayed-type hypersensitivity skin testing. Skin tests for delayed hypersensitivity are useful in overall evaluations of immunocompetence and as part of the diagnostic workup in certain infectious diseases (e.g., tuberculosis).
      (1) The patient undergoes a battery of skin tests intended to evoke a response to one or more antigens. Multiple antigens may be tested simultaneously.
         (a) Available **antigens** include mumps virus, trichophytin (a fungal antigen), candidin (a yeast antigen to which most humans have been exposed), streptokinase–streptodornase (SKSD; a product of group A β-hemolytic streptococci), purified protein derivative (PPD; a skin test reagent for *Mycobacterium tuberculosis* infection), and diphtheria toxoid (inactivated toxin from the diphtheria bacillus).
         (b) As with serum antibody assays, whether a response occurs depends on what antigens the patient has encountered during his or her lifetime.
      (2) For each test, the patient is given an intradermal injection of the material, and the injection site is observed for the next 3 days.
      (3) A positive test result typically is indicated by an erythematous, indurated lesion that peaks after 48 hours.
         (a) This reaction is due to the infiltration of cells (lymphocytes and macrophages) into the area, which causes it to harden.
         (b) Usually the erythema is larger than the induration, but it is the indurated area that is measured.
   b. Lymphocyte proliferation assays
      (1) These assays test T cell function in terms of **response to a mitogen** by determining the amount of radioactive tritium incorporated into the DNA of the cell [see IV B 3 d (2) (a)].

Table 8-2. Immunologic Specificity of Selected Anti–T Cell Serums

Antibody Against	Cells Detected	Normal Blood Values (%)
CD2*	T cells and natural killer (NK) cells	85 +
CD3†	T cells	75
CD4	Helper and inducer T cells	50
CD8	Suppressor and cytotoxic T cells	25

*CD = cluster of differentiation molecules, which are membrane components of various cells of the body that aid in identification of cellular function.

†Called the pan-T reagent because it reacts with all peripheral blood T cells; CD3 antigen is complexed with the T cell antigen receptor in the T cell membrane.

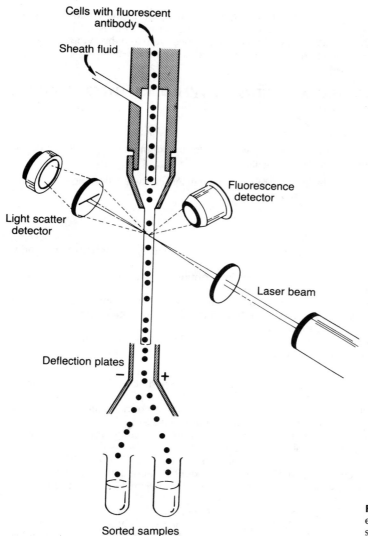

Cells with fluorescent antibody

Sheath fluid

Fluorescence detector

Light scatter detector

Laser beam

Deflection plates

− +

Sorted samples

Figure 8-5. Principle of the fluorescence-activated cell sorter (FACS; see text for description).

    (2) A specific antigen such as PPD could also be used in individuals known to be reactive to that particular substance.

  c. Mixed lymphocyte culture (This and other procedures used before tissue transplantation to test histocompatibility between donor and recipient are discussed in Chapter 12 III C.)

    (1) These assays depend on the fact that the patient's T cells have different histocompatibility antigens than do target cells from a nonrelated donor.

    (2) The target cells are treated with a drug (e.g., mitomycin C) or with irradiation to prevent DNA synthesis and proliferation. The patient's T cells then are mixed with the treated target cells.

    (3) The patient's cells will recognize the target cells as foreign and should begin proliferation, which can be measured by the addition of tritiated thymidine.

    (4) The degree of incompatibility between donor and recipient can be estimated by the amount of radioactivity taken up by the lymphocytes.

  d. Cell-mediated cytotoxicity assays

    (1) These tests are used to determine the functional integrity of cytotoxic T lymphocytes and also of natural killer (NK) cells.

    (2) The effector cells are incubated with the "target," which can be another lymphocyte, a tumor cell, or other human cells in culture. After a few hours' incubation, a dye such as eosin or trypan blue is added to the cell mixture.

(3) The end product of the test is a dead target cell with a porous membrane. The pores are created by perforin molecules released by the cytotoxic cells [see Chapter 1 II G 1 c; Chapter 9 V B 5 b (1)]; they allow the dye to penetrate into the cytoplasm so that the dead cells can be microscopically observed and counted.

V. IDENTIFICATION OF SPECIFIC ALLERGENS IN IMMEDIATE HYPERSENSITIVITY (TYPE I) REACTIONS

A. General considerations

1. A thorough patient history can be extremely valuable for the identification of allergens, particularly if environmental agents are involved.

2. A trial exposure may confirm the etiology of a type I hypersensitivity reaction; however, more precise techniques often must be used.

B. In vivo tests

1. **Skin tests**
   a. The potential allergens may be administered either cutaneously (**scratch test**) or intradermally.
   b. Multiple allergens may be tested simultaneously. Antihistaminic drugs must be discontinued 24 hours or more prior to skin testing.
   c. A positive test is characterized by the appearance, within seconds or minutes, of a typical **wheal (edema) and flare (erythema) reaction** in the skin at the site of allergen administration, due to the local release of mediators.
   d. False-positive and false-negative results are possible. Histamine or a histamine liberator may be administered as a positive control.

2. **Passive transfer tests**
   a. **Passive cutaneous anaphylaxis (PCA)** may be used in experimental animals, such as the guinea pig, to test serum for **cytotropic antibody**.
      (1) Serum is injected intradermally in the shaved skin of a normal animal; 3 to 6 hours later, antigen plus Evans blue dye is injected intravenously.
      (2) A positive reaction is characterized by bluing of the skin at the injection site due to increased capillary permeability and leakage of dye into the tissues.
   b. The **Prausnitz-Küstner (PK) reaction** is comparable to PCA but can be used in humans. However, the PK reaction is not used to any great extent because of the risk of transferring hepatitis and because tests that measure total and specific IgE are now available (see V C, below).
      (1) A small amount of serum from an allergic patient is injected intradermally into a nonallergic person. The serum contains IgE specific for a given allergen.
      (2) The IgE fixes to the skin and mast cells of the recipient during the next 12 to 24 hours, after which antigenic challenge (injection of the allergen into the same site) produces a typical wheal and flare reaction.

C. In vitro IgE assays. Either total IgE or specific IgE levels may be measured.

1. **Radioimmunosorbent test (RIST).** This technique is used to measure **total IgE concentration**. In this case, the IgE serves as **antigen**.
   a. Sheep or rabbit antibody to human IgE is coupled to a solid phase, such as a paper disk, and the serum to be examined is then added. The IgE in the serum reacts specifically with the coated disk.
   b. Unbound IgE is removed by washing, after which radiolabeled antibody to human IgE is added; the labeled antibody couples to the IgE bound to the disk.
   c. After rewashing, the radioactivity of the complex on the disk is measured. The bound radioactivity is directly proportional to the amount of IgE in the serum sample.

2. **Radioallergosorbent test (RAST).** This technique is used to measure **specific IgE levels**.
   a. A specific allergen (e.g., ragweed pollen antigen) is coupled to a solid phase, such as a cellulose particle or paper disk. The serum to be examined is then reacted with the solid phase–allergen complex, and if IgE specific for ragweed is present it will fix to the solid phase.

b. Unbound IgE is removed by washing, after which radiolabeled antibody to human IgE is reacted with the solid phase.

c. After rewashing, the radioactivity of the particles is measured to give the serum level of IgE specific for ragweed antigen.

VI. DETECTION OF IMMUNE COMPLEXES. Several types of assay are available for detecting immune complexes in serum and other biological fluids.

A. C1q binding assays. Complement component C1q has an affinity for immune complexes.

1. C1q solid-phase binding assay

a. Serum to be tested is incubated in a polystyrene tube that has been coated with C1q. After incubation, the sample is washed out.

b. The amount of immune complex bound to C1q is measured by using radiolabeled antibody to immunoglobulin.

2. C1q liquid-phase binding assay

a. Radiolabeled C1q is added to the serum being tested.

b. About 1 hour later, the bound C1q is removed from the free C1q by precipitation with polyethylene glycol.

c. The radioactivity level of the bound C1q corresponds to the C1q binding capacity and indicates the amount of immune complexes.

B. Raji cell binding assay

1. Raji cells (a human lymphoblastoid cell line) are well suited for the detection of immune complexes because:

a. They can bind immune complexes through C3 receptors.

b. They lack surface immunoglobulin.

2. Immune complexes bound to the surface of the Raji cells can be assayed by the addition of radiolabeled anti-IgG antibody.

3. After washing to remove unbound anti-IgG, the cells are quantitated for radioactivity.

VII. PRODUCTION AND USE OF MONOCLONAL ANTIBODIES

A. Present and potential uses of monoclonal antibodies

1. Monoclonal antibodies are becoming increasingly useful in **laboratory procedures**.

a. For example, fluorescent monoclonal antibodies are being used to assay specific T cell subsets by flow cytometric techniques (see IV C 1 b).

b. A constant and uniform source of antibody with a single specificity, instead of the usual mixture produced by the immune system, not only affords a powerful research tool but can be expected to provide quicker and more accurate identification of viruses, bacteria, and cancer cells.

2. The **long-range promise** of monoclonal antibodies is that they will be **therapeutically useful**.

a. Monoclonal antibodies are being tried experimentally in the **treatment of cancers,** primarily as **carriers** of anticancer agents such as radioisotopes or cytotoxic agents.

b. In addition, they may represent an alternative source of immunogens for **human anti–idiotypic antibody vaccines** (see Chapter 7 IV B 2 a). Monoclonal antibodies are very pure proteins, and if one carried an idiotype that resembled the epitope of the original immunogen (i.e., an **anti–idiotypic antibody**), it could substitute for the original immunogen in a vaccine.

B. Production of monoclonal antibodies by the murine hybridoma technique. Hybridomas are artificially created cells that produce pure or monoclonal antibodies.

1. A mouse is injected with antigen, and **plasma cells** from its spleen are **fused** with mouse cells of a cancerous type known as **plasmacytoma,** or **myeloma, cells**.

a. The cells are cultured at high dilutions to allow only one fused cell per culture dish.

    b. Only hybrid (fused) cells replicate because plasma cells are end cells (which do not multiply), and the plasmacytoma cells employed are deficient in hypoxanthine–guanine phosphoribosyltransferase (HGPRT), which makes them susceptible to metabolic poisoning by appropriate alterations in the media.

  2. Each hybrid cell formed by this technique has two important **properties**:
    a. It produces the single type of antibody molecule of its spleen-cell parent.
    b. It continually grows and divides, like its plasmacytoma-cell parent.

  3. The clone of hybrid cells that produces the desired antibody is identified and is then grown as a **continuous cell line,** from which large amounts of the pure or monoclonal antibody can be harvested.

STUDY QUESTIONS

Directions: Each of the numbered items or incomplete statements in this section is followed by answers or by completions of the statement. Select the **one** lettered answer or completion that is **best** in each case.

1. In the fluorescent treponemal antibody absorption (FTA–ABS) test, used to diagnose syphilis, the patient's serum is added to a slide containing

(A) *Treponema pallidum* organisms
(B) fluorescein-tagged antibody to *T. pallidum*
(C) fluorescein-tagged antibody to human gamma globulin
(D) fluorescein isocyanate
(E) complement and sheep red blood cells (SRBCs)

2. What is included in the indicator system of a complement fixation test?

(A) Specific antibody and complement
(B) Specific antigen and complement
(C) Red blood cells and hemolysin
(D) The patient's heat-inactivated serum
(E) Guinea pig serum

3. Which of the following procedures gives the most sensitive measure of antibody?

(A) Precipitation
(B) Agglutination
(C) Radial immunodiffusion
(D) Radioimmunoassay (RIA)
(E) Immunoelectrophoresis

4. In enumerating immune cells, the important marker in the cytoplasm of the pre-B cell is immunoglobulin heavy (H) chain

(A) α
(B) δ
(C) ε
(D) γ
(E) μ

5. In the direct immunofluorescence identification of a specific infectious agent (e.g., *Treponema pallidum* or *Streptococcus pyogenes*), fluorescein may be conjugated to

(A) the microorganism
(B) sheep red blood cells (SRBCs)
(C) antibody specific to human gamma globulin
(D) antibody specific to the microorganism
(E) antibody specific to complement

6. The radioimmunosorbent test (RIST) is a technique used to measure

(A) cellular antigens
(B) both antigen and antibody activity
(C) allergens in foods
(D) specific IgE levels
(E) total IgE concentration

7. The functional capability of T cells can be assayed by

(A) mixed lymphocyte culture
(B) fluorescent antibody assay with CD8 antiserum
(C) lipopolysaccharide mitogenic response
(D) erythrocyte (E)-rosette test
(E) fluorescent antibody assay with CD3 antiserum

8. In radioimmunoassay (RIA), it is essential that the substance to be detected

(A) can induce specific antibodies
(B) is protein in nature
(C) can be labeled with fluorescein isocyanate
(D) does not contain tritiated thymidine

1-A	4-E	7-A
2-C	5-D	8-A
3-D	6-E	

9. The functional integrity of phagocytic cells can be assessed by all of the following methods EXCEPT

(A) microbicidal assay
(B) nitroblue tetrazolium (NBT) test
(C) chemotaxis assay
(D) erythrocyte–antibody–complement (EAC) rosette test
(E) phagocytic index determination

10. Raji cells are well suited for use in an assay that detects immune complexes because these cells lack

(A) bound C1q
(B) free C1q
(C) C3 receptors
(D) surface immunoglobulin

ANSWERS AND EXPLANATIONS

1. The answer is A *[III B 2 b (1)]*.
In the fluorescent treponemal antibody absorption (FTA–ABS) test, *Treponema pallidum,* the etiologic agent of syphilis, is fixed to a slide which is then flooded with the patient's serum. If the patient's serum contains antibodies to *T. pallidum,* these antibodies will react with the spirochetes on the slide. The reaction can be visualized under a fluorescence microscope if fluorescein- labeled anti–human gamma globulin is added to the slide. The FTA–ABS test is an indirect immunofluorescence technique. Direct and indirect immunofluorescence techniques conjugate fluorescent dyes, such as fluorescein isocyanate, to antibody molecules in order to identify antigens.

2. The answer is C *[III A 3 b]*.
The indicator system in a complement fixation test consists of sheep red blood cells (SRBCs) plus antibody (hemolysin) specific for SRBCs. Complement fixation requires both a test system and an indicator system. The test system contains antibody, antigen, and a source of complement (e.g., guinea pig serum). To ascertain that the complement in the test system has been fixed (consumed), it is necessary to add a second set of reagents, the indicator system, which must react to the presence of active complement in a visible way. When complement has not been fixed, the SRBCs will be lysed if they are first sensitized to complement lysis by anti-SRBC antibody, such as hemolysin.

3. The answer is D *[III E 1 a; Table 8-1]*.
Radioimmunoassay (RIA) and enzyme-linked immunosorbent assay (ELISA) are the most sensitive of the methods available for the detection of antigens and antibodies. Precipitation is among the least sensitive tests, followed by (in order of increasing sensitivity) immunoelectrophoresis, radial immunodiffusion, and bacterial agglutination.

4. The answer is E *[IV B 2]*.
The pre-B cell has μ heavy (H) chain in its cytoplasm but no IgM in its membrane. Pre-B cells are enumerated by incubating a suspension of viable cells with fluorescein-labeled anti–human μ chain antiserum. At this point, the antibody is unable to enter the cell cytoplasm. After the cells are washed and fixed on a slide, the membrane is permeable, and rhodamine (red)-labeled anti–human μ chain serum is added to label any μ chain in the cytoplasm.

5. The answer is D *[III B 1]*.
In direct immunofluorescence, the fluorescein is conjugated directly onto the antibody that will react with the specific pathogen. Fluorescein-tagged anti–human gamma globulin is used in indirect tests. Some procedures employ two labeled antibodies—one fluorescein-conjugated and a second labeled with rhodamine, which fluoresces red. Thus, different cellular structures or organisms can be visualized at the same time.

6. The answer is E *[V C 1]*.
The radioimmunosorbent test (RIST) is used to measure total IgE concentration, and is useful in identifying individuals at risk for immediate hypersensitivity (type I) reactions. Specific IgE levels are measured by the radioallergosorbent test (RAST), in which particular allergens are complexed to insoluble carrier materials. These tests permit measurement of picogram quantities or less of immunogenic or haptenic substances. Both antigen and antibody activity can be measured by the enzyme-linked immunosorbent assay (ELISA). Cellular antigens are identified by means of agglutination reactions. Allergens in foods could be quantitated by a radioimmunoassay (RIA) procedure if the capture molecule was an allergen-specific antibody; however the RIST test "captures" serum IgE.

7. The answer is A *[IV C 2 c]*.
Of the tests listed in the question, only the mixed lymphocyte culture will reflect the **functional** status of T cells. The mixed lymphocyte culture, fluorescent antibody assay with CD3 or CD8 antiserum, and erythrocyte (E)-rosette test all will measure some T cell characteristic. CD8 is the membrane marker seen on suppressor and cytotoxic T cells (Ts and Tc cells); CD3 is on all peripheral T cells. T cells form E rosettes when they are mixed with sheep red blood cells (SRBCs); the E-rosette test is used to quantitate T cells regardless of their subtype. Lipopolysaccharide from the cell walls of gram-negative bacteria (endotoxin) is a potent B cell mitogen and is used to assay the ability of B cells to proliferate.

8. The answer is A *[III E 1].*
In a radioimmunoassay (RIA), the material being assayed must be immunogenic, since an essential ingredient in the procedure is specific antibody. Further, the immunogen must be labeled with radioactive materials without undergoing any immunologic alterations that would interfere in its reactivity with its homologous antibody. Fluorescein is not used in RIA; it is used to label antibodies for visualizing pathogens or detecting DNA antibodies, and in the fluorescent cell sorter technique for enumeration of T cell subsets. An antigen containing tritiated thymidine would not emit gamma rays and hence would not be confused with the iodine-125 (^{125}I) detected in the RIA.

9. The answer is D *[IV A; B 1 b].*
The erythrocyte–antibody–complement (EAC) rosette assay is a measure of the number of B cells in a specimen. B cells have membrane receptors for the Fc portion of antibody as well as a receptor for C3b, and hence will react with erythrocytes coated with these molecules. Intracellular destruction of bacteria by phagocytic cells can be measured by the microbicidal assay. The nitroblue tetrazolium (NBT) test measures hexose monophosphate (HMP) shunt activity that occurs during phagocytosis. Chemotactic responsiveness, an important attribute of phagocytic cells, is usually measured by enumerating cells that have migrated through a membrane.

10. The answer is D *[VI B 1].*
Raji cells are well suited for detection of immune complexes because they lack surface immunoglobulin. The Raji cell binding assay is based on the ability of immune complexes to bind to Raji cells, a human lymphoblastoid cell line, through C3 receptors. When bound to the surface of the Raji cells, immune complexes can be assayed by the addition of radiolabeled anti-IgG antibody.

Immunologic Mechanisms of Tissue Damage

I. INTRODUCTION—OVERVIEW

A. Hypersensitivity reactions

1. Although the immune system generally is protective, the same immunologic mechanisms that defend the host may at times result in severe damage to tissues and occasionally may cause death.

2. **Gell and Coombs** have classified these damaging immunologic reactions into four major **types of hypersensitivity reactions**:
   a. Type I—immediate hypersensitivity reactions
   b. Type II—cytotoxic reactions
   c. Type III—immune complex–mediated reactions
   d. Type IV—cell-mediated reactions

B. Plasma cell dyscrasias (paraproteinemias, monoclonal gammopathies)

1. In these diseases, a single clone of plasma cells overproduces an immunoglobulin or fragments of an immunoglobulin; the overproduced protein is called a **paraprotein**.

2. Plasma cell dyscrasias also may cause tissue damage.

II. IMMEDIATE HYPERSENSITIVITY (TYPE I) REACTIONS

A. Definition

1. Immediate hypersensitivity reactions are initiated by antigens reacting with cell-bound antibody, usually IgE.

2. Immediate hypersensitivity may manifest in many ways, depending on the target organ or tissue, and may range from life-threatening anaphylactic reactions to the lesser annoyances of atopic allergies (e.g., hay fever, food allergies).

B. Pathogenic mechanisms

1. Immediate hypersensitivity reactions involve the release of pharmacologically active mediators from mast cells or basophils, a mechanism which is triggered by antigens reacting with preformed, cell-bound IgE molecules.

2. **Allergens**
   a. Strictly speaking, allergens are antigens that induce the production of specific IgE antibodies in humans. By extension, the term "allergen" is also used at times to refer to antigens that produce other types of hypersensitivity reactions.
   b. Allergens include such diverse substances as:
      (1) Plant pollens (e.g., ragweed) and mold spores (e.g., *Alternaria, Aspergillus*)
      (2) House dust, the most likely antigenic component of which is the house dust mite
      (3) Animal hair, dander, and feathers
      (4) Foods (e.g., milk, wheat, eggs, fish, nuts, chocolate)
      (5) Foreign serums and hormones

(6) Insect venoms (e.g., bee, wasp)

(7) Drugs and chemicals (e.g., antibiotics, antiseptics, anesthetics, vitamins)

3. **IgE (reagin).** Although other immunoglobulin classes have been implicated in immediate hypersensitivity reactions in various species (including humans), the primary antibody responsible for such reactions in humans is IgE.

   a. Structural and chemical properties of IgE are discussed in Chapter 3 III E.

   b. IgE production

     (1) IgE is produced by plasma cells in the mucosa of the respiratory and gastrointestinal tracts.

       (a) In the mesenteric lymph nodes, there are as many B lymphocytes bearing surface IgE as bear surface IgG.

       (b) IgE-producing plasma cells are also present in the tonsils and adenoids, and in bronchial and gut-associated lymphoid tissues (GALT), although they are outnumbered by IgA secretors.

     (2) IgE production in the gut could have a **protective role** against intestinal parasites.

       (a) Local IgE could stimulate eosinophils (and perhaps macrophages and platelets) to exert cytotoxic effects on some common parasites.

       (b) Eosinophils have IgE receptors, and eosinophilia is commonly associated with parasitic diseases such as schistosomiasis and trichinosis.

     (3) Regulation of IgE production appears to be under the control of **helper T (Th) cells** and the lymphokines they produce.

       (a) IgE is not produced in athymic animals, nor in response to thymus-independent antigens.

       (b) The two subpopulations of Th cells [see Chapter 5 III B 3 b (3)] have opposing effects on IgE production by B cells.

         (i) Th2 cells produce interleukin-4 (IL-4), which induces class switching from IgM to IgE.

         (ii) Th1 cells produce gamma interferon, which blocks the IL-4 effect.

     (4) A subtle defect in **suppressor T (Ts) cells** is thought to lead to the increased IgE response in the atopic individual.

4. **Mediators of atopic disease**

   a. Release of mediators

     (1) If the initial exposure to an allergen results in the production of specific IgE and its ultimate fixation to mast cells and basophils, subsequent exposure to the allergen triggers an antigen–antibody reaction on the cell membrane.

     (2) A critical step is the bridging of adjacent membrane-bound IgE molecules by the allergen: this initiates degranulation and release of mediators stored in mast cells and basophils.

     (3) Mediator release requires energy and occurs in the following sequence:

       (a) There is an initial influx of calcium into the mast cell.

       (b) An intracellular serine protease is activated.

       (c) Intracellular cyclic adenosine 3,5-monophosphate (cAMP) levels fall.

       (d) Mediator-rich cytoplasmic granules migrate to the cell surface.

       (e) Exocytosis occurs, and the granule contents are released to the exterior of the cell.

   b. Sources of mediators

     (1) Some mediators derived from mast cells and basophils (Table 9-1) are stored within the cell in a preformed state.

     (2) Others are synthesized upon allergen contact.

       (a) Platelet-activating factor (PAF) is generated from a stored precursor.

       (b) Other synthesized mediators are **arachidonic acid derivatives**.

         (i) Following degranulation, changes in the cell membrane allow phospholipase A2 to release arachidonic acid.

         (ii) This is subsequently degraded, via lipoxygenase or cyclooxygenase, to leukotrienes or prostaglandin and thromboxane mediators, respectively.

     (3) Bradykinin is not a basophil or mast cell product. It is a nonapeptide (a chain of nine amino acids) derived from serum α_2-macroglobulin through the action of the enzyme **kallikrein**.

       (a) Bradykinin, like **slow-reacting substance of anaphylaxis (SRS-A),** causes smooth muscle contraction and increases vascular permeability in a slow, prolonged manner.

Table 9-1. Mast Cell and Basophil Mediators of Atopic Disease

Mediators	Effects	Comments
Preformed mediators		
Histamine	Smooth muscle contraction (e.g., bronchospasm)	Probably the most important mediator in anaphylaxis
	Increased capillary permeability	
	Increased nasal secretions	
	Increased airway resistance	
	Chemokinesis	
Heparin	Anticoagulation	Complexed to histamine in cell
Serotonin (5-hydroxytryptamine)	Smooth muscle contraction	Important in anaphylaxis in animals other than humans
	Increased capillary permeability	
ECF-A	Chemotaxis of eosinophils	
	Control of allergic reactions by releasing arylsulfatase B (inactivates SRS-A) and histaminase (inactivates histamine)	
NCF-A	Chemotaxis of neutrophils	
Proteases	Activation of complement cascade, generating C3a and C5a (anaphylatoxins causing mast cell degranulation)	
	Hydrolysis of plasma kininogen, releasing bradykinin	
Synthesized mediators		
PAF	Platelet aggregation	An acetyl glyceryl ether phosphoryl choline; inactivated by phospholipases
	Release of vasoactive amines	
	Increased vascular permeability	
	Smooth muscle contraction	
	Bronchoconstriction	
	Neutrophil chemotaxis	
SRS-A	Smooth muscle contraction	Lipoxygenase metabolite of arachidonic acid; probably a major factor in asthmatic bronchospasm
	Increased capillary permeability	
LTB4		
LTC4, LTD4	Chemotaxis of basophils	
Prostaglandins and thromboxanes	Mucus secretion in airways	Cyclooxygenase metabolite of arachidonic acid
PGE₁, PGE₂	Strong bronchodilation	
	Strong vasodilation	
PGI₂ (prostacyclin)	Disaggregation of platelets	

ECF-A = eosinophil chemotactic factor of anaphylaxis; LT = leukotrienes; NCF-A = neutrophil chemotactic factor of anaphylaxis; PAF = platelet-activating factor; PG = prostaglandin; SRS-A = slow-reacting substance of anaphylaxis.

        (b) It also increases mucus secretion and activates phospholipase A2 to augment arachidonic acid metabolism.

    c. Fate of mediators. Mediators are rapidly degraded in the body by various enzymes (e.g., histaminase).

  5. Genetic factors. These appear to play a role in **atopic allergies**.

    a. Hay fever, asthma, and food allergies, for example, show a familial tendency; there is a strong probability (about 75%) that children of two atopic parents will also be atopic.

      (1) Population studies suggest that total IgE levels are regulated by a single gene not linked to the major histocompatibility gene complex (MHC; see Chapter 12 II B).

      (2) However, specific IgE responses to particular allergens do have a **linkage with particular human leukocyte antigens (HLAs)**.

        (a) An IgE response to one of the ragweed allergens, Ra5, has a high association with HLA-DR2/Dw2.

        (b) An IgE response to ryegrass allergens is associated with HLA-DR3/Dw3.

b. The strong hereditary association noted in atopic allergies was once thought to be restricted to humans but has since been described in other animal species.

C. Clinical features

1. **Tests** for identifying specific allergens are described in Chapter 8 V.

2. **Symptoms and signs** of immediate hypersensitivity reactions vary greatly in severity and character, depending on the target organ or tissue and on whether the condition is anaphylactic or atopic.

   a. **Features of anaphylaxis**
      (1) Anaphylaxis is an immediate hypersensitivity response that is inducible in a normal host of any given species upon appropriate antigenic exposure (called **sensitization**).
      (2) The response may be either **systemic (anaphylactic shock)** or **local,** but in all species it is characterized primarily by smooth muscle contraction and increased capillary permeability.
      (3) The primary **target organ,** or **shock organ,** varies from species to species; examples include lung (in guinea pigs and humans), heart (in rabbits), and liver (in dogs).
      (4) The immediate hypersensitivity response in the guinea pig is a classic presentation of convulsions, itching, sneezing, urination, defecation, and death within minutes due to severe bronchoconstriction, smooth muscle contraction, and trapping of air in the lungs.

   b. **Features of atopy**
      (1) Atopy is an immediate hypersensitivity response that occurs only in genetically predisposed hosts upon sensitization to specific allergens. This condition differs from anaphylaxis in that it cannot be induced in normal hosts.
      (2) As in anaphylactic reactions, the response in atopic reactions is characterized by smooth muscle contraction and by increased capillary permeability with resultant local edema.
      (3) Specific **types of atopic reactions** include bronchial asthma, allergic rhinitis (hay fever), urticaria (hives), angioedema, and atopic dermatitis (eczema).

3. **Incidence of disease** (Table 9-2)
   a. **Anaphylactic shock** occurs in approximately 20,000 individuals each year in the United States, causing 200 to 400 deaths.
   b. Over 25% of the adult population were recently reported to have **anti–insect venom IgE,** suggesting that sting anaphylaxis should be considered in cases of unexpected death, particularly in summer.
   c. **Atopic reactions** are more common.
      (1) Approximately 5% of the population of the United States have **asthma,** and the death rate in 1987 was 4360. Asthma is slightly more common in boys than in girls (3:2).
      (2) About 10% of the population of the United States suffer from **hay fever.**
      (3) **Atopic dermatitis** is less common, affecting 1% to 2%.

D. Therapeutic measures

1. **Avoidance.** The most direct way to manage allergic disease is through environmental control; that is, avoidance of the responsible allergen (or allergens). This can be accomplished quite easily with food allergies but may be difficult with inhalant allergens.

Table 9-2. Impact of Selected Allergic Conditions on the Population of the United States

Allergic Condition	Estimated Number Affected
Allergic rhinitis	19.6 million persons
Chronic sinusitis	32.5 million persons
Contact dermatitis and eczema	5.8 million office visits annually
Allergy immunotherapy	5.4 million administrations to children annually
Skin rashes and allergic skin reactions	12 million office visits annually
Asthma	9 to 12 million persons with active disease
Anaphylaxis and allergic reactions	1 to 2 million episodes annually

From *Report of the NIAID Task Force on Immunology and Allergy.* NIH Publication No. 91-2414. Washington DC, U.S. Public Health Service, National Institutes of Health, September 1990, p. 67.

2. **Hyposensitization** involves injecting the patient, over a period of time, with gradually increasing doses of the responsible allergen. This form of immunotherapy is aimed at stimulating the production of **IgG blocking antibody,** which binds the offending allergen and prevents its combining with IgE on the mast cell membrane.

3. **Drug treatment** involves the administration of agents designed to reverse various allergic mechanisms (Figure 9-1). This may be achieved by:
   a. **Blocking mediators from binding** to target tissue (e.g., by using antihistaminics such as diphenhydramine)
   b. **Stabilizing granules or cell membranes** (corticosteroids may act here)
   c. **Blocking the release of mediators** by either:
      (1) Inhibiting calcium influx (e.g., by using cromolyn sodium)
      (2) Stimulating adenylate cyclase, the enzyme that converts adenosine triphosphate (ATP) to cAMP (e.g., by using epinephrine)
      (3) Preserving the needed levels of cAMP by inhibiting phosphodiesterase, an enzyme that converts cAMP to AMP (an effect of theophylline in vitro; however, the clinical significance is unclear)

III. CYTOTOXIC (TYPE II) REACTIONS

A. Definition. Cytotoxic reactions are initiated by antibody—usually IgG or IgM—reacting with cell-bound antigen.

B. Pathogenic mechanisms

1. Cytotoxic reactions primarily involve either of two mechanisms:
   a. The combination of IgG or IgM antibodies with epitopes on cell surface or tissue
   b. The adsorption of antigens or haptens to tissues or to the cell membrane, with subsequent attachment of antibodies to the adsorbed antigens

2. Either mechanism may lead to one of the following destructive processes:
   a. Lysis or inactivation of target cells via activation of **complement**

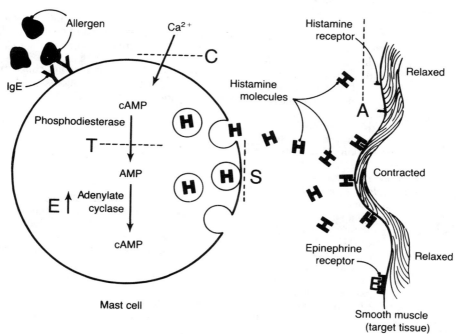

Figure 9-1. The steps in atopic disease development and their blockage by therapeutic measures. (See text for details.) The *dashed lines* indicate a blocking effect. A = antihistaminic; C = cromolyn; E = epinephrine; H = histamine molecules; S = steroids (e.g., cortisone), T = theophylline.

    b. Phagocytosis of target cells, with or without complement activation
    c. Lysis or inactivation of target cells by antibody-dependent cell-mediated cytolysis (ADCC), through the action of **natural killer (NK) cells**

C. Clinical features. The many **types of cytotoxic reactions** can be grouped according to the nature of the target cell or the tissue damage that occurs in the reaction.

    1. Red blood cell lysis. This probably is the most important clinical phenomenon associated with cytotoxic reactions. The following are classic examples.

      a. Transfusion reactions

        (1) Transfusion reactions may be classified as nonimmunologic (e.g., due to air embolism or circulatory overloading) or as immunologic.

        (2) Immunologically mediated transfusion reactions may occur by two different mechanisms: rapid intravascular destruction of transfused red blood cells or extravascular destruction of antibody-sensitized red blood cells, primarily by the reticuloendothelial system (RES).

          (a) Intravascular hemolysis of red blood cells usually is associated with **ABO system incompatibility**.

            (i) The ABO blood group system consists of genetically determined antigens on the red blood cell surface (see Chapter 12 III B).

            (ii) It is important to match donor blood to recipient blood, because transfusing blood into a person who has antibodies to the donor's red blood cells can produce a transfusion reaction.

            (iii) In this reaction, erythrocyte-bound anti-A or anti-B antibodies activate complement, with almost immediate lysis of the transfused red cells.

          (b) Extravascular hemolysis of red blood cells almost invariably is associated with **Rh incompatibility**.

            (i) Several distinct Rh antigens exist on the red blood cell membrane. These antigens strongly stimulate antibody formation when introduced into the blood of persons who lack the antigens. The Rh antigen most commonly involved is $Rh_o(D)$.

            (ii) Unlike anti-A and anti-B antibodies, anti-Rh antibodies do not cause complement-mediated intravascular hemolysis. Instead, there is antibody-mediated opsonization and phagocytosis of sensitized red blood cells by peripheral blood granulocytes and monocytes, and by macrophages of the RES.

          (c) Clinical consequences

            (i) Symptoms of transfusion reactions include fever, back pain, chills, malaise, hypotension, nausea, and vomiting. These manifestations are more pronounced in reactions that are due to intravascular hemolysis than in those due to extravascular hemolysis.

            (ii) Acute renal failure is a serious complication of intravascular hemolytic transfusion reactions.

        (3) Prevention of transfusion reactions includes careful blood typing and cross-matching.

      b. Hemolytic disease of the newborn

        (1) Etiology and pathogenesis

          (a) Hemolytic disease of the newborn (**erythroblastosis fetalis**) occurs when an Rh-negative mother gives birth to an Rh-positive infant, the Rh antigen having been acquired from an Rh-positive father. The most commonly involved antigen is $Rh_o(D)$.

          (b) In order for this condition to occur, the mother must be sensitized to blood group antigens on the infant's red blood cells.

            (i) The major risk of sensitization occurs during delivery, when large amounts of cord blood enter the mother's circulation.

            (ii) However, sensitization may occur during pregnancy, if fetal blood leaks into the maternal circulation (a small amount of transplacental blood leakage is normal).

          (c) After sensitization, IgG antibodies to the $Rh_o(D)$ antigen are produced. These antibodies may cross the placenta and destroy fetal cells.

(d) The first child usually is not affected, but the chance of sensitization increases with subsequent pregnancies.

(2) Symptoms. Affected infants develop anemia and jaundice, usually during the first 24 hours of life; hepatosplenomegaly and (in untreated infants) bilirubin encephalopathy also occur.

(3) Management. In severe cases, infants require exchange transfusion.

(4) Prevention. Hemolytic disease of the newborn is best avoided by preventing maternal sensitization to fetal Rh antigens or by inhibiting the production of antibodies to those antigens.

(a) Administering **anti-Rh$_o$ IgG antibodies (RhoGAM)** to an Rh-negative mother within 72 hours after delivery of an Rh-positive infant will prevent sensitization, probably via rapid destruction and clearance of Rh-positive cells from the circulation.

(b) The anti-Rh$_o$ IgG is a blocking agent; it does not induce immune tolerance to the Rh$_o$(D) antigen. Therefore, it must be given after each pregnancy.

c. Autoimmune hemolytic disease. Warm-antibody hemolytic anemia, cold-antibody hemolytic anemia, and paroxysmal cold hemoglobinuria are discussed in Chapter 10 II N.

2. White blood cell lysis

a. Systemic lupus erythematosus (SLE; see Chapter 10 II B). SLE can be considered a mixed disease—that is, both **type II and type III**.

(1) In SLE several types of antibodies are present in the serum.

(2) These include antinuclear antibodies, antibodies to membrane and cytoplasmic components, and antibodies cytotoxic to blood cells (lymphocytes, red blood cells, platelets).

b. Granulocytopenia. Cytotoxic reactions involving antibodies to neutrophils or to drugs adsorbed to neutrophil surfaces can result in granulocytopenia and a consequent phagocytic defect, leading to increased susceptibility to infection.

c. Idiopathic thrombocytopenic purpura (ITP; see Chapter 10 II O). ITP is characterized by the presence of platelet-specific IgG antibodies, which can lead to various bleeding disorders.

3. Nephrotoxic nephritis

a. This **experimental glomerulonephritis** can be induced in rats by injection of heterologous antibodies against glomerular basement membrane or by active immunization with antigens isolated from glomerular basement membrane.

b. The disease is characterized by proteinuria, impaired glomerular filtration, neutrophil infiltration of glomeruli, and antibody deposition in a linear pattern along the glomerular basement membrane, which is visible on immunofluorescence imaging.

c. Goodpasture's syndrome (see Chapter 10 II L) is a similar clinical condition that occurs in humans.

4. Immunization of experimental animals with **acetylcholine receptors** produces a condition of muscular weakness that closely resembles **myasthenia gravis** (see Chapter 10 II H).

5. Bullous diseases. In bullous diseases such as pemphigus vulgaris and bullous pemphigoid (see Chapter 10 II P), antibody and complement are deposited in squamous intercellular spaces and along the basement membrane of the skin.

D. Therapeutic measures

1. Therapy for cytotoxic reactions includes treatment of the underlying cause as well as the manifestations of the reaction.

2. Examples of therapeutic measures include the following:

a. Suppression of the immune response by means of corticosteroids, with or without cytotoxic immunosuppressive drugs (e.g., cyclophosphamide and azathioprine), or by splenectomy

b. Removal of offending antibodies via exchange transfusion (in the case of hemolytic disease of the newborn) or plasmapheresis (in the case of Goodpasture's syndrome)

c. Withholding the offending drug (in the case of a drug-induced syndrome such as ITP or drug-induced hemolytic disease)

d. Nephrectomy (in the case of Goodpasture's syndrome)

IV. IMMUNE COMPLEX–MEDIATED (TYPE III) REACTIONS

A. Definition

1. Immune complex–mediated reactions are initiated by antigen–antibody (i.e., immune) complexes that either are formed locally at the site of tissue damage or are deposited there from the circulation.

2. Immune complex disorders are characterized by the presence of antigen–antibody complexes in vascular and glomerular basement membranes.

3. Symptoms depend on the location of the immune complex deposition, and can include arthritis, nephritis, vasculitis, or skin lesions.

B. Pathogenic mechanisms

1. The pathogenesis of immune complex disorders involves an interplay of antigen, antibody, complement, and neutrophils.
   a. The first step is the formation of **soluble immune complexes,** which generally occurs when there is a large **excess of antigen**.
      (1) Virtually any antigen that induces a detectable antibody response will serve; autoantigens are commonly involved.
         (a) A number of common complex-inducing antigens are mentioned in section IV C.
         (b) In addition, the following microbial antigens can induce significant immune complex–caused tissue damage: *Mycobacterium leprae, Treponema pallidum, Plasmodium* and *Trypanosoma* species, and Epstein-Barr, hepatitis B, and dengue hemorrhagic fever viruses.
      (2) The antibodies involved are primarily precipitating IgG and IgM capable of fixing complement.
   b. Only **small immune complexes** cause damage because, being very small, these immune complexes escape phagocytosis. They penetrate the endothelium of blood vessel walls (probably with the aid of vasoactive amines released from platelets and basophils) and are deposited on the vascular basement membrane.
   c. **Complement** is activated, with the release of C3a and C5a.
      (1) These anaphylatoxins increase the permeability of the vascular endothelium.
      (2) C5a is also chemotactic for neutrophils, which then infiltrate the area and release lysosomal enzymes that destroy the basement membrane.

2. **Large immune complexes** are destroyed by phagocytosis.
   a. The complexes are first bound to red blood cells through complement receptors in the cell membrane.
   b. The red cells circulate to the liver where the immune complexes are removed by the RES.

C. Clinical features. The following are classic examples of immune complex–mediated reactions.

1. **Arthus reaction.** This necrotic dermal reaction is considered to be a **local immune complex–deposition** phenomenon. It was observed first in rabbits, but similar reactions are observed in other animals, including humans.
   a. The Arthus reaction is seen in rabbits that have been repeatedly injected subcutaneously with antigen (e.g., normal horse serum).
   b. The rabbits tolerate the first few doses without any local reactions; however, the injections induce the formation of antibodies specific for horse serum proteins.
   c. With subsequent exposures foci of erythema, edema, and necrosis are noted at the injection sites. Microscopic examination of tissue reveals an accumulation of neutrophils plus a vasculitis related to destruction of the basement membrane of blood vessel walls.

2. **Serum sickness.** This syndrome follows the injection of foreign serum into humans. It is considered to be a **systemic immune complex–deposition** phenomenon.
   a. Serum sickness was first seen following the administration of diphtheria antitoxin (prepared in horses) to humans.
   b. As in the Arthus reaction, the primary damage observed in serum sickness appears to be a vasculitis associated with destruction of vascular basement membrane.
   c. The syndrome is characterized by fever, rash, splenomegaly, lymphadenopathy, arthritis, and glomerulonephritis.

(1) The hallmark of **immune complex glomerulonephritis** is its **granular ("lumpy bumpy") appearance** as detected by direct immunofluorescence using tagged antibody specific for immunoglobulin or complement.

(2) This technique can differentiate immune complex glomerulonephritis from **autoimmune** or **idiopathic injury** to the glomerular basement membrane, in which a **smooth linear pattern** of immunoglobulin deposition is observed.

3. Poststreptococcal glomerulonephritis. The immune complex glomerulonephritis that can follow a streptococcal pharyngitis is characterized by proteinuria and hematuria with red blood cell casts in the urine.

   a. Antibody, complement, and bacterial antigen are present in the renal vasculature.

   b. As with serum sickness glomerulonephritis, poststreptococcal glomerulonephritis has a **lumpy bumpy appearance** under immunofluorescence.

4. Autoimmune disease. Endogenous antigen–antibody–complement complexes are involved in the pathogenesis of certain autoimmune diseases, such as rheumatoid arthritis and SLE (see Chapter 10 II A, B).

5. Hypersensitivity pneumonitis (extrinsic allergic alveolitis). Both **type III and type IV** reactions appear to play a role in this granulomatous interstitial lung disease (see V C 3).

D. Therapeutic measures. Therapy for immune complex–mediated reactions includes:

   1. Reduction of inflammation by means of aspirin, antihistaminics, and corticosteroids

   2. Suppression of the immune response by means of corticosteroids and cytotoxic immunosuppressive drugs (cyclophosphamide, azathioprine)

   3. Removal of offending complexes via plasmapheresis

V. CELL-MEDIATED (TYPE IV) REACTIONS: DELAYED HYPERSENSITIVITY AND CELL-MEDIATED CYTOTOXICITY

A. Overview

   1. Cell-mediated specific immune reactions are independent of antibody and complement; rather, they are dependent upon functioning **T cells.**

   a. This was originally demonstrated by showing that delayed hypersensitivity could be **transferred** from sensitized animals to nonsensitized animals (including humans) with antigen-reactive T cells, but not with serum containing antibodies.

   b. Delayed hypersensitivity can also be transferred by a small molecule called **transfer factor,** a dialyzable extract of lymphocytes (see Chapter 7 IV B 3).

   2. Cell-mediated immunity has two **facets: delayed-type hypersensitivity** and **cytotoxic T (Tc) cell responses,** each initiated by a different type of sensitized (antigen-reactive) T cell.

   a. The effector cells that are responsible for delayed-type hypersensitivity reactions (**Tdth cells**) recruit other cells (e.g., macrophages) that actually do most of the damage.

   b. The effector cells that are responsible for cell-mediated cytotoxic reactions (**Tc cells**) are themselves cytotoxic, both directly and through the release of cytotoxic lymphokines.

   3. In contrast to antibody-mediated immune reactions, which are seen in minutes after antigen exposure, both delayed hypersensitivity reactions and cell-mediated cytotoxic reactions are **delayed in time course**.

   a. Delayed hypersensitivity reactions manifest as inflammation at the site of antigen exposure, usually peaking 24 to 48 hours after exposure.

   b. Tc cell reactions have a similar time course.

B. Pathogenic mechanisms

   1. The effector cells of cell-mediated immune reactions. As discussed in Chapter 1, immune functions are mediated by numerous types of cells. Only those functions mediated by sensitized T cells are addressed here.

   a. There are two **types of effector T cells**:

   (1) Tdth cells

   (a) Tdth cells recognize foreign antigens, primarily those of intracellular pathogens.

> **(b)** They confer resistance by secreting gamma interferon and other lymphokines, thereby activating macrophages to cytotoxic activity and enhancing other T and B cell responses.
>
> **(2) Tc cells, often called cytolytic T lymphocytes (CTLs)**
>> **(a)** Tc cells recognize foreign antigens on most cells of the body.
>> **(b)** They confer resistance in two ways:
>>> **(i)** Secretion of gamma interferon, which induces other cells to produce antiviral proteins (see Chapter 1 II F 2 c and Table 9-3 footnote)
>>> **(ii)** Direct destruction of target cells (e.g., grafted tissue, tumors, and virus-infected cells) by release of perforin, with subsequent cytolysis

b. The **key to differentiating** the activity of **Tc cells** from **Tdth cells** is that Tc cells are directly cytotoxic, whereas Tdth cells act primarily through recruitment of other cells.

c. Tdth cells can be distinguished serologically from Tc cells by their **CD** (cluster of differentiation) surface antigens (see Table 5-2).
> **(1)** **Tdth** cells are **CD4$^+$** (i.e., they carry the CD4 surface antigen).
> **(2)** **Tc** cells are **CD8$^+$**.

2. Induction of T cell–mediated immune reactions. Cell-mediated reactions are induced by the uptake and processing of antigen and the activation of T cells (see Chapter 5 III B 2, 3).

a. There are several different **types of antigen-processing cells**.
> **(1)** Antigen-processing cells for **B cells** and for **CD8$^+$ cells** are usually **macrophages**.
> **(2)** However, macrophages do not normally have much class II antigen in their membranes.
> **(3)** Hence, a delayed-type hypersensitivity reaction is probably initiated by the interaction of **Tdth CD4$^+$ cells** with epitope–class II MHC complexes on **dendritic cells,** which constitutively express high concentrations of class II molecules.

b. Antigen-processing cells and T cells can interact only if the two participants are **MHC-identical**.
> **(1)** **CD4$^+$** cells recognize antigen in conjunction with **class II** MHC molecules (e.g., HLA-DR).
> **(2)** **CD8$^+$** cells recognize antigen in conjunction with **class I** MHC molecules (HLA-A, -B, and -C).

c. Under the influence of antigen and MHC gene products, antigen-reactive (sensitized) Tdth and Tc cells are produced.

d. Role of Th cells in delayed hypersensitivity
> **(1)** The Th population of CD4$^+$ cells aids in the development of CD8$^+$ cells by releasing **lymphokines** (interleukins) that augment proliferative and maturational signals generated by antigen contact (Table 9-3).
> **(2)** Lymphokines produced by Th cell subpopulations aid in regulating humoral, as well as cell-mediated, immune responses [see Chapter 5 III B 3 b (3)].

3. Expression of delayed hypersensitivity

a. Upon interaction with homologous epitope (probably presented on the surface of dendritic cells), the Tdth subpopulation of CD4$^+$ cells responds by secreting lymphokines such as gamma interferon.

b. The lymphokines in turn activate nearby macrophages and recruit the immigration of more cells into the area.

c. **Activated macrophages** secrete a variety of biologically active compounds that cause inflammation and destroy bacteria, tumors, and other cells considered foreign by the immune apparatus:
> **(1)** Cytokines (see Table 9-3), among which are:
>> **(a)** Interleukins 1 and 6
>> **(b)** Tumor necrosis factor α (TNF-α)
> **(2)** Reactive oxygen metabolites such as superoxide anion, hydroxyl radical, and hydrogen peroxide (see Chapter 1 II D 5).
> **(3)** Proteases and other lysosomal enzymes

d. In addition, an **amplification loop** is activated.
> **(1)** The gamma interferon secreted by activated Tdth cells stimulates macrophages to express MHC class II proteins in their membranes.
> **(2)** The interferon-activated macrophages can now present epitopes to Tdth cells, with the resultant release of more gamma interferon and more efficient antigen presentation.

Table 9-3. Cytokines* of Importance in Expression of Immunity

Cytokine	Major Source	Targets	Effects
IL-1	Macrophages	Lymphocytes Macrophages	Activation Stimulation Pyrexia Acute-phase reaction[†] Increased cell adhesion
IL-2	Th cells	Lymphocytes Macrophages	Activation Activation Stimulation of lymphokine secretion
IL-4	Th cells	Macrophages	Activation Influence on immunoglobulin class switching
IL-5	Th cells	Stem cells	Differentiation (e.g., eosinophilia)
IL-6	Numerous	Macrophages	Stimulation Acute-phase reaction[†]
TNF-α	Macrophages	Macrophages Neutrophils Endothelial cells	Activation Activation Increased cell adhesion Cachexia
TNF-β[‡]	T cells	Tumor cells	Cytotoxicity
IFN-α	Leukocytes	Tissue cells	Block of viral replication
IFN-β	Fibroblasts	Tissue cells	Block of viral replication
IFN-γ	T cells	Macrophages NK cells Tissue cells	Activation[§] Activation Block of viral replication
MIF	Tdth cells	Macrophages	Inhibition of migration
MAF	Tdth cells	Macrophages	Activation
MCF	Tdth cells	Macrophages	Stimulation of chemotaxis
TF	Tdth cells	Lymphocytes	Transfer of cell-mediated immunity
LIF	Tdth cells	Neutrophils	Inhibition of migration
Perforin	Tc cells	Tissue cells Tumor cells	Lysis Lysis

IFN = interferon; IL = interleukin; LIF = leukocyte inhibition factor; MAF = macrophage-activating factor; MCF = macrophage chemotactic factor; MIF = migration-inhibiting factor; NK cells = natural killer cells; TF = transfer factor; TNF = tumor necrosis factor.

*Cytokines are soluble mediators with hormone-like actions. Cytokines produced by macrophages and other mononuclear phagocytes are called monokines; those produced by lymphocytes are called lymphokines.

†Acute-phase reaction = increased concentration of certain serum proteins (C-reactive protein, amyloid A, haptoglobin, ceruloplasmin, and many complement components) in response to acute inflammation.

‡TNF-β is also called lymphotoxin.

§The major activities of gamma interferon are as follows:
1. Inhibiting viral replication
2. Inducing the expression of class II major histocompatibility complex (MHC) molecules on tissue cells, allowing these cells to become active in antigen presentation
3. Increasing the expression of Fc receptors on macrophages
4. Activating macrophages to heightened microbicidal and tumoricidal activity
5. Inhibiting cell growth
6. Enhancing the activity of NK cells
7. Influencing class switching in immunoglobulin synthesis

    e. Lymphokines as mediators of delayed hypersensitivity. It is not known how many biochemically distinct lymphokines exist; however, the following are among those generally recognized.

        (1) Migration-inhibiting factor (MIF) inhibits migration of macrophages.

        (2) Macrophage-activating factor (MAF) enhances the microbicidal and cytolytic activity of macrophages.

        (3) Macrophage chemotactic factor stimulates infiltration of macrophages.

        (4) Transfer factor can transfer cell-mediated immunity from sensitized to nonsensitized individuals (see Chapter 7 IV B 3).

(5) **Leukocyte-inhibiting factor (LIF)** inhibits random migration of neutrophils.
(6) **IL-2** is a mitogenic factor: it stimulates the growth of activated T cells.
(7) **TNF-β (lymphotoxin)** has the ability to lyse certain tumor cells.
(8) **Gamma interferon** has numerous functions (see Table 9-3 footnote).

4. **Expression of Tc cell cytotoxicity**
   a. Tc cells destroy only those target cells which they recognize antigenically.
      (1) When a Tc cell encounters a cell, it explores the other cell's surface for an epitope that its T cell receptor can recognize.
      (2) If recognition occurs, the Tc cell is activated to release cytotoxic proteins from its intracytoplasmic granules.
   b. The effector molecules released by Tc cells are more cytotoxic than those of Tdth cells and commonly lead directly to cell lysis.
      (1) The most important of the Tc cell's cytotoxic proteins is **perforin,** which resembles the complement component C9, both functionally and in amino acid sequence.
         (a) Like C9 (see Chapter 4 III B 4), perforin inserts itself into target cell membranes and polymerizes, forming transmembrane channels that allow the influx (and egress) of essential ions and low-molecular-weight metabolites.
         (b) Perforin is a highly hydrophobic molecule that integrates very rapidly into the membrane of target cells. Hence, its diffusion is limited and lysis of "innocent bystander" cells is minimal.
         (c) The perforin-induced channels cause the target cell to lose electrolytes, imbibe water, swell, and burst.
      (2) **Other molecules** released from these intracytoplasmic granules include serine proteases, proteoglycans, and molecules that resemble TNF.
      (3) The fragmentation of target-cell DNA suggests that another significant product of the Tc cell might be an endonuclease; alternatively, an endogenous endonuclease may be activated during the lytic process.
   c. After the Tc cell delivers its lethal "hit," it detaches from the target and searches out another victim.

C. Clinical features

1. **The role of T cell–mediated immunity in disease**
   a. **Delayed hypersensitivity and Tc cell reactions** can be **protective** as well as damaging. They provide resistance to:
      (1) Chronic intracellular bacterial infections (e.g., tuberculosis and brucellosis)
      (2) Fungal infections (e.g., blastomycosis and histoplasmosis)
      (3) Viral infections (e.g., herpes and mumps)
      (4) Protozoan infections (e.g., leishmaniasis)
      (5) Tumors (cytotoxic antibody is also involved at times)
   b. Tc cells also play a role in the **rejection of grafted tissues and organs**. (Humoral immunity is also involved at times in allograft rejection.)
   c. In addition, sensitized T lymphocytes provide the basic **mechanism of tissue injury** in the following diseases:
      (1) **Contact dermatitis,** a delayed hypersensitivity reaction that occurs in response to exposure of the skin to certain allergens
      (2) Some **autoimmune diseases,** in which Tc cells play a major role in pathogenesis (see Chapter 10 I A 3)
   d. Major clinical characteristics of four types of hypersensitivity reactions involving Tdth lymphocytes are presented in Table 9-4.

2. The **tuberculin skin test reaction** is the classic clinical example of delayed hypersensitivity.
   a. A small amount of antigen—usually purified protein derivative (PPD) of tuberculin—is injected intradermally into a sensitized person.
   b. The reaction appears slowly, about 12 to 24 hours after the injection, and reaches maximal reactivity 24 to 48 hours after injection.
      (1) Initially, there is erythema and a neutrophil infiltrate.
      (2) Later, a mononuclear cell (lymphocyte and macrophage) infiltrate causes induration in the region of the injection.

Table 9-4. Major Clinical Features of Delayed Hypersensitivity Reactions

Feature	Type of Reaction			
	Cutaneous Basophil Hypersensitivity	**Contact Dermatitis**	**Tuberculin Reaction**	**Granulomatous Reaction**
Antigens	Soluble proteins	Poison ivy, simple chemicals (e.g., nickel)	Mycobacterial proteins	Immune complexes or intracellular parasites
Time of onset (days)	1	2	1–2	21–28
Skin lesion	Edema	Eczema	Induration	Induration
Systemic manifestations	No	No	Yes	Yes
Histologic pattern	Basophils, macrophages, lymphocytes	Lymphocytes, macrophages	Lymphocytes, macrophages	Lymphocytes, macrophages, epithelial cells, giant cells; fibrosis*, necrosis*

*May or may not be seen.

3. Hypersensitivity pneumonitis (extrinsic allergic alveolitis)
 a. These generic terms refer to the parenchymal reaction that develops in the lung on repeated inhalation of particulate allergens; a list of some of these, with the names of their associated diseases, is presented in Table 9-5.
 b. Pathogenesis
  (1) Patients often have antibodies to the offending substances, with deposition of antigen–antibody complexes in target (lung) tissue during the early phase of the disease; this suggests that a **type III reaction** occurs during the **induction of sensitization**.
  (2) Evidence suggests that in addition to immune complexes, **delayed hypersensitivity (type IV) reactions** also play a role in the pathogenesis of hypersensitivity pneumonitis, particularly in the **chronic disease process**.
 c. Symptoms. Fever, chills, chest pain, cough, and dyspnea occur 4 to 8 hours after exposure. In severe, chronic cases, irreversible lung damage (fibrosis) may occur.

4. Cutaneous basophil hypersensitivity (Jones-Mote reaction)
 a. These terms refer to a group of delayed-onset, T cell–mediated reactions that have been experimentally induced in humans as well as in animals.
 b. These reactions mimic delayed hypersensitivity reactions in that they are T cell–mediated and transferred passively with lymphocytes.
 c. However, they differ in significant ways. For example, basophils comprise 50% of the cell exudate, the lesions lack the induration seen in classic delayed hypersensitivity reactions, and cutaneous basophil hypersensitivity usually is seen soon after immunization and is short-lived.

Table 9-5. Allergens Associated with Hypersensitivity Pneumonitis

Allergen	Source	Disease
Thermophilic actinomycetes	Hay, grains	Farmer's lung
	Bagasse	Bagassosis
Bacillus subtilis	Wall plaster	Domestic hypersensitivity pneumonitis
Aspergillus species	Barley	Malt worker's lung
	Compost	Compost lung
Penicillium casei	Cheese	Cheese worker's lung
Wheat weevil	Infested flour	Wheat miller's lung
Isocyanates	Industrial	Chemical worker's lung
Coffee bean protein	Coffee bean dust	Coffee worker's lung
Rat urine protein	Laboratory rats	Laboratory worker's lung

5. **Modulation of cell-mediated hypersensitivities.** Numerous agents affect delayed-type hypersensitivity and Tc cell activity by either enhancing or suppressing reactivity.
   a. **Enhancing agents**
      (1) The **thymic hormones** thymosin and thymopoietin promote the development of immunocompetent T cells and T cell differentiation, respectively.
      (2) **Levamisole** is an immunostimulating agent in experimental animals and humans, although it is not approved for use in humans in the United States.
         (a) The drug inhibits Ts cells.
         (b) It also appears to restore T cell–mediated immune mechanisms, and may enhance macrophage–T cell interaction and macrophage activity.
   b. **Suppressant agents**
      (1) Agents that suppress cell-mediated immunity include **corticosteroids** (e.g., cortisone), **antibodies** (e.g., antilymphocyte serum and antithymocyte serum), and **cytotoxic immunosuppressive drugs** (e.g., azathioprine, cyclosporine, and cyclophosphamide).
      (2) These agents and their mechanisms of action are discussed in Chapter 6 II B 2.

VI. PLASMA CELL DYSCRASIAS

A. Overview

1. Plasma cell dyscrasias represent a group of diseases characterized by the overproduction of immunoglobulins, or their fragments, by a single clone of plasma cells. The abnormal monoclonal product is called **paraprotein** or **M component**.

2. The most important of the plasma cell dyscrasias is multiple myeloma; also notable are Waldenström's macroglobulinemia, benign monoclonal gammopathy, primary amyloidosis, and heavy chain diseases.

3. **Therapy** for plasma cell dyscrasias includes such procedures as:
   a. Administration of prednisone, with or without cytotoxic drugs (e.g., melphalan or cyclophosphamide)
   b. Removal of the excess protein (e.g., IgM in Waldenström's macroglobulinemia) via plasmapheresis

B. Multiple myeloma

1. This plasma cell tumor in bone marrow overproduces a single class of immunoglobulin; most cases involve IgG.
   a. The most characteristic feature of multiple myeloma is the demonstration of an abnormal protein (called **paraprotein** or **M component**) in the blood, urine, or both. The M component consists of intact monoclonal antibodies (usually IgG or IgA), heavy (H) chains, or light (L) chains, alone or in any combination.
   b. In some cases a substance called **Bence Jones protein** (a dimer of L chains) is found in the urine.

2. The **clinical features and complications** of multiple myeloma vary widely. Some of the more common manifestations include:
   a. Bone pain and pathologic fractures
   b. Bone marrow infiltration by an abundance of abnormal plasma cells, with resultant normochromic normocytic anemia
   c. Renal abnormalities, possibly resulting in chronic renal failure
   d. Fatigue and weakness

C. Waldenström's macroglobulinemia

1. Waldenström's macroglobulinemia is a lymphocytic lymphoma characterized by overproduction of lymphocytes and plasma cells.

2. The most distinguishing feature of this disorder is a high level of **monoclonal IgM** in the serum. Bence Jones proteins also may be seen in the urine.

3. Because of the high serum IgM, patients have a hyperviscosity of the blood, which may be severe. Anemia, lymphadenopathy, and chronic lymphocytic leukemia also are common clinical features.

D. Benign monoclonal gammopathy

1. This condition is seen in older individuals (usually over age 70), who reveal an increased serum concentration of monoclonal protein—usually IgG, but occasionally IgM—but are otherwise normal.

2. There usually are no other manifestations of disease. However, some patients are at risk for developing multiple myeloma.

E. Amyloidosis

1. Amyloidosis is a disease characterized by deposition of an abnormal protein (**amyloid**) in the vascular endothelium of various organs of the body. The clinical features depend on the site and extent of amyloid deposition.

2. **Two types** of amyloidosis have been defined.
   a. **Primary amyloidosis** is a plasma cell dyscrasia characterized by the accumulation of amyloid fibrils that are composed primarily of immunoglobulin L chain fragments and are therefore called **amyloid light chain (AL) protein**. This type of amyloidosis often is associated with multiple myeloma.
   b. **Secondary amyloidosis** refers to amyloidosis that accompanies or follows a chronic infection or inflammation. The amyloid fibrils in secondary amyloidosis, called **amyloid A (AA) protein,** bear no structural resemblance to the AL protein seen in primary amyloidosis.

F. Heavy chain diseases

1. These rare malignancies are characterized by a serum paraprotein consisting of incomplete H chains without L chains; γ, α, and μ heavy chain diseases have been described.

2. The abnormal H chain shows deletion of the hinge region, or partial deletion of the Fd portion, or a combination of both abnormalities.

STUDY QUESTIONS

Directions: Each of the numbered items or incomplete statements in this section is followed by answers or by completions of the statement. Select the **one** lettered answer or completion that is **best** in each case.

1. Immunotherapy for atopy induces formation of which of the following blocking antibodies?

(A) IgA
(B) IgD
(C) IgE
(D) IgG
(E) IgM

2. The pathogenesis of immune complex disorders involves an interplay of antigen, antibody, neutrophils, and which of the following complement-derived factors?

(A) C1s
(B) Cla4b
(C) C3b inactivator
(D) C3 activator
(E) C5a

3. What is the most direct method of treating atopic allergies?

(A) Hyposensitization
(B) Environmental control
(C) Administration of modified allergens
(D) Administration of antihistamines
(E) Administration of corticosteroids

4. Mediators of immediate hypersensitivity (type I) reactions are either preformed and stored in host cells or are newly formed from precursor constituents. Which one of the following is a preformed mediator of type I reactions?

(A) Platelet-activating factor (PAF)
(B) Anaphylatoxin I
(C) Slow-reacting substance of anaphylaxis (SRS-A)
(D) Serotonin (5-hydroxytryptamine)
(E) Myeloperoxidase

5. What is the major protein component of the amyloid deposits seen in patients with primary amyloidosis?

(A) Complement protein fragments
(B) Intact IgM
(C) Immunoglobulin light (L) chain fragments
(D) Aggregated IgG
(E) IgE heavy (H) chains

6. Which of the following disorders is characterized by overproduction of monoclonal IgG?

(A) Serum sickness
(B) Asthma
(C) Waldenström's macroglobulinemia
(D) Hypersensitivity pneumonitis
(E) Multiple myeloma

7. Tissue injury in cytotoxic (type II) hypersensitivity reactions is initiated by which of the following pathogenetic mechanisms?

(A) Antibody interfering with the functioning of biologically active substances
(B) Antigen reacting with cell-bound antibody
(C) Antibody reacting with cell-bound antigen
(D) Formation of antigen–antibody complexes
(E) Sensitized T cells reacting with specific antigens

8. The pathogenetic requirements for immune complex–induced glomerulonephritis include

(A) red blood cell and complement interaction
(B) lymphocytes
(C) neutrophils
(D) kidney-derived antigen
(E) large aggregated immune complexes

9. Allergic urticaria is best described as being a manifestation of

(A) an IgE-mediated disorder
(B) delayed hypersensitivity
(C) cytotoxic IgG antibodies
(D) cytotoxic T (Tc) cells
(E) an immune complex–mediated disorder

1-D	4-D	7-C
2-E	5-C	8-C
3-B	6-E	9-A

Directions: The group of items in this section consists of lettered options followed by a set of numbered items. For each item, select the **one** lettered option that is most closely associated with it. Each lettered option may be selected once, more than once, or not at all.

Questions 10–13

Match the pathogenetic factor below with the disorder with which it is most closely associated.

(A) Waldenström's macroglobulinemia
(B) Poststreptococcal glomerulonephritis
(C) Hemolytic disease of the newborn
(D) Food allergy
(E) Contact dermatitis
(F) Chronic granulomatous disease (CGD)
(G) Bagassosis (inductive phase)
(H) Amyloidosis

10. $Rh_o(D)$ antigen

11. Excess monoclonal IgM

12. Antigen-reactive T cells

13. IgE antibody

10-C   13-D
11-A
12-E

ANSWERS AND EXPLANATIONS

1. The answer is D *[II D 2].*
Immunotherapy for atopy involves the deliberate injection of the offending allergen, beginning at a low dosage and increasing to a maintenance dosage (i.e., the highest dose the patient can tolerate). The procedure stimulates production of IgG blocking antibody, which binds the allergen and forms complexes that are removed by the reticuloendothelial system (RES), thus preventing the allergen from reaching and combining with the IgE on basophils and mast cells.

2. The answer is E *[IV B 1 c].*
In immune complex disorders, antigen–antibody (immune) complexes are formed either locally or in the circulation and are deposited in the vascular or glomerular basement membrane, causing inflammation by the following sequence of events: the antigen–antibody complexes, once deposited, fix complement component C1q, thus activating the classic complement pathway. C5a is generated, which is chemotactic for neutrophils; neutrophils then infiltrate the area and release lysosomal enzymes that destroy the surrounding tissue.

3. The answer is B *[II D 1].*
The most direct method of managing atopic allergies is through environmental control (i.e., avoidance of the specific allergen or allergens responsible for the allergic reaction). Atopic allergies are immediate hypersensitivity reactions that occur only in genetically predisposed hosts upon sensitization to specific allergens. Other forms of management of atopic allergies include immunotherapy, which can be accomplished through hyposensitization or administration of modified allergens, and drug treatment (e.g., with antihistamines, corticosteroids, or epinephrine).

4. The answer is D *[II B 4 b; Table 9-1].*
Immediate hypersensitivity (type I) reactions involve the release of pharmacologically active substances (mediators) from mast cells or basophils, a mechanism that is triggered by antigens reacting with cell-bound IgE. Some type I mediators are stored within the mast cells and basophils in a preformed state; others are newly synthesized upon initiation of the immediate hypersensitivity response. Preformed mediators include histamine (probably the most important), eosinophil chemotactic factor of anaphylaxis (ECF-A), and serotonin (5-hydroxytryptamine). Mediators that are synthesized and released after the antigen–antibody reaction include slow-reacting substance of anaphylaxis (SRS-A), platelet-activating factor (PAF), bradykinin, and prostaglandins. The anaphylatoxins are products of the complement cascade; myeloperoxidase is an antibacterial enzyme found in lysosomes and in tears and other secretions.

5. The answer is C *[VI E 2 a].*
Primary amyloidosis is a plasma cell dyscrasia characterized by the deposition of amyloid fibrils in the vascular endothelium; the amyloid fibrils (termed amyloid light chain, or AL, proteins) are composed primarily of immunoglobulin light (L) chain fragments. Secondary amyloidosis is amyloidosis that is associated with chronic infection or inflammation; the amyloid fibrils in secondary amyloidosis (termed amyloid A, or AA, proteins) bear no structural resemblance to those seen in primary amyloidosis.

6. The answer is E *[VI B 1].*
Multiple myeloma is one of several plasma cell dyscrasias—diseases in which a single clone of plasma cells overproduces an immunoglobulin or an immunoglobulin fragment. Most cases of multiple myeloma involve plasma cell tumors of bone marrow that overproduce IgG.

7. The answer is C *[III A, B 1].*
The same immunologic mechanisms that defend the host may at times cause severe damage to tissues. These damaging immunologic reactions (also called hypersensitivity reactions) have been classified into four types according to the mechanism of tissue injury. Immediate hypersensitivity (type I) reactions are initiated by antigen reacting with cell-bound antibody—usually IgE. Cytotoxic (type II) hypersensitivity reactions are initiated by antibody—usually IgG or IgM—reacting with cell-bound antigen. Immune complex–mediated (type III) reactions are initiated by antigen–antibody complexes that form locally or are deposited from the circulation. Delayed hypersensitivity (cell-mediated; type IV) reactions are initiated by sensitized (antigen-reactive) T cells reacting with specific antigens. A fifth mechanism of tissue injury exists, in which antibody interferes with the functioning of biologically active substances (e.g., clotting factors and intrinsic factors); this has sometimes been referred to as a type V reaction.

8. The answer is C *[IV B 1].*

The pathogenetic requirements for immune complex–induced glomerulonephritis include neutrophils and complement, as well as antibody and antigen (any of several antigens may be involved; they need not be derived from the kidney). The small size of the immune complex is critical to its pathogenicity; complexes that are small are not cleared from the circulation readily, and are deposited on blood vessel walls. Such immune complexes form in a region of antigen excess and are soluble, escape phagocytosis, penetrate the vascular endothelium, and lodge on the basement membrane. Activation of complement attracts neutrophils, which release lysosomal enzymes that destroy basement membrane. Studies have shown that in humans, red blood cells participate in clearing immune complexes from the circulation: complexes that have been coated with C3b attach to C3b receptors on red blood cells, are transported to the liver and spleen, and then are removed from the red blood cells by phagocytes.

9. The answer is A *[II A 1, B 1, 3].*

Allergic urticaria (hives) is one of the milder manifestations of immediate hypersensitivity—specifically, atopic allergy. A more serious, sometimes life-threatening, form of immediate hypersensitivity is systemic anaphylaxis. Although other immunoglobulin classes have been implicated in immediate hypersensitivity reactions, the primary antibody responsible for such reactivity in humans is IgE.

10–13. The answers are: 10-C *[III C 1 b],* **11-A** *[VI C 2],* **12-E** *[V C 1 c],* **13-D** *[II A 2, B 2 b]*

Hemolytic disease of the newborn occurs when an Rh-negative mother gives birth to an Rh-positive infant, the Rh antigen having been acquired from an Rh-positive father. The most commonly involved antigen is $Rh_o(D)$. For this condition to occur, the mother must be sensitized to blood group antigens of the infant's blood; sensitization usually occurs during a previous delivery. After sensitization, IgG antibodies to the acquired antigen are produced, which may cross the placenta and destroy fetal cells.

Waldenström's macroglobulinemia is a lymphocytic lymphoma characterized by overproduction of lymphocytes and plasma cells. The most distinguishing feature of this disorder, however, is the high level of monoclonal IgM molecules in the serum, which causes moderate to severe hyperviscosity of the blood. Plasmapheresis (plasma exchange) is used to treat the symptoms of the hyperviscosity syndrome (i.e., fatigue, confusion, increased bleeding tendency).

Delayed hypersensitivity (cell-mediated; type IV) reactions are T cell–dependent reactions manifesting as inflammation at the site of antigen exposure. Tissue damage results from the interaction between sensitized (antigen-reactive) T cells and specific antigen; antibody and complement are not required for these reactions. Contact dermatitis is a form of delayed hypersensitivity, which occurs in response to antigen exposure on skin. Delayed hypersensitivity reactions also occur in response to tumors as well as viral, bacterial, fungal, and parasitic infections. The secondary phase of hypersensitivity pneumonitis disease has a T cell component (e.g., bagassosis), but in the early (inductive) phase, immune complexes predominate.

Food allergy is an immediate, or type I, (IgE-mediated) hypersensitivity reaction. Immediate hypersensitivity reactions are initiated by antigens reacting with cell-bound IgE antibody. The reaction may manifest in many ways, ranging from life-threatening systemic anaphylaxis to the lesser annoyance of atopic allergies, such as food allergies, allergic rhinitis (hay fever), and urticaria (hives).

10
Autoimmune Diseases

I. GENERAL CONSIDERATIONS. Autoimmune responses are immune responses of an individual to antigens present in the individual's own tissue. Autoimmune diseases affect more than 20 million Americans.

A. Etiology

1. A defect in the mechanisms underlying self-recognition (autotolerance, self-tolerance) can result in autoimmune responses.

2. Autoimmune responses can be mediated by humoral factors (circulating antibodies, immune complexes) or cellular factors [delayed hypersensitivity, cytotoxic T (Tc) cell–mediated] (see Table 10-2).
   a. Most autoimmune diseases have associated autoantibodies.
      (1) These are thought to be etiologically involved and to be the cause of the damage, namely Gell and Coombs types II and III hypersensitivity reactions.
      (2) However, the autoantibodies may merely reflect the damage done to an organ, and as such would be of diagnostic but not etiologic interest.
   b. The autoimmune diseases that involve nervous tissue (the encephalomyelitides and Guillain-Barré syndrome) are thought to be due to Gell and Coombs type IV hypersensitivity reactions. Guillain-Barré syndrome may also have an antibody component.
   c. Some autoimmune diseases (dermatomyositis, Hashimoto's thyroiditis, diabetes mellitus) are "mixed," with both an antibody and a T cell component.
   d. The pathogenesis of **multiple sclerosis** is still unclear, but the finding that patients have a defect in suppressor T (Ts) cells and excessive numbers of activated T cells in the blood and spinal fluid supports the theory of a defect in immune regulation.

3. **Possible mechanisms**
   a. The basic process most likely involves recruitment of a helper/inducer T cell which cooperates with preexisting autoreactive B cells or Tc cell precursors to induce a self-destructive immune response.
   b. The immunologic imbalance may arise from one or more of the following:
      (1) An excess of self-reactive helper T (Th) cell activity
         (a) The Th cell hyperactivity may be induced, for example, by the following.
            (i) Altered forms of self-antigen
            (ii) Antigen that cross-reacts with self-antigen due to epitope similarity
            (iii) **Molecular mimicry,** in which self-antigens and foreign materials such as viruses or bacteria share identical epitopes
         (b) Altered forms or cross-reacting antigens might be produced by coupling of a virus or a chemical or drug (e.g., hydralazine) to self-antigen.
         (c) The modified chemical–host or viral–host antigens would then trigger a self-reactive Th cell and elicit autoantibody production.
      (2) If the requisite self-reactive Th cell activity was somehow bypassed
         (a) Such bypass may occur via polyclonal B cell activation.
         (b) Possible activating materials include bacterial lipopolysaccharide, Epstein-Barr virus, or purified protein derivative (PPD) of tuberculin.
      (3) A deficiency of Ts cells, which normally down-regulate the immune response to self-antigen

(4) Release of sequestered antigen (e.g., from the lens of the eye or from sperm)
  (a) Sequestered antigens are not ordinarily available for recognition by the immune system.
  (b) Release might occur via such means as trauma or infection.

4. Genetic predisposition. There is clearly a role for genetic factors in autoimmune disease.
  a. The familial incidence that is seen is believed to be largely genetic rather than environmental.
  b. It is thought to be associated with those major histocompatibility complex (MHC) genes that code for the class II antigens that are so important in the presentation of antigens during the induction of an immune response.
    (1) Most autoimmune diseases appear to be associated with human leukocyte antigens (HLAs) DR2, DR3, DR4, and DR5 (see Table 12-1).
    (2) Over 90% of patients with ankylosing spondylitis have the HLA-B27 antigen while only 8% of the normal population do—a high concordance indeed.

5. Other factors affecting incidence
  a. Autoimmune diseases tend to occur at a higher frequency in females than in males (Table 10-1).
    (1) For example, the incidence of systemic lupus erythematosus (SLE) in women is four to six times that in men, and rheumatoid arthritis is three to four times more common in females.
    (2) The reason for this is still not certain, but it seems possible that sex hormones may play a role [see II B 2 g (3)].
  b. The frequency of autoimmune diseases increases with age. Very few autoimmune diseases occur in children and adolescents; most first appear in the 20- to 40-year age group.

B. Clinical categories

  1. Autoimmune diseases have been divided into two clinical types, **organ-specific** and **systemic,** based on the distribution of lesions (Table 10-2).

  2. Systemic autoimmune diseases are sometimes called **collagen vascular diseases,** indicating the widespread distribution of lesions in connective tissues and the vascular system.

C. Diagnosis

  1. General signs of autoimmune disease that may be of diagnostic importance include the following:
    a. Elevated serum gamma globulin levels
    b. The presence of various autoantibodies
    c. Depressed levels of serum complement
    d. Immune complexes in serum
    e. Depressed levels of Ts cells
    f. Lesions detected on biopsy (e.g., glomerular lesions) resulting from deposition of immune complexes

  2. Diagnostic tests are designed to detect antibodies specific to the particular antigen involved in the disease. Certain facts should be pointed out, however.
    a. Patients with autoimmune disease may have more than one autoantibody and, in fact, may suffer from multiple autoimmune diseases.
      (1) Some 10% of patients with autoimmune thyroiditis also suffer from pernicious anemia, and 30% will have antibodies to gastric parietal cells.

Table 10-1. Sex Ratio and Incidence of Certain Autoimmune Diseases

Disease	Female:Male	Estimated Incidence*
Rheumatoid arthritis	3:1	1000
Systemic lupus erythematosus (SLE)	4:1	100
Multiple sclerosis	1:1	100
Sjögren's syndrome	9:1	0.5–1
Polymyositis–dermatomyositis	2:1	0.5–1
Ankylosing spondylitis	1:9	0.5–1

*Per 100,000 United States population.

Table 10-2. Tissue Distribution and Presumed Immune Mediation in Representative Autoimmune Diseases

Disease	Presumed Mediation	Tissue Involvement
Systemic		
Rheumatoid arthritis	H	Joints and vascular bed
Systemic lupus erythematosus (SLE)	H	Kidney, skin, central nervous system, cardiovascular system
Organ- or tissue-specific		
Sjögren's syndrome	H	Lacrimal and salivary glands
Addison's disease	H	Adrenal glands
Acute disseminated encephalomyelitis	T	Nervous system
Guillain-Barré syndrome	T	Nervous system
Multiple sclerosis	T	Nervous system
Myasthenia gravis	H	Nervous system
Hashimoto's thyroiditis	H,T	Thyroid
Primary myxedema	H	Thyroid
Graves' disease	H	Thyroid
Diabetes mellitus	H,T	Pancreas
Goodpasture's syndrome	H	Lung and kidney
Pernicious anemia	H	Stomach
Atrophic gastritis	H	Stomach
Crohn's disease	H	Ileum and colon
Autoimmune hemolytic diseases	H	Red blood cells
Idiopathic thrombocytopenic purpura (ITP)	H	Platelets
Pemphigus	H	Skin
Pemphigoid	H	Skin
Dermatomyositis	H,T	Skin and muscle

H = humoral (circulating antibodies, immune complexes); T = T cell–mediated.

    (2) Fully 50% of individuals with pernicious anemia will have antibodies reactive with thyroid antigens.

    (3) Nearly 50% of patients with Sjögren's syndrome suffer from rheumatoid arthritis or other autoimmune arthritic diseases.

    (4) Patients with SLE may have 10 to 15 autoantibodies of differing specificities.

  b. While SLE is associated primarily with antinuclear antibodies, and rheumatoid arthritis primarily with rheumatoid factor, both kinds of antibodies may be found in both diseases (Table 10-3).

  c. Autoantibodies are not unique to autoimmune disease (e.g., antinuclear antibodies may be found in tuberculosis, in histoplasmosis, and in malignant lymphoma and other neoplasias).

D. Therapy. Therapy for autoimmune disease involves several approaches.

  1. In certain organ-specific diseases metabolic control may suffice.

    a. In thyrotoxicosis (Graves' disease), antithyroid drugs such as propylthiouracil or methimazole may be prescribed. Surgical or radionuclide (iodine-131; I^{131}) ablation of the gland is also effective.

    b. Vitamin B_{12} is given to patients with pernicious anemia.

  2. Agents such as nonsteroidal anti-inflammatory drugs (e.g., aspirin, indomethacin), steroidal anti-inflammatory drugs (e.g., cortisone, which may also be immunosuppressive), and immunosuppressive cytotoxic drugs (e.g., cyclophosphamide, azathioprine) are useful in treating disease symptoms. The latter agents are used only in advanced disease.

  3. Anticholinesterase drugs and thymectomy are of value in myasthenia gravis.

  4. Plasmapheresis, or plasma exchange therapy, appears to be of value in certain diseases (e.g., Guillain-Barré disease, SLE, and Goodpasture's syndrome).

    a. Plasmapheresis is beneficial by removing offending antibodies and immune complexes.

    b. The plasma removed is replaced with normal serum albumin or fresh frozen plasma.

  5. Splenectomy is of value in hemolytic diseases and idiopathic thrombocytopenic purpura (ITP).

II. REPRESENTATIVE AUTOIMMUNE DISEASES

A. Rheumatoid arthritis is a chronic inflammatory joint disease, with systemic involvement as well.

1. **Clinicopathologic features**
   a. An unknown etiologic agent initiates a nonspecific immune response. An inflammatory joint lesion that begins in the synovial membrane can become proliferative, destroying adjacent cartilage and bone and resulting in joint deformity.
   b. **General symptoms** include weight loss, malaise, fever, fatigue, and weakness.
   c. Serum protein electrophoresis may show hypergammaglobulinemia and hypoalbuminemia.
   d. The disease primarily affects females and is associated with HLA-DR4, which may confer genetic susceptibility.

2. **Immunologic findings**
   a. **Rheumatoid factor.** A hallmark of rheumatoid arthritis is the presence of rheumatoid factor, an immunoglobulin (mainly IgM but also IgG and IgA) produced by B cells and plasma cells in the synovial membrane.
      (1) Rheumatoid factor is present in the serum of most patients (90% or more) with established rheumatoid arthritis, and these patients generally have more severe disease than do patients without rheumatoid factor.
      (2) IgM and IgG rheumatoid factors are the primary components of immunoglobulin production in the rheumatoid synovial membrane.
      (3) Rheumatoid factor has antibody specificity for the Fc fragment of IgG. IgG is apparently altered in some way to appear as "nonself," perhaps by binding to another antigen.
   b. **Immune complexes**
      (1) The synovial fluid of patients with rheumatoid arthritis contains immune complexes consisting of rheumatoid factor, IgG, and complement.
      (2) These complexes can trigger an immune response in two ways.
         (a) **Immune complex activation of complement**
            (i) Rheumatoid factor combines with IgG away from its antibody combining site, leaving the IgG molecule free to combine with its homologous antigen or with more antibodies to form large complexes.
            (ii) These aggregates can reach a size large enough to activate both the classic and alternative complement pathways, with production of neutrophil chemotactic factors (C5a).
         (b) **Immune complex ingestion**
            (i) An inflammatory response is amplified as aggregates of IgG rheumatoid factor are phagocytized by macrophages (which release cytokines) and by neutrophils (which release digestive enzymes). Neutrophils that have engulfed immune complexes are called **rheumatoid arthritis (RA) cells**.
            (ii) Compared to serum levels of IgG, synovial levels of IgG (but not IgM) rheumatoid factor are relatively reduced, suggesting that phagocytosis of IgG rheumatoid factor may have a specific role in the inflammatory response.
   c. **Antinuclear antibodies.** These are also present in some patients with rheumatoid arthritis (see Table 10-3).

B. Systemic lupus erythematosus is a chronic, inflammatory, multiorgan disorder that predominantly affects young women of childbearing age.

1. **Clinicopathologic features**
   a. **General symptoms** include malaise, fever, lethargy, and weight loss.
   b. Multiple tissues are involved, including the skin, mucosa, kidney, brain, and cardiovascular system.

Table 10-3. Incidence of Antinuclear Antibodies and Rheumatoid Factor in Various Autoimmune Diseases

Disease	Incidence	
	Antinuclear Antibodies	**Rheumatoid Factor**
Systemic lupus erythematosus (SLE)	90% +	20%
Rheumatoid arthritis	20%	90% +
Sjögren's syndrome	70%	75%

(1) The most characteristic feature is the **butterfly rash,** an erythematous rash that occurs over the nose and cheeks. Other skin lesions (e.g., discoid, psoriasiform, maculopapular, and bullous) have also been described.

(2) Renal involvement occurs in 50% of patients with SLE. Diffuse proliferative glomerulonephritis and membranous glomerulonephritis are common manifestations.

(3) Central nervous system manifestations appear in 50% of patients and include depression, psychoses, seizures, and sensorimotor neuropathies.

c. At least 5000 Americans die of SLE each year, but the majority of cases are controlled by medical treatment. Death usually results from renal failure or from infection brought on by immunosuppressive therapy.

2. Immunologic findings

a. The lupus erythematosus (LE) cell phenomenon. The discovery of this phenomenon led to the current understanding of the immunologic basis of SLE.

(1) When peripheral blood from a patient is incubated at 37° C for 30 to 60 minutes, the lymphocytes swell and extrude their nuclear material.

(2) The nuclear material is opsonized by anti-DNA antibody and complement, and is then phagocytized by neutrophils (now called **LE cells**).

b. Antinuclear antibodies. The detection of antinuclear antibodies by indirect immunofluorescence is of diagnostic importance in SLE. **Antibodies to DNA** are either IgG or IgM; three primary types can be detected:

(1) Antibodies to single-stranded DNA (ssDNA)

(2) Antibodies to double-stranded DNA (dsDNA)

(a) Antibodies to dsDNA are complement-fixing antibodies.

(b) They are most closely associated with active SLE and the glomerulonephritis that is triggered by the deposition of immune complexes (consisting of DNA, antibody, and complement) on the basement membrane of blood vessels of renal glomeruli.

(3) Antibodies that react with both ssDNA and dsDNA

c. Other autoantibodies

(1) Some patients with SLE also form antibodies against RNA, red blood cells, platelets, mitochondria, ribosomes, lysosomes, thromboplastin, or thrombin.

(2) Some patients demonstrate a positive test for rheumatoid factor (see II A 2 a and Chapter 8 III D 2 a).

d. Genetic aspects. Autoantibody formation is in part genetically determined.

(1) Patients with the HLA-DR2 gene are more likely to produce anti-dsDNA antibodies.

(2) Those with HLA-DR3 produce anti–SS-A (Ro) and anti–SS-B (La) autoantibodies. (SS = Sjögren's syndrome; Ro, La, and Sm = patients in whom the antibodies were first identified.)

(3) Those with HLA-DR4 or HLA-DR5 produce anti-Sm and anti-RNP (ribonucleoprotein) autoantibodies.

e. Altered serum levels. Most patients show hypergammaglobulinemia and reduced serum complement levels (particularly C3 and C4) due to increased complement utilization caused by immune complex formation.

f. T cell changes. There is a drop in the number of T cells and a subsequent impaired ability to develop delayed hypersensitivity. Antibodies cytotoxic for T cells correlate with this T cell deficiency.

g. Animal model

(1) Mice of the NZB/NZW strain spontaneously develop disease with essentially all of the features of SLE (e.g., LE cells, antinuclear antibodies, immune complex glomerulonephritis, T cell deficiency).

(2) They show a deficiency of Ts cells that is associated with the presence of thymocytotoxic antibodies in the serum.

(3) Estrogens enhance anti-DNA antibody formation and increase the severity of renal disease in experimental animals, while androgens have an opposite effect, suggesting that hormones may be involved in the predominance of SLE in women.

C. Sjögren's syndrome (sicca syndrome) is a chronic inflammatory disease that affects the exocrine glands; the primary targets appear to be the lacrimal and salivary glands.

1. Clinicopathologic features

a. The disease is characterized by dry eyes (keratoconjunctivitis sicca) and dry mouth (xerostomia). Dryness of the nose, larynx, and bronchi is also seen. In females, who constitute the majority of patients, the vaginal mucosa is also dry.

    b. Sjögren's syndrome is usually associated with another connective tissue disease such as rheumatoid arthritis or SLE.

  2. Immunologic findings. Numerous features suggest an immunologic etiology.

    a. Patients demonstrate hypergammaglobulinemia, suggesting excessive B cell activity, and several types of autoantibodies, such as rheumatoid factor, antinuclear antibodies, and antibody to salivary duct epithelium.

    b. Salivary and lacrimal glands are infiltrated with plasma cells, B cells, and T cells. Some patients show a quantitative and qualitative T cell suppression in peripheral blood.

D. Acute disseminated encephalomyelitis may occur following vaccination (e.g., rabies immunization) or viral infection (e.g., measles, influenza).

  1. Clinicopathologic features

    a. Symptoms and signs

      (1) Symptoms of encephalomyelitis include headache, backache, stiff neck, nausea, low-grade fever, malaise, and weakness or paralysis of extremities.

      (2) Vaccination with attenuated viruses (e.g., measles, rubella) may produce symptoms such as elevated body temperature, convulsions, drowsiness that may progress to a comatose state, and paralysis of extremities, particularly the legs.

      (3) Survivors of the acute stages of disease usually experience no permanent neurologic disorders, although mental retardation, epileptic seizures, or even death can result.

    b. Pathologic examination reveals perivascular accumulation of macrophages, lymphocytes, and some neutrophils throughout the gray or white matter of the brain with variable demyelination.

  2. Immunologic findings. These suggest that the disease represents a cell-mediated allergic response to **basic protein of myelin** similar to that seen in experimental allergic encephalomyelitis (see II E). Antibodies to basic protein of myelin do not seem to be involved.

E. Experimental allergic encephalomyelitis is the experimental model for postvaccinal and postinfectious encephalomyelitis. It can be induced in animals (e.g., guinea pigs) by the injection of either homologous or heterologous brain or spinal cord extracts emulsified in complete Freund's adjuvant.

  1. Clinicopathologic features

    a. Within 2 to 3 weeks after sensitization, animals start to lose weight and then develop impaired righting reflex, ataxia, flaccid paralysis of the hind legs, urinary incontinence, and fecal impaction. Most animals ultimately die; however, some recover completely.

    b. Histologic lesions consist of perivascular accumulation of lymphocytes, mononuclear cells, and plasma cells throughout the brain and spinal cord and demyelination of nerve tissue.

  2. Immunologic findings

    a. The encephalitogenic factor appears to be certain polypeptide sequences of **myelin basic protein**.

    b. Although both B cells and T cells respond to basic protein, the T cell appears to be responsible for the lesion (demyelination).

      (1) Animals demonstrate classic cutaneous delayed hypersensitivity to basic protein, and the disease can be passively transferred with lymphoid cells.

      (2) Antibodies to basic protein are formed but they correlate poorly with disease and cannot passively transfer the disease.

F. Guillain-Barré syndrome (acute idiopathic polyneuritis) commonly occurs after an infectious disease (e.g., measles, hepatitis) or after vaccination (e.g., influenza); it affects all age groups.

  1. Clinicopathologic features

    a. Symptoms include progressive weakness, first of the lower extremities and then of upper extremities and respiratory muscles; the weakness can lead to paralysis. Most patients recover normal function in 6 to 10 months.

    b. Examination of peripheral nerve tissue reveals a perivascular mononuclear cell infiltrate and demyelination.

2. Immunologic findings
a. Experimental model
    (1) A similar disease can be produced in experimental animals by injection of peripheral nerve extracts, or peptides derived therefrom, incorporated in complete Freund's adjuvant.

    (2) The experimental disease appears to be T cell–mediated, as evidenced by sensitivity of lymphocytes to nerve extracts, release of lymphokines from sensitized lymphocytes, and passive transfer of disease with sensitized cells.

    (3) Antinerve antibodies can be detected but seem to play no role in pathogenesis.

b.
The **human disease** has several of the same immunologic features as the experimental animal model: lymphocytes sensitive to peripheral nerve extracts, lymphokine production, and antinerve antibodies.

G. Multiple sclerosis is a relapsing neuromuscular disease with exacerbations between periods of remission.

1. Clinicopathologic features
a. Symptoms include motor weakness, ataxia, impaired vision, urinary bladder dysfunction, paresthesias, and mental aberrations.

b. Inflammatory lesions (sclerotic plaques) are confined to the myelin in the central nervous system and consist of mononuclear cell infiltrates and demyelination.

2. Immunologic findings
a. The cause of multiple sclerosis remains unknown, but the clustering character of cases suggests an infectious agent.

    (1) Epidemiologic studies have revealed high-risk and low-risk areas of the world, suggesting a possible role for a transmissible agent.

    (2) Also of interest in this regard is the finding that patients tend to have elevated levels of antibodies to measles virus in their serum and spinal fluid; however, the exact role of measles virus is unknown. There is, in fact, evidence that other viral agents may also be involved.

b. Evidence that susceptibility may be genetically determined is suggested by a close association with HLA-DR2 and HLA-DQw1.

c. Most patients show increased concentrations of IgG in the spinal fluid. The spinal fluid: serum immunoglobulin ratio is elevated, and there is evidence that local IgG synthesis occurs in nerve tissue, based on the oligoclonal pattern seen on electrophoresis.

d. Patients tend to show suppressed levels of circulating T cells and increased levels of B cells. This may explain the decrease in the delayed hypersensitivity response to measles observed in patients.

H. Myasthenia gravis is a chronic disease resulting from faulty neuromuscular transmission.

1. Clinicopathologic features
a. The disease is characterized by muscle weakness and fatigability, particularly of the ocular, pharyngeal, facial, laryngeal, and skeletal muscles.

b. Muscle weakness and neuromuscular dysfunction result from depletion of acetylcholine receptors at the myoneural junction.

2. Immunologic findings
a. Experimental model
    (1) Injection of experimental animals with purified **acetylcholine receptor** incorporated in complete Freund's adjuvant induces experimental myasthenia gravis that closely mimics human disease.

    (2) Serum from animals with experimentally induced disease, as well as serum from human patients, will passively transfer the syndrome to normal animals.

b. About 60% to 80% of patients have an enlarged thymus, and 80% to 90% of patients have antibodies (frequently an IgG3 isotype) against the acetylcholine receptor. It is apparently this antibody that binds to acetylcholine receptors at the myoneural junction, causing endocytosis of the receptors.

c. Although there is evidence that cellular immunity may also be involved (e.g., lymphocyte stimulation by purified acetylcholine receptor and passive transfer with lymphoid cells), it would appear that the antibody response is more intimately involved.

    d. Complement-binding immune complexes may cause further problems at the myoneural junction.

I. Chronic thyroiditis (Hashimoto's thyroiditis) is a disease of the thyroid that mainly affects women age 30 to 50 years.

  1. Clinicopathologic features

    a. The thyroid gland may be enlarged (**goiter**) and firm or hard. Histologic examination reveals a lymphocyte and plasma cell infiltrate, disappearance of colloid, and varying amounts of fibrosis.

    b. As the disease progresses, signs of hypothyroidism may be seen; for example, low values of circulating thyroid hormones and decreased thyroidal uptake of radioiodine.

  2. Immunologic findings

    a. Various antibodies to thyroid-specific antigens can be demonstrated.

      (1) Antibody to thyroglobulin will precipitate this antigen and will agglutinate tanned red blood cells coated with thyroglobulin (passive hemagglutination). Anti-thyroglobulin antibodies may also be detected via radioimmunoassay (RIA), immunofluorescence, and enzyme-linked immunosorbent assay (ELISA).

      (2) Antibody to thyroid microsomal antigen can be detected by complement fixation and hemagglutination tests.

      (3) Antibody to a second colloid antigen has been detected but is not well characterized.

    b. Experimental model

      (1) Animals (e.g., rabbit, guinea pig, rat, mouse) injected with homologous or autologous thyroid extract incorporated in complete Freund's adjuvant develop lesions and other features similar to those seen in human disease.

      (2) A delayed hypersensitivity reaction to thyroid extract can also be demonstrated.

    c. The relative importance of T cells and B cells in the pathogenesis of disease is not yet clearly resolved. Both cell types may be essential for maximum effect. Antibody-dependent cell-mediated cytotoxicity (ADCC; see Chapter 1 II G 2) may also be involved.

J. Graves' disease (thyrotoxicosis, hyperthyroidism) results from the overproduction of thyroid hormone (thyroxine).

  1. Clinicopathologic features. Patients demonstrate fatigue, nervousness, increased sweating, palpitations, weight loss, and heat intolerance.

  2. Immunologic findings

    a. An increase in the number of peripheral B cells correlates with the severity of the disease.

    b. Patients also show a decrease in the percentage of T cells in blood, mainly Ts cells.

    c. Current evidence suggests that patients produce several antibodies to **thyrotropin receptors**.

      (1) One type of antibody blocks the binding of thyroid-stimulating hormone (TSH) to thyroid epithelial cells.

      (2) A second antithyroid antibody causes thyroid cells to proliferate.

      (3) The third type, referred to as **thyroid-stimulating antibody,** reacts with TSH receptors on the thyroid cell membrane and mimics the action of the pituitary hormone thyrotropin. The result of this interaction is overproduction of thyroid hormone and hyperthyroidism.

    d. Since thyroid-stimulating antibodies are IgG, they can cross the placenta and cause hyperthyroidism in the newborn. The condition resolves spontaneously as the maternal IgG is catabolized by the infant over a period of several weeks.

    e. Increased frequencies of HLA-Bw35 and HLA-DR3 have been found.

K. Insulin-dependent diabetes mellitus (IDDM; type I diabetes, juvenile diabetes) results from immunologic destruction of the insulin-producing beta cells of the islets of Langerhans in the pancreas.

  1. Clinicopathologic features

    a. The disease affects about 1 person out of every 500 in the population. It has its peak onset between ages 10 and 15 years.

    b. The inability to synthesize insulin makes the patient susceptible to wide fluctuations in blood glucose levels.

    c. Acute manifestations of insulin insufficiency include ketoacidosis, polyuria, polydipsia, and polyphagia.

    d. Chronic hyperglycemia and associated abnormal metabolic events lead to cardiovascular disease, neuropathies, kidney problems, and cataracts.

    e. Patients with IDDM are refractory to dietary control and oral hypoglycemic drugs, and require daily insulin injections.

  2. Immunologic findings

    a. Affected individuals produce antibodies to insulin and to cytoplasmic constituents of beta cells.

    b. Cytotoxicity of T cells for islet cells has also been reported.

    c. The islets are infiltrated with B and T cells, and are eventually destroyed.

    d. The onset of disease is often preceded by a viral infection: mumps, cytomegalovirus, influenza, rubella, and coxsackievirus have been implicated.

      (1) Mumps and coxsackievirus can destroy islet cells in vitro.

      (2) A B4 coxsackievirus, isolated from the pancreas of a diabetic child, has produced a similar disease in experimental animals.

    e. Individuals with HLA-DR3 and HLA-DR4 haplotypes have an increased risk of developing IDDM.

    f. Variations in β-chain alleles of a HLA-DQ antigen distinguish susceptible from resistant individuals.

      (1) Serine, valine, or alanine at amino acid position 57 seems to confer susceptibility.

      (2) Aspartic acid at position 57 (asp57) is correlated with protection. The mechanism of this effect is obscure. Suggested theories have included the following.

        (a) The epitope that includes the asp57 resembles the antigen (self or viral) that triggers the autoimmune response, and thus induces autotolerance.

        (b) Asp57 adversely affects epitope presentation to T cells because it is located in the peptide-binding groove of the class II MHC molecule.

L. Goodpasture's syndrome is a rare, progressive disease of the lungs and kidneys. The disease occurs in all age groups, affecting mainly young men. The prognosis is poor.

  1. Clinicopathologic features

    a. Classic symptoms include pulmonary hemorrhage, hemoptysis, hematuria, and glomerulonephritis.

    b. Pulmonary infiltrates may show on x-rays.

  2. Immunologic findings

    a. Immunofluorescence reveals linear deposits of immunoglobulin (usually IgG) and complement on alveolar and glomerular **basement membranes**.

    b. The IgG appears to represent an antibody specific for an antigen shared by kidney and lung basement membranes.

    c. Some cases have characteristics suggestive of an immune complex phenomenon.

M. Pernicious anemia results from defective red blood cell maturation due to faulty absorption of vitamin B_{12}. Normally, dietary B_{12} is transported across the small intestine into the body as a complex with **intrinsic factor** (which is synthesized by parietal cells in the gastric mucosa). In patients with pernicious anemia, the process is blocked.

  1. Clinicopathologic features

    a. The hallmark of the disease is the progressive destruction of gastric glands, associated with a loss of parietal cells. The consequent lack of intrinsic factor leads to failure of B_{12} absorption.

    b. The gastric mucosa is infiltrated with mononuclear leukocytes and neutrophils.

    c. Defective red blood cell maturation leads to megaloblastic anemia, with attendant weakness, loss of appetite, fatigability, pallor, and weight loss.

    d. Neurologic damage can occur due to B_{12} deficiency, and may be irreversible.

    e. Patients with pernicious anemia have an increased incidence of stomach cancer.

  2. Immunologic findings

    a. Patients produce antibodies (mainly IgG) to three different gastric **parietal cell antigens,** all of which are cell-specific. In addition, antibody to **intrinsic factor** is produced.

    b. Antibody to intrinsic factor may block the attachment of B_{12} to intrinsic factor or may bind to intrinsic factor or to the intrinsic factor–B_{12} complex.

   c. Some patients also show cell-mediated immunity to intrinsic factor and parietal cell antigen.

N. Autoimmune hemolytic diseases. These include warm-antibody hemolytic anemia (the most common type of autoimmune hemolytic disease), cold-antibody hemolytic anemia, and paroxysmal cold hemoglobinuria.

  1. Clinicopathologic features. Classic symptoms include fatigue, fever, jaundice, and splenomegaly referable to the presence of antibodies directed against self red blood cell antigens and the resultant anemia.

  2. Immunologic findings
    a. Warm-antibody hemolytic anemia
     (1) Warm antibodies are so-called because they show optimum reactivity at 37° C. They are primarily IgG, are poor at complement fixing, and can be detected on the red blood cell surface by the antiglobulin (Coombs) test.
     (2) Various patterns of red blood cell coating can be detected in different patients: cells can be coated with IgG alone, IgG plus complement, or complement alone.
     (3) The warm antibody is directed primarily against **Rh determinants,** and antibody-coated red cells appear to be opsonized for phagocytosis primarily in the spleen.
    b. Cold-antibody hemolytic anemia
     (1) Cold antibodies show optimum reactivity at 4° C. They are primarily of the IgM class, fix complement, and agglutinate red blood cells directly, without the requirement for Coombs antiglobulin.
     (2) The IgM is specific against red blood cell **antigens I or i.**
     (3) Cold agglutinins may also be detected secondary to infections (e.g., mycoplasmal pneumonia).
    c. Paroxysmal cold hemoglobinuria is a rare syndrome associated with **Donath-Landsteiner antibody,** a cold antibody of the IgG class directed against red blood cell **antigen P.**
     (1) The antibody is biphasic in that it sensitizes cells in the cold, usually below 15° C, and then hemolyzes them when the temperature is elevated to 37° C.
     (2) Patients demonstrate symptoms (e.g., fever, pain in extremities, jaundice, hemoglobinuria) following exposure to cold.

O. Idiopathic thrombocytopenic purpura, which may be either acute or chronic, results from antibody-mediated platelet destruction. In children, it is sometimes preceded by a viral infection.

  1. Clinicopathologic features
    a. Patients demonstrate petechiae and various bleeding problems in their gums, gastrointestinal tract, and genitourinary tract.
    b. The peripheral blood platelet counts are profoundly suppressed (i.e., less than 100,000/ml), as is platelet survival time.

  2. Immunologic findings
    a. IgG antibodies specific for platelets can be demonstrated.
     (1) Antibody-coated platelets are sequestered and destroyed by macrophages primarily of the spleen and liver.
     (2) Since routine simple laboratory techniques are not sensitive enough to detect antibodies, more sophisticated tests must be used (e.g., ELISA or radiolabeled Coombs antiglobulin test).
    b. Thrombocytopenia may sometimes be drug-induced.
     (1) Causative drugs include sulfonamides, antihistamines, quinidine, and quinine.
     (2) Drug–antibody complexes are adsorbed onto the platelet surface, with subsequent complement activation. Treatment consists of withholding the drug.

P. Bullous (vesicular) diseases are chronic dermatologic problems that result when destruction of intercellular bridges (**desmosomes**) interferes with cohesion of the epidermis, leading to the formation of blisters (**bullae**).

  1. Clinicopathologic features
    a. Pemphigus vulgaris is an erosive disease of the skin and mucous membranes, with intraepidermal blisters.
    b. Bullous pemphigoid is a bullous disease of the skin and mucosa, usually seen in middle-aged and older people. The blisters form beneath the epidermis at the dermal–epidermal junction.

   2. Immunologic findings
   a. Pemphigus vulgaris skin lesions, when examined by immunofluorescence, show deposition of antibody (mainly IgG) and complement components in squamous intercellular spaces.
   b. Bullous pemphigoid lesions, by immunofluorescence examination, demonstrate deposition of antibody and complement along skin basement membrane. Circulating anti-basement membrane antibodies can also be detected.

Q. Polymyositis–dermatomyositis is an acute or chronic inflammatory disease of the muscles and skin.

   1. Clinicopathologic features. Patients demonstrate weakness of striated muscle, with some muscle pain and tenderness, plus a characteristic skin rash.

   2. Immunologic findings
   a. Hypergammaglobulinemia is common, along with deposition of immunoglobulin and complement in the vessel walls of the skin and muscle.
   b. Cellular immunity may also play a role in pathogenesis, as judged from studies showing cellular passive transfer and lymphokine release by T cells.

STUDY QUESTIONS

Directions: Each of the numbered items or incomplete statements in this section is followed by answers or by completions of the statement. Select the **one** lettered answer or completion that is **best** in each case.

1. All of the following are signs of diagnostic importance in autoimmune disease EXCEPT

(A) lesions detected on biopsy
(B) immune complexes in serum
(C) depressed levels of serum complement
(D) depressed levels of suppressor T (Ts) cells
(E) depressed serum gamma globulin levels

2. The Donath-Landsteiner antibody is characteristic of

(A) warm-antibody hemolytic anemia
(B) cold-antibody hemolytic anemia
(C) paroxysmal cold hemoglobinuria
(D) idiopathic thrombocytopenic purpura (ITP)
(E) pernicious anemia

3. Antinuclear antibodies and rheumatoid factor are commonly associated with all of the following conditions EXCEPT

(A) rheumatoid arthritis
(B) Sjögren's syndrome
(C) systemic lupus erythematosus (SLE)
(D) idiopathic thrombocytopenic purpura (ITP)

4. Organ-specific autoimmune diseases include all of the following EXCEPT

(A) thyroiditis
(B) systemic lupus erythematosus (SLE)
(C) pernicious anemia
(D) multiple sclerosis
(E) myasthenia gravis

5. A T cell response to basic protein of myelin appears to be responsible for the pathogenesis of

(A) Guillain-Barré syndrome
(B) Graves' disease
(C) acute disseminated encephalomyelitis
(D) myasthenia gravis
(E) multiple sclerosis

6. The chronic inflammation characteristic of Sjögren's syndrome affects multiple body systems, including primarily the

(A) lacrimal glands
(B) salivary glands
(C) both
(D) neither

7. All of the following statements about the warm antibody involved in autoimmune hemolytic disease are correct EXCEPT that it

(A) causes agglutination at 37° C but not at 4° C
(B) primarily consists of IgG
(C) fixes complement poorly
(D) demonstrates specificity for Rh red blood cell antigens
(E) can be detected by Coombs antiglobulin reagent

8. Autoimmune diseases can be characterized by all of the following EXCEPT

(A) a tendency to occur more frequently in women
(B) hypergammaglobulinemia
(C) familial incidence
(D) autoantibodies in the serum
(E) elevated serum complement levels

9. Renal failure is a common cause of death in patients with

(A) Sjögren's syndrome
(B) rheumatoid arthritis
(C) rheumatic fever
(D) pemphigus vulgaris
(E) systemic lupus erythematosus (SLE)

1-E	4-B	7-A
2-C	5-C	8-E
3-D	6-C	9-E

10. Rheumatoid factor is an antibody directed against determinants on the immunoglobulin molecule's

(A) γ chain
(B) μ chain
(C) J (joining) chain
(D) λ chain
(E) κ chain

Directions: The group of items in this section consists of lettered options followed by a set of numbered items. For each item, select the **one** lettered option that is most closely associated with it. Each lettered option may be selected once, more than once, or not at all.

Questions 11–14

For each characteristic of an autoimmune disease listed below, select the disease most closely associated with it.

(A) Amyotrophic lateral sclerosis
(B) Systemic lupus erythematosus (SLE)
(C) Sjögren's syndrome
(D) Guillain-Barré syndrome
(E) Hemolytic anemia
(F) Rheumatoid arthritis
(G) Goodpasture's syndrome

11. Dry eyes and dry mouth

12. Peripheral neuritis

13. Antibody specific for an antigen shared by the kidney and lung

14. Butterfly rash

10-A   13-G
11-C   14-B
12-D

ANSWERS AND EXPLANATIONS

1. The answer is E *[I C 1].*
Elevated, not depressed, serum gamma globulin levels are one of several general signs of autoimmune disease that may be of diagnostic importance. Other signs include depressed levels of serum complement or suppressor T (Ts) cells, lesions detected on biopsy, and the presence of immune complexes in the serum.

2. The answer is C *[II N 2 c].*
Paroxysmal cold hemoglobinuria is a rare type of autoimmune hemolytic disease that is associated with the Donath-Landsteiner antibody, a cold antibody of the IgG class directed against red blood cell antigen P. Cold-antibody hemolytic anemia involves antibodies of the IgM class that are optimally reactive in the cold. Warm-antibody hemolytic anemia involves primarily IgG antibodies that are optimally reactive at 37° C. Idiopathic thrombocytopenic purpura (ITP) results from antibody-mediated platelet destruction. Pernicious anemia results from defective red blood cell maturation due to immunologically mediated faulty absorption of vitamin B_{12}.

3. The answer is D *[Table 10-3].*
In idiopathic thrombocytopenic purpura (ITP), IgG antibodies specific for platelets cause the platelets to be destroyed by macrophages of the spleen and liver. While systemic lupus erythematosus (SLE) is primarily associated with antinuclear antibodies and rheumatoid arthritis with rheumatoid factor, both antibodies may be found in both diseases as well as in other collagen vascular disorders such as Sjögren's syndrome.

4. The answer is B *[Table 10-2].*
Systemic lupus erythematosus (SLE) is a systemic autoimmune disease. Some autoimmune diseases are organ-specific: the immune response is directed against just one organ or tissue type, as in Hashimoto's thyroiditis (target = thyroid), pernicious anemia (target = gastric tissue), multiple sclerosis (target = basic protein of myelin), and myasthenia gravis (target = acetylcholine receptor). Other autoimmune diseases are systemic: the target antigens are widespread throughout the body, as in SLE (target = cell nuclear material) and rheumatoid arthritis (target = IgG). In the case of organ-specific disease, the lesions are generally restricted because the antigen in that organ is the target of the immunologic attack. In systemic autoimmune diseases, lesions affect more tissues because antigen–antibody complex deposition is more disseminated.

5. The answer is C *[II D 2].*
In acute disseminated encephalomyelitis, both in humans and in the experimental animal model, there is perivascular accumulation of lymphocytes and other cells throughout nervous tissue, along with variable demyelination. The latter appears to be triggered via a T cell–mediated response to basic protein of myelin.

6. The answer is C *[II C].*
Sjögren's syndrome is characterized by dry eyes (keratoconjunctivitis sicca) and dry mouth (xerostomia). Salivary and lacrimal glands are infiltrated with plasma cells, B cells, T cells, suggesting an immunologic etiology. Patients also demonstrate hypergammaglobulinemia and several types of autoantibodies such as rheumatoid factor, antinuclear antibodies, and antibody to salivary duct epithelium.

7. The answer is A *[II N 2 a].*
The so-called "warm" antibody of autoimmune hemolytic disease will react with red blood cells at 4° C or at 37° C, although the antibody shows optimal reactivity at 37° C. By contrast, the "cold" isoagglutinins react optimally at 4° C. The most common type of autoimmune hemolytic disease involves the so-called warm antibodies, which are primarily IgG, are poor at complement fixation, and can be detected by the antiglobulin (Coombs) test. Warm antibody is directed primarily against Rh antigens on the red blood cells.

8. The answer is E *[I A 4 a, 5 a, C 1 a–c].*
Complement levels are usually depressed in autoimmunity, not elevated, due to the presence of immune complexes in the serum. Most autoimmune diseases are more common in females; for example, approximately 85% of patients with systemic lupus erythematosus (SLE) are women. This implies that sex hormones may play a precipitating (estrogens) or controlling (androgens) role. Certain autoimmune diseases

have an increased incidence in association with particular HLA antigens, especially antigens coded for in the HLA-DR locus. Most diagnostic tests rely on examination of serum for decreased complement and suppressor T (Ts) cell levels and for increases in immune complexes and gamma globulin.

9. The answer is E *[II B 1 c].*
Systemic lupus erythematosus (SLE) is a chronic inflammatory systemic (multiorgan) disease triggered by the deposition of immune complexes on the basement membrane of blood vessels. Renal failure is a common cause of death since the immune complex deposition occurs in blood vessels of the renal glomeruli, leading to glomerulonephritis.

10. The answer is A *[II A 2 a (3)].*
Rheumatoid factor is an antibody that has specificity for the IgG heavy chain. Rheumatoid factor is usually of the IgM class; however, rheumatoid factors have also been described that are IgG or IgA. These molecules occur in a high percentage (70% to 90%) of patients with rheumatoid arthritis. Other autoimmune diseases [e.g., systemic lupus erythematosus (SLE), Sjögren's syndrome] can also induce rheumatoid factor in the patient's serum. Rheumatoid factor is also found in patients with leprosy, tuberculosis, and other nonautoimmune diseases.

11–14. The answers are: 11-C *[II C 1]*, **12-D** *[II F]*, **13-G** *[II L 2 b]*, **14-B** *[II B 1 b (1)].*
Sjögren's syndrome is a chronic inflammatory disease that primarily affects secretory glands such as the lacrimal and salivary glands, producing dry eyes (keratoconjunctivitis sicca) and dry mouth (xerostomia).

Guillain-Barré syndrome (acute idiopathic polyneuritis) manifests as progressive weakness, first of the lower extremities and then of the upper extremities and respiratory muscles. Peripheral nerve tissue shows perivascular mononuclear cell infiltrate and demyelination.

Goodpasture's syndrome is a relatively rare disorder with symptoms referable to both the lungs (e.g., pulmonary hemorrhage) and kidneys (e.g., glomerulonephritis). The IgG deposited on alveolar and glomerular basement membranes appears to be specific for an antigen shared by the kidneys and lungs.

Systemic lupus erythematosus (SLE) is a chronic inflammatory multiorgan (systemic) disease that primarily affects females. A characteristic feature is the erythematous butterfly rash that occurs on the face of some patients. Death usually results from renal failure or infection.

11
Immunodeficiency Disorders

I. **GENERAL CONSIDERATIONS.** In view of the complex nature of the immune response, it is not surprising that a wide array of immunodeficiencies exist. An estimated 1 in every 500 people in the United States is born with an immune system defect. Many more will acquire a transient or permanent immunologic impairment that may have serious consequences.

A. Clinical evaluation

1. Immunodeficiency disorders are heralded primarily by recurrent infections, chronic infections, unusual (opportunistic) infecting agents, and a poor response to antimicrobial treatment. Occasionally other manifestations such as hepatosplenomegaly or diarrhea are seen (Table 11-1).

2. When an immunodeficiency syndrome is suspected in a given individual because of persistent and recurrent infections, the workup of the patient includes an evaluation of the native and acquired immune capabilities (see Chapter 8 IV).

B. Management of the immunodeficient patient

1. Therapy of the patient with immunodeficiency disease has two goals:
   a. Minimize the occurrence and impact of infections. This is accomplished by:
      (1) **Avoidance** of individuals with contagious diseases
      (2) Close **monitoring** of the patient for infections
      (3) Prompt and vigorous use of **antibiotics** when appropriate
      (4) Active (or passive) **immunization** as it may be possible in the individual patient
   b. Replace the defective component of the immune system by passive transfer or transplantation.
      (1) Pooled **gamma globulin** is useful in the treatment of certain immunoglobulin deficiencies (e.g., Bruton's hypogammaglobulinemia).
      (2) Infusions of **thymic hormones or cytokines** such as interleukin-2 (IL-2) and gamma interferon may be helpful in certain diseases (e.g., DiGeorge syndrome).
      (3) **Transfusions** that may be of value include:
         (a) Neutrophils in the treatment of phagocytic defects
         (b) Irradiated erythrocytes in the treatment of adenosine deaminase (ADA) deficiency
      (4) **Transplantation** of fetal thymus or of bone marrow stem cells may be used in attempts at reconstitution of immune competence.

2. Other aspects of management are mentioned below under specific disorders.

II. **PHAGOCYTIC CELL DEFECTS.** Although defects can occur in most phagocytic cells, emphasis is given here to neutrophils (polymorphonuclear leukocytes).

A. Quantitative defects

1. In **neutropenia** or **granulocytopenia,** the total number of normal circulating cells is suppressed, due either to decreased production or increased destruction.
   a. **Decreased production of neutrophils** can be caused by:
      (1) Administration of bone marrow depressant drugs (e.g., nitrogen mustard)
      (2) Leukemia

Table 11-1. Clinical Features Associated with Impaired Immune Function

---

Highly suggestive features
Infections, recurrent or chronic, characterized by:
    Unusual etiologies (opportunists)
        Normal flora
        Common environmental organisms
    Slow recovery or poor response to treatment

Features frequently seen
Chronic diarrhea
Eczema
Failure to thrive
Hepatosplenomegaly
Autoantibodies or autoimmune disease

---

    (3) Inherited conditions in which there appears to be defective development of all bone marrow stem cells, including myeloid precursors (e.g., reticular dysgenesis)
    (4) Spontaneously arising autoantibody that inhibits granulopoiesis
  b. Increased destruction of neutrophils can be caused by:
    (1) Autoimmune phenomena following the administration of certain drugs (e.g., quinidine and oxacillin) that may induce antibodies capable of opsonizing normal neutrophils
    (2) Hypersplenism characterized by exaggeration of the destructive functions of the spleen, with resultant deficiency of peripheral blood elements

  2. Asplenia, either congenital, surgical, or due to organ destruction by malignancy or sickle cell disease, can result in an increased incidence of infections, particularly septicemia due to *Streptococcus pneumoniae.*

B. Qualitative defects. In qualitative disorders, the phagocytic cells fail to engulf and kill microorganisms. The defect may reside in any of the phagocytic activities: chemotaxis, ingestion, or killing and digestion.

  1. Chronic granulomatous disease (CGD) is characterized by recurrent infections with various microorganisms, both gram-negative (e.g., *Escherichia, Serratia,* and *Klebsiella*) and gram-positive (e.g., *Staphylococcus*).
    a. Clinical and immunologic features
      (1) CGD is primarily an X-linked recessive disorder, and onset is in the first 2 years of life. Between 200 and 250 cases have been reported in the United States.
      (2) Granuloma formation occurs in many organs, and it appears to reflect the body's attempt to mount a T cell response, with increased gamma interferon production and macrophage activation, to compensate for the inability of the neutrophils to kill the organism.
      (3) There is an enzymatic inability to generate toxic oxygen metabolites during the oxygen consumption activity of the hexose monophosphate (HMP) shunt.
        (a) This is due to a defect in neutrophilic **cytochrome b,** which is part of an enzyme complex with the reduced form of nicotinamide-adenine dinucleotide phosphate (NADPH) oxidase that catalyzes the one-electron reduction of oxygen (O_2) to superoxide (O_2^-).
        (b) The result is suppression of intracellular killing of ingested microorganisms.
        (c) In most cases of X-linked CGD, the defect involves a gene located in band p21 of the X chromosome.
          (i) The gene normally encodes the 91-kDa component of the cytochrome b heterodimer.
          (ii) In X-linked CGD, the gene may be either absent or mutated, so that the RNA product is either not transcribed or is unstable.
      (4) Two other neutrophil enzymes are intact and generate other antimicrobial compounds.
        (a) Superoxide dismutase converts superoxide anions to hydrogen peroxide.
        (b) Myeloperoxidase generates hypochlorite from hydrogen peroxide and chloride ions.
      (5) B cell and T cell function and complement levels are generally normal.
    b. Diagnosis. This depends on the in vitro demonstration of defective killing by neutrophils.

   c. Treatment
   (1) Treatment involves the use of antibiotics appropriate for the infectious agent.
   (2) Temporary maintenance with neutrophil infusions from a family member may be of value.
   (3) Gamma interferon may stimulate the production of superoxide anions and may restore microbicidal activity to the neutrophils.
2. **Glucose-6-phosphate dehydrogenase (G6PD) deficiency** is an X-linked immunodeficiency disease with a clinical picture similar to that of CGD; in G6PD deficiency, however, hemolytic anemia is also present. The disorder is believed to result from the deficient generation of NADPH, needed as a reducing equivalent for the oxidase.
3. **Myeloperoxidase deficiency** is found in some patients with recurrent microbial infections.
   a. Myeloperoxidase is an important microbicidal agent contained in normal neutrophils.
   b. Superoxide and hydrogen peroxide are formed in these patients in normal amounts, but because the myeloperoxidase enzyme is lacking, neutrophil killing is impaired [see II B 1 a (4) (b)].
   c. A susceptibility to *Candida albicans* and *Staphylococcus aureus* infections is the chief problem in these patients.
   d. Treatment is with appropriate antimicrobial agents.
4. **Chédiak-Higashi syndrome** is a relatively rare disease of humans and of a variety of animals (e.g., mink, cattle, mice).
   a. Clinical and immunologic features
   (1) Chédiak-Higashi syndrome is characterized by partial albinism and recurrent severe pyogenic infections, primarily streptococcal and staphylococcal. Prognosis is poor: most patients die in childhood.
   (2) The patient's neutrophils contain abnormal giant lysosomes. These can apparently fuse with the phagosome but are impaired in their ability to release their contents, resulting in a delayed killing of ingested microorganisms.
   b. Diagnosis. Neutrophil chemotaxis and killing are abnormal, natural killer (NK) cell activity is decreased, and lysosomal enzyme levels are depressed. Oxygen consumption, hydrogen peroxide formation, and HMP activity are normal.
   c. Treatment. This involves the use of antibiotics appropriate for the type of infection.
5. **Job's syndrome**
   a. Clinical features. Job's syndrome is characterized by recurrent "cold" (i.e., lacking the normal inflammatory response) staphylococcal abscesses, chronic eczema, and otitis media.
   b. Immunologic features and diagnosis
   (1) Neutrophils demonstrate normal ingestion and killing activity but defective chemotaxis.
   (2) Serum levels of IgE are extremely high in association with increased specificity for staphylococcal antigens.
   (3) Eosinophilia may be present, and the number of suppressor T (Ts) cells may be reduced.
   c. Treatment. This involves the use of antibiotics appropriate for the infectious agent.
6. **"Lazy leukocyte" syndrome** is characterized by susceptibility to severe microbial infections.
   a. Clinical and immunologic features. Patients show neutropenia, defective chemotactic response by neutrophils (hence the name of the disorder), and an abnormal inflammatory response.
   b. Treatment. This involves the use of antibiotics appropriate for the infectious agent.
7. **Tuftsin deficiency** is a familial absence of **tuftsin,** a phagocytosis-promoting serum tetrapeptide that is cleaved from an immunoglobulin-like molecule, leukokinin, in the spleen. Tuftsin also is absent in asplenic individuals. Tuftsin-deficient patients have severe systemic infections with *C. albicans, S. aureus,* and *S. pneumoniae.*
8. **Leukocyte adhesion deficiency** is another rare immunodeficiency disorder. It is characterized by recurrent bacterial and mycotic infections and impaired wound healing.
   a. Immunologic features
   (1) Patients' leukocytes have defects of adhesion to endothelial surfaces and to each other (aggregation), as well as poor chemotactic and phagocytic activities.
   (2) The leukocytes lack membrane proteins that are important in adhesion of leukocytes to other cells of the body [e.g., leukocyte function–associated antigen-1 (LFA-1, also identified as CD11a)].

      (3) There is also depressed cytotoxicity mediated by neutrophils, NK cells, and T lymphocytes.

    b. Treatment. This involves the use of antimicrobials appropriate for the infectious agent.

III. B CELL DEFICIENCY DISORDERS (Table 11-2)

  A. Bruton's X-linked hypogammaglobulinemia manifests as recurrent bacterial infections that do not induce immunoglobulin synthesis. Cellular immunity is normal in these patients.

    1. Clinical features. Infections (e.g., sinusitis, pneumonia, meningitis) caused by organisms such as *Streptococcus, Haemophilus, Staphylococcus,* and *Pseudomonas* begin when the infant is 5 to 9 months of age.

    2. Immunologic findings include:
      a. Low serum levels of all classes of immunoglobulins
      b. Lack of circulating B cells
      c. Lack of germinal centers and plasma cells in lymph nodes
      d. Absent or hypoplastic tonsils and Peyer's patches
      e. Intact T cell functions

Table 11-2. Key Features of Selected B Cell and T Cell Immunodeficiency Diseases

Disease	Cellular Defect	Functions Affected
B cell disorders		
X-linked agammaglobuline-mia	Pre-B cell maturation	All antibodies
Common variable hypogam-maglobulinemia	B cell maturation	Various antibodies
Transient hypogammaglobu-linemia of infancy	Unknown; Th cell maturation in some patients	IgG, IgA
Selective IgM deficiency	Th cell maturation	IgM
Selective IgA deficiency	IgA B cell maturation	IgA
Secretory component deficiency	Mucosal epithelial cell	sIgA
T cell disorders		
DiGeorge syndrome	Dysmorphogenesis of third and fourth pharyngeal pouches	T cells
Chronic mucocutaneous candidiasis	No T cell receptor for *Candida* antigens	T cells
Bare lymphocyte syndrome	No class II MHC antigen on T cells	T cells
Combined B and T cell disorders		
SCID		
X-linked form	T cell maturation	T cells and antibody
Autosomal recessive form	T and B cell maturation	T cells and antibody
ADA deficiency	Toxic metabolite accumulation	T cells and antibody
PNP deficiency	Toxic metabolite accumulation	T cells and antibody
Nezelof's syndrome	Unknown	T cells and antibody
Reticular dysgenesis	Hematopoietic stem cell maturation	T cells and antibody
Immunodeficiency associated with other defects		
Ataxia–telangiectasia	B and T cells; suspected defect in DNA repair	T cells and antibody [with abnormal gait (ataxia), vascular malformations (telangiectasia)]
Wiskott-Aldrich syndrome	Glycosylation of membrane proteins	T cells and antibody (with thrombocytopenia and eczema)

ADA = adenosine deaminase; MHC = major histocompatibility complex; PNP = purine nucleotide phosphorylase; SCID = severe combined immunodeficiency disease; sIgA = secretory IgA; Th = helper T cell.

3. Immunogenetic features
   a. The genetic defect has been mapped to the long arm of the X chromosome.
   b. The disease is presumably due to a block in the maturation of pre-B cells into lymphocytes with surface IgM.
      (1) The protein product of the gene has not been identified, but it appears to be involved in light (L) chain gene rearrangement or expression (see Chapter 3 IV B 3).
      (2) Patients' pre-B cell V/D/J rearrangement and μ chain production are normal (see Chapter 3 IV B 4).
4. Treatment consists of intramuscular or intravenous injections of pooled human gamma globulin, usually administered monthly. Fresh frozen plasma may also be used. Obviously, avoidance of infection and use of appropriate antibiotics are also essential.

B. Transient hypogammaglobulinemia of infancy results when the onset of immunoglobulin synthesis, particularly IgG synthesis, is delayed beyond the norm. The cause is unknown but may be associated with a temporary deficiency of helper T (Th) cells.

1. Clinical and immunologic features
   a. Most infants go through a period of hypogammaglobulinemia between the fifth and sixth months of life. Many normal children experience recurrent respiratory infections.
   b. A few infants will have a developmental delay in the ability to synthesize IgG.
      (1) Infants with this disorder suffer recurrent pyogenic gram-positive infections of, for example, the skin, meninges, or respiratory tract.
      (2) The situation cures itself, usually by 16 to 30 months of age.

2. Treatment involves administering antibiotics, gamma globulin, or both.

C. Common variable hypogammaglobulinemia (acquired hypogammaglobulinemia) resembles Bruton's disease (see III A) except that symptoms (e.g., repeated sinopulmonary infections) first appear when the patient is 20 to 30 years of age.

1. Immunologic findings. The disorder is characterized by a high incidence of autoimmune disease.
   a. Although the number of circulating B cells is normal, the ability to synthesize or secrete immunoglobulin is defective, and serum levels of immunoglobulins are low.
      (1) The defect may be due to a population of Ts cells that suppress B cell maturation.
      (2) Alternatively, there may be a defect in Th lymphocyte triggering of the B cells.
   b. Cell-mediated immune functions are usually intact, but they may be defective in some patients.

2. Treatment is the same as that for Bruton's disease.

D. Selective immunoglobulin deficiency (dysgammaglobulinemia) describes a decrease in the serum level of one or more immunoglobulins, but not all immunoglobulins, with normal or increased levels of the others.

1. Clinical features
   a. Selective IgA deficiency, which affects about 1 in 700 individuals of Caucasian descent, is both the most common form of this disorder and the most common primary immunodeficiency.
   b. Clinical findings include recurrent sinopulmonary infection, gastrointestinal disease, autoimmune disease, malignancy, and allergy. However, many individuals may be asymptomatic.

2. Immunologic findings
   a. Serum levels of IgA are low, but levels of IgG and IgM are normal or increased.
   b. IgA-bearing B cells are present in normal numbers, but they are defective in their ability to synthesize or release IgA, possibly due to the presence of hyperactive Ts cells or excessive numbers of Ts cells.

3. Treatment consists of appropriate antibiotics. Gamma globulin should not be administered, since it might stimulate the formation of antibodies to IgA, which could trigger an anaphylactic transfusion reaction.

IV. T CELL DEFICIENCY DISORDERS (see Table 11-2)

A. **DiGeorge syndrome** is the eponymic name for **congenital thymic hypoplasia,** a disorder due to embryonic maldevelopment.

1. **Etiology**
   a. DiGeorge syndrome is due to faulty development of the third and fourth pharyngeal pouches during embryogenesis, with resulting absence or hypoplasia of both the thymus and parathyroid glands.
   b. The basis for the developmental abnormality is not known. Some cases are associated with maternal alcoholism, and there appears to be an autosomal inheritance pattern in others.

2. **Clinical features**
   a. Thymus aplasia (or hypoplasia) results in cellular immunodeficiency with profoundly impaired T cell function, as manifested by recurrent infection with viral, fungal, protozoan, and certain bacterial agents.
   b. Hypoparathyroidism leads to hypocalcemic tetany.
   c. The facial appearance is abnormal, with a fish-shaped mouth and low-set ears.
   d. Cardiac anomalies are usually present.

3. **Immunologic findings**
   a. Lymphocytopenia is usual in these patients. T cells [i.e., erythrocyte-rosetting (E-rosetting) cells and cells that respond to phytohemagglutinin (PHA)] are diminished in number.
   b. Delayed hypersensitivity reactions and the ability to reject allografts are impaired.
   c. Most patients have normal immunoglobulin levels. However, in some patients the levels of circulating antibody are low, at least to certain antigens, due to low numbers of Th cells.

4. **Treatment**
   a. Transplantation of a thymus from an aborted fetus can result in permanent reversal of the syndrome, with the production of functioning T cells. The fetus should not be older than 14 weeks' gestation to avoid graft-versus-host (GVH) disease.
   b. Hypocalcemia can be controlled by administration of calcium and vitamin D.
   c. Most patients improve with age, even without a thymus transplant, and are relatively normal by the age of 5 or 6. Probably, extrathymic sites serve as areas for T cell maturation, or typical thymic and parathyroid tissues develop ectopically.

B. **Chronic mucocutaneous candidiasis** is a syndrome of skin and mucous membrane infection with *C. albicans*. It is associated with a unique defect in T cell immunity.

1. **Immunologic findings**
   a. The total lymphocyte count appears to be normal, and the presence of T cells is confirmed through their response to PHA and E-rosette tests.
   b. However, the T cells show an impaired ability to produce macrophage migration-inhibiting factor (MIF) in response to *Candida* antigen, although their response to other antigens may be normal. Likewise, the delayed hypersensitivity skin reaction to *Candida* antigen is negative.
   c. The antibody response to *Candida* antigen is normal. Some patients produce autoantibodies associated with idiopathic endocrinopathies.

2. **Treatment.** Attempts at therapy with various antifungal agents and with thymus transplantation have met with varying degrees of success. The patient must be carefully observed for the onset of endocrine dysfunction, particularly Addison's disease, which is the major cause of death.

C. **Bare lymphocyte syndrome** is a recently described form of autosomal recessive immunodeficiency in which the expression of class II major histocompatibility complex (MHC) gene products on the T cell surface is deficient.

1. Class II MHC antigens are required for the presentation of antigen during the induction of an immune response [see Chapter 5 IV E 1 a (1)].

2. The consequence of deficient class II MHC antigen expression is a failure of antigen presentation, with resultant abnormal antibody and cell-mediated immune responses.

V. COMBINED B CELL AND T CELL DEFICIENCY DISORDERS (see Table 11-2)

A. Severe combined immunodeficiency disease is an X-linked recessive or autosomal recessive disease that involves a combined defect in both humoral and cell-mediated immunity. Patients usually die within the first or second year of life from overwhelming microbial infection.

1. Immunologic findings

    a. Classically, SCID is associated with lymphopenia and hypoplasia of the thymus gland, as demonstrated on x-ray.

    b. There is an absence of T cells and an inability to mount a humoral immune response.

    c. The autosomal recessive form of the disease often involves an **enzyme deficit**.

        (1) About 50% of patients with the autosomal recessive form of the disease (about 20% of the total) have a **deficiency of ADA**.

            (a) ADA is widely distributed in mammalian tissues but is particularly abundant in lymphocytes.

            (b) Its deficiency leads to the accumulation of metabolites that are toxic to lymphocytes because they block DNA synthesis.

        (2) Another form of SCID is due to deficiency of **purine nucleotide phosphorylase (PNP),** an enzyme involved in purine catabolism. This defect also leads to the accumulation of metabolites toxic to DNA synthesis.

2. Treatment

    a. Specific antibiotics and gamma globulin are helpful, but successful immunologic reconstitution demands transplantation of histocompatible bone marrow.

    b. Transplantation of fetal liver and thymus has also shown promise.

    c. The ADA-deficiency variant of SCID may be treated with irradiated erythrocytes.

B. Nezelof's syndrome encompasses several disorders which show rather consistent immunologic features. The disorders lack uniformity in their clinical presentation, but all patients are susceptible to recurrent microbial infections of diverse etiology.

1. Immunologic findings

    a. There is a marked deficiency of T cell immunity.

    b. B cell deficiency varies: there may be low, normal, or elevated levels of specific immunoglobulin classes (**dysgammaglobulinemia**). The antibody response to specific antigens is usually low or absent.

2. Treatment. Fetal thymus transplantation or thymic hormone administration has had partial success. Aggressive treatment of infections with specific antibiotics and gamma globulin is useful.

C. Wiskott-Aldrich syndrome comprises a triad of features: thrombocytopenia, which is present at birth; eczema, usually present at the age of 1 year; and recurrent pyogenic infections, starting after 6 months of age.

1. Immunologic findings

    a. The serum IgM level is low, with normal levels of IgG and elevated levels of IgA and IgE; isohemagglutinin levels are low or absent.

    b. B cells are normal in number; the B cell deficit seems to be associated with a failure to make an antibody response to polysaccharide antigens.

    c. T cell immunity is usually intact in the early phases of the disease but wanes as the disease progresses.

2. Treatment involves vigorous use of antibiotics and bone marrow transplantation.

D. Ataxia–telangiectasia is an autosomal recessive disease that involves the nervous, endocrine, and vascular systems.

1. Clinical features

    a. Ataxia–telangiectasia is characterized by uncoordinated muscle movements (**ataxia**) and by dilatation of small blood vessels (**telangiectasis**) that is readily observed in the sclera of the eye.

    b. It first appears in the very young (less than 2 years of age) and is associated with repeated sinopulmonary infections.

2. Immunologic findings
   a. There is selective IgA deficiency, with variable abnormalities affecting other immunoglobulins and, occasionally, an inhibited antibody response to certain antigens.
   b. T cell deficiency is variable.

3. Treatment of sinopulmonary infection with antibiotics is essential. Fetal thymus and bone marrow transplants are of uncertain value.

VI. SECONDARY IMMUNODEFICIENCY.
Several conditions are associated with secondary immunodeficiency, which can lead to an increased susceptibility to opportunistic infection that may be either transient or permanent.

A. Measles and other viral infections can affect the body's defenses in several ways.

   1. They can induce a transient suppression of delayed hypersensitivity. The number of circulating T cells is decreased, and lymphocytic response to antigens and mitogens is reduced. Similar effects may be seen following **measles immunization**.

   2. Viral infections can also adversely affect macrophages (see Chapter 6 Table 6-1).

B. Acquired immune deficiency syndrome (AIDS) is caused by a retrovirus, designated **human immunodeficiency virus (HIV)**.

   1. Clinical features
      a. AIDS is contracted primarily, but not exclusively, by male homosexuals, intravenous drug abusers, individuals who receive transfusions, and infants born of infected mothers.
      b. Patients demonstrate pronounced suppression of the immune system and develop severe, life-threatening opportunistic infections (e.g., with *Pneumocystis, Mycobacterium, Toxoplasma,* or *Candida* species).

   2. Immunologic findings
      a. The virus has a tropism for cells bearing the **CD4 surface marker** (see Chapter 5 III B 2 a).
         (1) This causes a reduction in the level of Th cells (identified by their binding of CD4 antibody).
         (2) The result is a marked lymphopenia and a reversal of the ratio of Th cells to Ts cells (identified by binding with CD8 antibody) to less than 0.5 (the normal Th:Ts ratio is more than 1.5).
      b. T lymphocytes cannot produce the normal amount of IL-2, and the activity of NK cells is reduced.
      c. The response of peripheral blood lymphocytes to PHA and to specific antigens is impaired.
      d. Specific antibody production is also impaired.

   3. Treatment
      a. Zidovudine (azidothymidine, AZT) has been shown to confer significant clinical benefit in all stages of HIV infection.
         (1) AZT interferes with DNA synthesis and blocks viral replication; however, drug-resistant strains are being observed.
         (2) Recently, alpha interferon has been used with AZT with encouraging results.
         (3) Dideoxyinosine (DDI), a nucleoside analog that interferes with DNA synthesis, has recently been approved for use in patients who are unable to tolerate AZT or whose disease progresses with AZT treatment. The value of DDI has not yet been proven.
      b. Drugs that **mimic the CD4 target** show promise, and **recombinant CD4** has been shown to inhibit HIV replication in vitro.
      c. Antimicrobial agents are of value in the management of opportunistic infections and may significantly prolong the life of AIDS patients.

VII. COMPLEMENT DEFICIENCY
(see also Chapter 4 I D 4). Deficiencies of complement components or functions have been associated with increased incidence of infections and autoimmune diseases [e.g., systemic lupus erythematosus (SLE); see Chapter 10 II B].

A. C1 esterase inhibitor (C1 INH) deficiency is linked with **hereditary angioedema,** a disorder that is characterized by transient but recurrent localized edema.

1. The defect leads to uncontrolled C1s activity and resultant production of a kinin that increases capillary permeability.

2. The skin, gastrointestinal tract, and respiratory tract may be affected. Laryngeal edema may be fatal.

B. C1q deficiency is reported to be associated with hypogammaglobulinemia, SCID, and repeated infections. The level of C1q in affected individuals appears to be about 50% of normal.

C. C2 and C4 deficiencies can cause a disorder similar to SLE, possibly due to a failure of complement-dependent mechanisms to eliminate immune complexes.

D. C3 deficiency can result in severe life-threatening infections, particularly with *Neisseria meningitidis* and *S. pneumoniae*. Absence of the C3 component means that the chemotactic fragment C5a will not be generated. C3b will not be deposited on membranes, with resultant impaired opsonization.

E. C5 deficiency leads to increased susceptibility to bacterial infection associated with impaired chemotaxis.

F. C6, C7, and C8 deficiencies can lead to increased susceptibility to meningococcal and gonococcal infections, since complement-mediated lysis is a major control mechanism in immunity to *Neisseria* organisms.

STUDY QUESTIONS

Directions: Each of the numbered items or incomplete statements in this section is followed by answers or by completions of the statement. Select the **one** lettered answer or completion that is **best** in each case.

1. Bruton's hypogammaglobulinemia is indicative of a deficiency of what cell type?

(A) B cell
(B) Macrophage
(C) T cell
(D) Monocyte
(E) Neutrophil

2. Job's syndrome is thought to be due to

(A) a B cell deficit
(B) suppressed IgE production
(C) a defect in macrophage killing
(D) a defect in neutrophil chemotaxis
(E) suppressed IgA production

3. Chronic granulomatous disease (CGD) is due to which of the following immunodeficiency conditions?

(A) Hypocomplementemia
(B) A defect in T cell number
(C) A defect in T cell function
(D) A defect in B cell function
(E) A defect in neutrophil function

4. Transplantation of the thymus gland from an aborted fetus to an immunodeficient neonate has been beneficial in which of the following immunodeficiency disorders?

(A) Chédiak-Higashi syndrome
(B) DiGeorge syndrome
(C) Bruton's hypogammaglobulinemia
(D) Hereditary angioedema

5. A 4-year-old child suffering from repeated infections with staphylococci and streptococci was found to have normal phagocytic function and delayed hypersensitivity responses. Lymph node biopsy would probably reveal

(A) depletion of thymus-dependent regions
(B) intact germinal centers
(C) hyperplastic degeneration
(D) lack of plasma cells

6. All of the following are neutrophil defects that could result in immunodeficiency EXCEPT

(A) impaired chemotaxis
(B) insufficient hexose monophosphate (HMP) shunt (glucose) metabolism
(C) suppression of intracellular killing
(D) abnormal complement levels
(E) defective opsonization

7. Chronic granulomatous disease (CGD) is characterized by all of the following conditions EXCEPT

(A) delayed chemotactic response
(B) recurrent bacterial infections
(C) hepatosplenomegaly
(D) defective oxidative burst by neutrophils
(E) reduced NADPH level

1-A	4-B	7-A
2-D	5-D	
3-E	6-D	

Directions: The group of items in this section consists of lettered options followed by a set of numbered items. For each item, select the **one** lettered option that is most closely associated with it. Each lettered option may be selected once, more than once, or not at all.

Questions 8–12

For each characteristic listed below, select the immunodeficiency disorder that is most closely associated with it.

(A) Acquired immune deficiency syndrome (AIDS)
(B) Common variable hypogammaglobulinemia
(C) C2 deficiency
(D) Ataxia–telangiectasia
(E) Reticular dysgenesis
(F) Bruton's disease
(G) Chronic granulomatous disease (CGD)
(H) DiGeorge syndrome

8. Selective IgA deficiency plus variable T cell deficiency

9. Marked lymphopenia associated with reversal of helper:suppressor T cell (Th:Ts) ratio

10. Clinical features similar to those of systemic lupus erythematosus (SLE)

11. Defective development of all bone marrow stem cells

12. Normal numbers of circulating B cells but defective synthesis or secretion of immunoglobulin

8-D   11-E
9-A   12-B
10-C

ANSWERS AND EXPLANATIONS

1. The answer is A *[III A]*.
Patients with Bruton's hypogammaglobulinemia are deficient in B cells and plasma cells, and hence have low serum levels of all classes of immunoglobulins. T cells and phagocytes are normal in number and function.

2. The answer is D *[II B 5]*.
Job's syndrome (hyper-IgE syndrome) is characterized by "cold" staphylococcal abscesses, chronic eczema, and extremely high serum levels of IgE. It is related to defective neutrophil chemotaxis. The ingestion and killing of microorganisms by neutrophils appear to be normal.

3. The answer is E *[II B 1]*.
Chronic granulomatous disease (CGD) reflects an inability of neutrophils to respond to phagocytosis with the normal oxidative burst; apparently it is due to a reduction in intracellular reduced nicotinamide-adenine dinucleotide phosphate (NADPH). There is also decreased superoxide anion production due to a defect in cytochrome b. The result is suppression of intracellular killing of ingested microorganisms. B cell, T cell, and natural killer (NK) cell functions, as well as complement levels, are generally normal. The mortality rate can be reduced considerably by early diagnosis and aggressive therapy.

4. The answer is B *[IV A 4 a]*.
Patients with DiGeorge syndrome (congenital thymic hypoplasia) are markedly deficient in thymic tissue due to faulty development of the third and fourth pharyngeal pouches during embryogenesis. This results in profoundly impaired T cell numbers. Treatment via fetal thymus transplantation can result in permanent reversal and the production of functioning T cells.

5. The answer is D *[III A 2 c]*.
The child described in the question probably has Bruton's X-linked hypogammaglobulinemia, which manifests as recurrent infections with such organisms as staphylococci and streptococci and is associated with a B cell deficiency. Features of the disease include lack of germinal centers and plasma cells in lymph nodes, low serum levels of immunoglobulins, intact T cell and phagocytic function, and absent or hypoplastic tonsils and Peyer's patches.

6. The answer is D *[II B 1 a (5)]*.
In qualitative immunodeficiency disorders affecting phagocytes, the serum levels and functions of B cells, T cells, and complement are generally normal. Neutrophil immunodeficiency could be due to a defect in any of the processes involved in neutrophil protective action. A defect in chemotaxis could cause immune deficiency by blocking the ability of phagocytes to migrate to the site of inflammation. A defect in opsonization, in phagocytosis, or in degranulation of the lysosome would also constitute defective neutrophil function. If hexose monophosphate (HMP) shunt activity is insufficient, there would not be the energy in the cell required for chemotaxis or for new membrane synthesis, which is an essential part of phagocytosis. Intracellular killing defects could be due to the absence of enzymes which are needed for killing, or to the absence of oxygen-dependent or oxygen-independent microbicidal activities.

7. The answer is A *[II B 1]*.
In chronic granulomatous disease (CGD), chemotactic responses are normal. CGD is an immunodeficiency syndrome with onset in the first 2 years of life; it is inherited primarily as an X-linked trait. Characteristics include recurrent bacterial infections, hepatosplenomegaly, lymphadenopathy, and granuloma formation, which appears to reflect faulty phagocytosis. Neutrophils fail to respond to phagocytosis with the normal oxidative burst, apparently because of a reduction in the level of intracellular reduced nicotinamide-adenine dinucleotide (NADH) or its phosphate (NADPH).

8–12. The answers are: 8-D *[V D]*, **9-A** *[VI C]*, **10-C** *[VII C]*, **11-E** *[II A 1 a (3)]*, **12-B** *[III C]*.
Immune deficits in ataxia–telangiectasia include variable T cell deficiency, selective IgA deficiency with variable abnormalities in other immunoglobulins, and an occasional inhibited antibody response to certain antigens. Ataxia–telangiectasia is an inherited immune deficiency characterized by uncoordinated muscle movements (ataxia) and dilatated small blood vessels in the sclera of the eye (telangiectasia).

Acquired immune deficiency syndrome (AIDS) is caused by a retrovirus, human immunodeficiency virus (HIV), which causes a marked reduction in helper T (Th) cells and a marked reversal of the helper: suppressor cell (Th:Ts) ratio to less than 0.5 (normally it is greater than 1.5). This leads to pronounced suppression of the immune system, with resultant susceptibility to opportunistic infections.

A deficiency in complement component C2 may manifest itself as a disorder similar to systemic lupus erythematosus (SLE), possibly due to failure of complement-dependent mechanisms to eliminate immune complexes.

Reticular dysgenesis, an inherited defect, results from defective development of all bone marrow stem cells, including myeloid precursors.

In common variable hypogammaglobulinemia, levels of circulating B cells are normal, but the ability to synthesize or to secrete immunoglobulin is defective. The defect may be due to a population of suppressor T (Ts) cells that suppress B cell maturation.

12
Transplantation Genetics and Immunology

$5)25$

I. INTRODUCTION

A. Types of grafts

1. **Syngrafts,** or **isografts,** involve the transfer of normal tissue between **genetically identical (syngeneic) individuals;** that is, between identical twins or animals of the same inbred line.

2. **Autografts** are grafts removed from and placed in the **same individual.**

3. **Allografts,** or **homografts,** involve the transfer of normal tissue between **allogeneic individuals;** that is, between genetically different **individuals of the same species.**

4. **Heterografts,** or **xenografts,** also called **xenogeneic grafts,** involve the transfer of tissue between **animals of two different species.**

B. Outcome

1. Generally, **isografts** and **autografts** survive for an indefinite period of time.

2. **Allogeneic** and **xenogeneic grafts** result in an immune rejection phenomenon of a lesser or greater degree, which may or may not be prevented or aborted by the use of immunosuppressive agents.

C. Organ transplantation in humans. The National Institutes of Health, in September 1990, reported the following statistics.

1. **Incidence**
   a. In 1988, more than 10,000 patients had organ transplants (Table 12-1).
   b. The demand for transplants far exceeds the number of organs available for transplantation. In mid-1989, more than 18,000 patients were awaiting transplant organs.

2. **Importance of kidney transplants**
   a. Kidneys are the organs most frequently transplanted (see Table 12-1).
   b. In 1987, nearly 158,000 Medicare patients had end-stage renal disease, for which the only available treatment alternatives are maintenance dialysis or a kidney transplant.

II. HISTOCOMPATIBILITY GENE COMPLEX

A. Characteristics of histocompatibility antigens

1. The **histocompatibility antigens** (synonymous with **transplantation antigens**) are antigens on tissues or cell surfaces that determine the compatibility or incompatibility of transplanted tissue.

2. It is these antigens that induce the immune response in the host that may cause the rejection of transplanted tissue.

3. The most important histocompatibility antigens are products of genes of the **major histocompatibility complex (MHC).**
   a. These antigens are termed **human leukocyte antigens (HLA)** because they are found in high concentrations on lymphocytes and other white blood cells.
   b. They also occur on other nucleated cells of the body (e.g., macrophages and hepatocytes).

Table 12-1. Incidence of Selected Organ Transplants, United States, 1988

Organ	Number of Transplants	Number of People Awaiting Transplants
Kidney	7278	15,721
Heart	1647	1227
Lung	31	77
Heart/lung	74	231
Liver	1680	734
Pancreas	243	298
Bone marrow	~2000	*

*Not available.
From *Report of the NIAID Task Force on Immunology and Allergy.* NIH Publication No. 91-2414. Washington DC, U.S. Public Health Service, National Institutes of Health, September 1990, p. 70.

    4. The **ABO antigens** of the red blood cell system also act as strong transplantation antigens. The compatibility of the red blood cell system cannot be violated with the expectation of graft survival.

    5. Minor histocompatibility antigens, such as those coded for on the Y chromosome, are infrequently the cause of graft rejection.

B. The major histocompatibility complex and histocompatibility genes

    1. The MHC is a closely linked complex of genes that govern the production of the major histocompatibility antigens.
      a. In **mice** this complex, termed **H-2,** is found on chromosome 17.
      b. In **humans,** the MHC resides on the short arm of chromosome 6. A portion of the MHC codes for the HLA histocompatibility antigens (Figure 12-1).

    2. A population varies considerably in its histocompatibility makeup because of the **multiplicity of HLA molecules.**
      a. Seven groups of HLA antigens are presently recognized.
        (1) HLA-A, HLA-B, and **HLA-C** are encoded by the HLA-A, B, and C loci of the MHC complex (see Figure 12-1).
        (2) HLA-DR, HLA-DQ, and **HLA-DP** are encoded by genes in three subregions (DR, DQ, and DP) of the HLA-D region of the MHC complex (see Figure 12-1).
        (3) In addition, there are some **HLA-D** antigens that are not the product of specific gene clusters; rather, they are the result of gene mixing between antigens encoded by the three major D subregion loci.
      b. There are also **three minor subregions** in the D region, termed **HLA-DX, HLA-DN** (formerly DZ), and **HLA-DO.**
        (1) HLA-DX has two loci coding for α and β chains.
        (2) DN and **DO** lie between the DP and DQ loci in the MHC complex. DN and DO each contain a single genetic locus; the functions of their gene products are not known at this time, and they are considered **pseudogenes.**
      c. Most of the HLA genes are highly **polymorphic;** that is, **multiple alleles** occur at a single HLA locus.
        (1) At present, locus HLA-A has 24 recognized alleles; loci DR, C, DQ, and DP have 20, 11, 9, and 6, respectively; and locus B has 52. There are also 26 possible D antigens. Thus, the number of potential antigen combinations in the population is astronomical (at least 24 x 20 x 11 x 9 x 6 x 52 x 26).
        (2) In the HLA-D subregions, especially HLA-DR, many of the HLA molecules have two or three functional β-chain genes (but only one α chain).
          (a) This allows a single cell to express more than two allelic forms of each DR molecule.
          (b) Additional variants are formed as hybrids of the α chain of one allele and the β chain of the other allele within an HLA-DR locus. Such hybridization leads to the formation of the HLA-D molecules [see II B 2 a (3)].
      d. The HLA genes are **codominant** in expression.
        (1) When an individual is heterozygous for a particular HLA locus (as in Figure 12-2, case B locus B), both alleles at that locus will be expressed. Therefore, in the heterozygote, both antigens encoded by these alleles are present on the tissue cells.

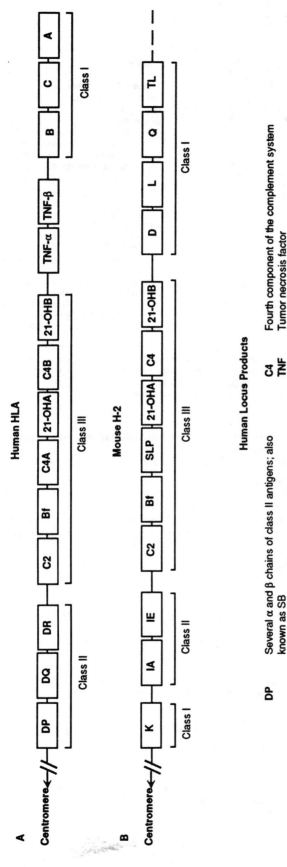

Human HLA

A

Centromere ← // — DP — DQ — DR — C2 — Bf — C4A — 21-OHA — C4B — 21-OHB — TNF-α — TNF-β — B — C — A

Class II | Class III | Class I

Mouse H-2

B

Centromere ← // — K — IA — IE — C2 — Bf — SLP — 21-OHA — C4 — 21-OHB — D — L — Q — TL — — —

Class I | Class II | Class III | Class I

Human Locus Products

DP	Several α and β chains of class II antigens; also known as SB
DQ	Several α and β chains of class II antigens; homologous to mouse IA
DR	Several α and β chains of class II antigens; homologous to mouse IE
21-OH	21-Hydroxylases of cytochrome P-450 system
Bf	Factor B of the complement system
C2	Second component of the complement system
C4	Fourth component of the complement system
TNF	Tumor necrosis factor
B	1 of ~ 50 allelic class I polypeptides; homologous to mouse H-2D
C	1 of ~ 8 allelic class I polypeptides; homologous to mouse H-2L
A	1 of > 20 allelic class I polypeptides; homologous to mouse H-2K

Figure 12-1. (A) Schematic map of the major histocompatibility gene complex (MHC) in humans and the gene products associated with each locus. The immune response (Ir)-associated genes are located in the HLA-D region, which contains the DP, DQ, and DR loci. There is not a single locus for each component, but rather there are clusters of several loci encoding the α and β chains of each of the class II antigens (see Figure 12-3). Genes for tumor necrosis factor (TNF) are between the class III and class I genes. (B) Map of the mouse H-2 region. Note the close homology with the human MHC. The Q and TL genes are, respectively, loci for antigens expressed on thymocytes and some lymph node cells, and a series of antigens expressed also on thymocytes and certain thymic leukemias. The class II region (IA–IE) contains several loci for Ir genes as well as loci controlling the mixed lymphocyte culture response and immune-associated (Ia) antigens. The murine SLP (sex-limited protein) encodes for a C4 protein in mouse serum. In both maps, the sizes of the genetic loci and the distances between loci are not drawn to scale.

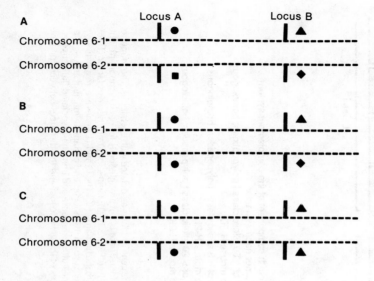

Figure 12-2. Schematic representation of codominant alleles. In the HLA complex on chromosome 6, each gene is codominant in expression; that is, in an individual having different alleles at corresponding loci of the two chromosomes, both alleles are expressed. ●, ■, ▲, ◆ represent HLA antigens expressed by each locus on both chromosomes. In case (A), four different antigens are expressed (● ■ ▲ ◆); in case (B), three antigens (● ▲ ◆) are expressed; and in case (C), two antigens are expressed (● ▲). The haplotype is the set of alleles present on a single chromosome; thus, in case (A) the haplotype of chromosome 6-1 is ● ▲ and the haplotype of chromosome 6-2 is ■ ◆. The ● ▲ haplotype is also found in chromosome 6-1 in case (B) and in both chromosomes in case (C).

(2) By contrast, in a homozygous individual, the alleles of the locus on both chromosomes are identical (as in Figure 12-2, case B locus A), and only one HLA antigen is specified.

(3) Usually, one individual will express a dozen or more different DR, DQ, and DP gene products per cell. This greatly expands the population of molecules that can act as epitope presenters in the process of MHC restriction (see II C 4 a).

C. MHC class I and class II antigens

1. **Classification.** The HLA molecules encoded by genes of the MHC fall into **two classes**.
   a. **HLA-A, HLA-B,** and **HLA-C** are **class I** antigens.
   b. **HLA-D, HLA-DP, HLA-DQ,** and **HLA-DR** antigens are **class II** antigens.

2. **Location.** Both class I and class II antigens are surface components of the cell.
   a. Class I antigens are found on all nucleated human cells and on platelets. (In the mouse the corresponding H-2 MHC antigens are also present on erythrocytes.)
   b. The class II antigens are found chiefly on the surfaces of immunocompetent cells, including macrophages, monocytes, resting T cells (in low amounts), activated T cells, and, particularly, B cells.

3. **Structure.** Class I and class II antigens are each composed of two polypeptide chains, α and β, held together by noncovalent bonds (Figure 12-3). The chains are 90% protein and 10% carbohydrate.
   a. **Class I antigens**
      (1) The α **chain** (44 kDa) has three domains, carries the antigenic specificity, and is anchored in the cell membrane.
      (2) The β **chain** (12 kDa) is a β_2-microglobulin (i.e., it is a small protein that migrates with the beta globulins in serum electrophoresis). It is not encoded by the MHC, it is not polymorphic, and it does not have a transmembrane region.
   b. **Class II antigens**
      (1) The α chain (34 kDa) and the β chain (29 kDa) each consist of two extracellular domains (α_1, α_2, and β_1, β_2, respectively), a connecting peptide, a transmembrane region, and a tail that lies within the cell cytoplasm.
      (2) Both chains are encoded in closely linked HLA-D region gene clusters.
      (3) Most of the HLA epitopes (i.e., the antigenic determinant regions) are found in the β chain.

4. **Functions**
   a. Both class I and class II MHC molecules are important in **controlling immunologic responses,** in a process known as **MHC restriction** (see Chapter 5 IV D, E, F 3).
      (1) The class II antigens have a role in **antigen presentation** by macrophages to many T cells and in T cell interaction with B cells.

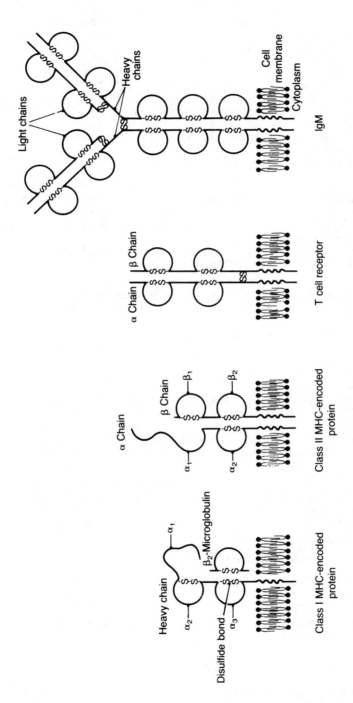

Figure 12-3. Molecular structures of the class I and class II proteins encoded by the major histocompatibility complex (MHC), the T cell receptor, and the monomeric immunoglobulin molecule. Note the structural similarity; the molecules also share similar sequences of amino acids. The molecules are characterized by loops (domains) made up of about 70 amino acids within each chain. (Adapted with permission from Marrack P, Kappler J: The T cell and its receptor. *Sci Am* 254:36–45, 1986.)

(2) Both class I and class II MHC antigens are involved in the **sensitization phase** of **cell-mediated cytotoxicity** (also called **cell-mediated cytolysis,** or **CMC**), which is mediated by **cytotoxic T (Tc) lymphocytes.**

    (a) Class I and class II antigens are both present on the antigen-presenting cell.

        (i) Class I antigens react with the CD8 molecule on the Tc cell precursor.

        (ii) Class II antigens react with the CD4 molecule on the helper T (Th) cell, thereby ensuring the presence of lymphokines that will enhance the proliferation and maturation of the Tc cell precursor.

    (b) Class I antigens are involved in MHC restriction of cell-mediated cytotoxicity primarily in the case of virus-infected cells [see Chapter 5 IV E 2 e (3)].

(3) MHC restriction is not found in hyperacute graft rejection nor in some antitumor processes, both of which are mediated by antibodies. It is also absent from the **effector phase** of acute and chronic graft rejection (see III E 2 c).

b. In addition to their regulatory role, class I and class II MHC antigens can serve as **targets of the immune response.**

    (1) In **cell-mediated cytotoxicity,** HLA alloantigens are targets recognized by Tc cells.

    (2) Therefore, they serve as important target antigens in **graft rejection.**

        (a) Class I HLA-A and HLA-B antigens and class II HLA-DR antigens are designated as **major transplantation antigens** because they are among the principal antigens recognized by the host during the process of graft rejection.

        (b) The cell-mediated cytotoxicity assay (see Chapter 8 IV C 2 d) is an in vitro correlate of graft rejection.

    (3) Class II antigens are thought to be the antigens principally responsible for the **graft-versus-host (GVH) reaction** (see III H 3).

5. Identification

a. The **mixed lymphocyte reaction** (see III C 3 and Chapter 8 C 2 c) is often used to identify and define **class II antigens.** The mixed lymphocyte reaction is an in vitro correlate of the GVH reaction.

b. The **lymphocytotoxicity test** (see III C 2) can identify **both class I and class II antigens.**

c. DR-encoded class II antigens can also be identified by serologic assays.

D. Other types of MHC molecules

1. Class III antigens

a. Some loci on chromosome 6 are associated with certain complement components (C2, C4, and factor B of the alternative pathway), with tumor necrosis factors α and β (TNF-α and TNF-β), and with two hydroxylase enzymes. (Figure 12-1 shows the location of the genes that encode these proteins.) These gene products are known as class III MHC antigens.

b. Class III antigens do not participate in MHC restriction or graft rejection.

2. Immune response (Ir) genes

a. Specific Ir genes are found in the MHC of inbred lines of animals, indicating that the response to particular antigens is genetically controlled. Thus, strain 2 guinea pigs and the F-1 hybrid respond to phenylated poly-L-lysine (DNP-PLL), whereas strain 13 does not.

b. In humans these genes occur in the HLA-D region and encode the DR, DP, and DQ antigens (class II antigens).

E. Diseases associated with MHC alleles

1. Many diseases have been found to have a statistical association with molecules of the MHC. For example, several autoimmune diseases, such as systemic lupus erythematosus (SLE), occur more frequently in individuals with the HLA-DR3 antigen (Table 12-2).

2. Most HLA-associated diseases are connected to haplotypes of HLA-B and HLA-D subregions (particularly DR and DQ).

III. CLINICAL TRANSPLANTATION IMMUNOLOGY

A. Overview of the donor–recipient workup. The compatibility of donor and recipient must be determined before a transplantation procedure, in order to optimize graft survival and minimize the likelihood of a rejection reaction.

1. First, **ABO blood group compatibility** is established (see III B 3).

Table 12-2. Association between HLA-DR Alleles and Selected Autoimmune Diseases

Disease	HLA Antigen	Relative Risk[*]
Multiple sclerosis	DR3	4.0
Systemic lupus erythematosus (SLE)	DR2	3.0
SLE	DR3	3.0
Myasthenia gravis	DR3	3.0
Rheumatoid arthritis	DR4	6.0
Hashimoto's thyroiditis	DR5	3.0

[*]Increase in risk for Caucasian individuals who bear the antigen as opposed to those who do not (e.g., a DR2-positive individual is four times more likely to develop multiple sclerosis than someone who is DR2-negative).

    2. Tissue typing to identify **histocompatibility (HLA) antigens** is then performed (see III C).

    3. Cross-matching is used to test the recipient's serum for **preformed antibodies** against the donor's HLA antigens (see III D).

    4. When the recipient's serum does not kill donor lymphocytes (as when the donor–recipient pair are HLA-identical siblings), the mixed lymphocyte reaction (see III C 3) may be used to determine if the donor cells stimulate blastogenesis in the recipient's lymphocytes.

B. Blood group antigens

    1. General considerations

        a. These very strong cell-surface antigens are found on many other tissues of the body as well as on the surface of red blood cells, and they represent very potent transplantation antigens because antibodies (**isohemagglutinins**) against the blood group antigens occur naturally in humans (see Table 12-3).

        b. Therefore, the donor's and the recipient's blood group must be established before a transplantation procedure as well as before a transfusion (see Chapter 9 III C 1 a).

    2. The four blood groups

        a. The four antigenic phenotypes (blood groups) of the ABO system are **A, B, AB,** and **O** (Table 12-3).

        b. The various phenotypes are determined by different **allelic combinations**. The ABO gene has three alleles, **A, B,** and **O; A** and **B** are dominant over O.

           (1) People in blood groups A or B can be either homozygous (AA, BB) or heterozygous (AO, BO).

           (2) Those in blood group O are homozygous (OO).

           (3) Those in blood group AB are heterozygous (AB).

    3. Tests for ABO blood group compatibility. Both recipient's and donor's blood types are established by agglutination tests.

        a. Red blood cells are tested with standard anti-A and anti-B antisera.

        b. The presence of preformed antibodies (anti-A or anti-B isohemagglutinins) is determined by assays employing standard A and B cells.

    4. Genetics of the ABO blood group system. The ABO antigens are under the influence of four loci, **ABO, H, Le** (for Lewis), and **Se** (for secretor).

        a. The **A and B alleles** control the formation of transferase enzymes that add specific monosaccharide units to an existing oligosaccharide core; A transferase adds N-acetyl-galactosamine, and B transferase adds galactose.

Table 12-3. ABO Blood Group Genetics and Occurrence

Phenotype	Genotype	Isohemagglutinin Present	Occurrence of Phenotype (%)[*]
A	AA or AO	Anti-B	40
B	BB or BO	Anti-A	10
O	OO	Both	45
AB	AB	Neither	5

[*]Figures represent percentage of United States population.

   b. The **H antigen** (so called because it is a heterophile antigen) is the oligosaccharide core that functions as the precursor to the A and B antigens. The H gene codes for an enzyme that is involved in the synthesis of the oligosaccharide core.
   c. The **O allele** is not a true gene, as it codes for no product. O cells do have the H antigen, however.
   d. The **Le gene,** like the H gene, segregates independently from A, B, and O. The Le gene codes for the Le antigen. This antigen appears to be a precursor of the H antigen.
   e. The **Se gene** is present in individuals who secrete the ABO blood group antigens. In most people, the ABO antigens are found in soluble form in body secretions such as saliva and urine, and in the serum. About 25% of the population are nonsecretors.

C. Histocompatibility testing

   1. **Sources of cells and typing sera**
      a. The best **cells** for detecting HLA antigens are lymphocytes obtained from the peripheral blood and from lymph nodes, spleen, or thymus. These cells are used because of their availability and because they have the highest concentration of HLA antigens on the cell surface.
      b. The **typing sera** used in the lymphocytotoxicity assay come from several sources:
         (1) Multiparous women
            (a) During pregnancy, fetal lymphoid cells can cross the placenta into the mother's circulation.
            (b) The fetal antigens that are derived from the father's genetic contribution will be foreign to the mother and will sensitize her, much like Rh sensitization (see Chapter 9 III C 1 b), although no fetal disease has been associated with HLA sensitization.
         (2) Patients who have received multiple transfusions: the white blood cells and platelets in the transfused blood provide the sensitizing antigens
         (3) Volunteers who have been sensitized by blood transfusions, white blood cell inoculations, or tissue grafts
         (4) Patients who have rejected a transplanted kidney

   2. **The lymphocytotoxicity test.** This test can identify both class I and class II antigens.
      a. Purified lymphocytes to be tested are incubated with a battery of antisera of known HLA specificity. If a test antiserum contains an antibody to one of the HLA antigens on the cell, the antibody will bind to the cell membrane.
      b. Complement is then added, and incubation is continued. If the cell has antibody bound to its membrane, it will be killed by complement activation.
      c. Trypan blue or eosin is then added, which is specifically taken up into damaged or dying cells.
      d. Because dead cells are stained, while live cells do not take up the dye, it can be demonstrated whether a particular test serum–complement combination is cytotoxic for the lymphocytes; thus, the HLA antigens on a cell can be determined by noting which antiserum caused cell lysis.

   3. **The mixed lymphocyte reaction (MLR; blastogenesis assay)**
      a. This assay uses DNA synthesis to detect the incompatibility of class II antigens—those dictated by HLA-D region genes. Over 60 antigens are encoded by this region, and all can be detected by mixed lymphocyte reactions.
      b. The test is a mitotic response of T cells to HLA antigens.
         (1) Lymphocytes are stimulated to divide (i.e., to undergo mitosis) when they interact with antigens such as HLA molecules on the membranes of other cells.
         (2) Small lymphocytes are transformed into blast cells in response to interaction with foreign HLA antigens.
         (3) To identify any HLA-D antigen, it is necessary to use lymphocytes that are sensitized to the antigen in question.
      c. **Procedure**
         (1) If the lymphocytes from a donor and a recipient are mixed in tissue culture, both sets of lymphocytes will undergo blastogenesis and proliferate if they are histoincompatible (a **two-way** test).
         (2) The mixed lymphocyte reaction is usually done in a **one-way procedure** (i.e., only one of the cell populations in the mixture can respond).

(a) Donor lymphocyte division is prevented by irradiating the cells or treating them with mitomycin C, which cross-links DNA. Thus, the donor cells cannot undergo blast transformation but can still act as stimulating cells.

(b) The recipient's cells will still undergo blastogenesis if there is HLA-D region incompatibility. Histocompatibility varies inversely with the number of blast cells produced.

d. If there are several potential donor–recipient pairs or several donors, the donor chosen should have lymphocytes that stimulate the recipient the **least**.

D. Cross-matching

1. The recipient's serum may have **preformed antibodies** against the donor's HLA antigens as a result of multiple blood transfusions, an earlier transplantation, or multiple pregnancies.

2. Cross-matching may be performed by complement-dependent lymphocytotoxicity (see III C 2), using the donor's lymphocytes as targets for the recipient's preformed antibodies.

    a. Samples of the patient's serum are collected over a period of time. All of the serum samples must be cross-matched against the donor's lymphocytes because the antibody titer may change over time and thus may be detectable in only one serum sample.

    b. If even one cross-matching kills the donor's lymphocytes, transplantation is not performed.

E. Host response to transplantation

1. Graft survival rates

    a. When kidney transplants come from HLA-identical siblings, the transplants have a 5-year survival rate of more than 80%.

    b. When two HLA antigens match, the graft survival rate is 70%.

    c. When more than two antigens are mismatched, the chances for graft survival are considerably lower.

    d. When kidney transplants come from cadavers, regardless of matching, the 5-year survival rate is 33% to 50%, although these figures are improving due to better patient management practices and the use of new immunosuppressive drugs.

2. Rejection reactions

    a. Types of reactions. At least three types of rejection reactions can take place following transplantation.

      (1) Hyperacute rejection. This rejection pattern may occur when the donor and recipient have not been matched for ABO blood group antigens or when the recipient has preformed antibodies to other donor antigens.

        (a) As soon as the vascular supplies between the recipient and the donor organ are linked, the antibodies start attacking the organ; they may sensitize donor cells to complement-mediated lysis or to destruction by phagocytic cells.

        (b) In certain cases, the organ will fail to show any blood flow. There is a rapid vascular spasm and vascular occlusion, and the organ will never be perfused by the recipient's blood.

      (2) Acute or accelerated rejection. Acute rejection is believed to be due to sensitized T lymphocytes.

        (a) This type of reaction occurs 10 to 30 days after transplantation. Since the recipient has not been previously sensitized, it takes time to develop sensitized lymphocytes, which then increase in number and attack the graft. This is the typical picture of a cell-mediated immune response.

        (b) The graft (especially around small blood vessels) is infiltrated with small lymphocytes and mononuclear cells, along with some granulocytes, causing destruction of the transplanted tissue.

        (c) If an antigenically identical graft is made in this sensitized recipient, it will undergo very rapid rejection, an event referred to as the **second-set phenomenon,** which is really an example of the anamnestic response.

      (3) Chronic rejection. This may be a cellular immune response, an antibody response, or a combination of the two.

        (a) In chronic rejection, there is a slow loss of tissue function over a period of months or years.

        (b) The antigens that evoke chronic rejection may be weak antigens of the HLA system or antigens in minor histocompatibility loci such as those on the Y chromosome.

b. Non–MHC restriction. The initial recognition of allogeneic (nonself) cells—that is, the recipient's immunologic recognition of the donor's cells—is **not** MHC restricted.
   (1) T lymphocytes can react with foreign HLA antigens without the necessity for presentation of the antigen in association with self class I MHC molecules.
   (2) This phenomenon, termed **alloreactivity,** is a reflection of the T lymphocytes' innate ability to recognize foreign MHC molecules.
      (a) These are the cells stimulated in the mixed lymphocyte reaction.
      (b) Alloreactive CD8$^+$ Tc cells are stimulated by target cells that bear class I MHC molecules.
      (c) Alloreactive CD4$^+$ Th cells are stimulated by target cells bearing class II MHC molecules.
   (3) If this alloreactivity did not exist, and rejection were MHC restricted, the mixed lymphocyte reaction would not take place. It has been estimated that as high as 10% of circulating T lymphocytes can react with any given allograft antigen.
c. MHC restriction may play a role in the **induction** of antigraft antibodies and Tc cells. Hence, MHC restriction contributes to graft rejection. However, the expression (or attack) phase of Tc activity must occur in the absence of self MHC molecules on the target cell. In fact, if the target cell were self, there would be no reaction against it.

F. Creation of immunologic tolerance and enhancement. These are established in the recipient in order to reduce the risk of graft rejection. Most of the procedures involved are experimental and have not yet found their way to human medicine.

1. **Development of immune tolerance**
   a. Tolerance to foreign histocompatibility antigens can be induced in fetal animals by injecting tissue containing these foreign antigens (see Chapter 6 III B 2).
   b. Tolerance may be induced in human transplantation recipients by large-volume transfusions of the donor's blood prior to the transplantation procedure.
   c. Immunologic tolerance, or, at least, graft-specific immunosuppression, may be the result of either:
      (1) Suppressor T (Ts) cell development
      (2) Th cell depletion
      (3) Terminal (exhaustive) differentiation of either B cells or precursors of Tc cells

2. **Immunologic enhancement**
   a. In contrast to immunologic tolerance, immunologic enhancement prolongs graft survival by means of specific antibodies, either passively administered or induced by immunization.
   b. These **graft-specific antibodies** interfere with the destructive action of Tc cells.
   c. The antibodies are most likely growth-promoting (as opposed to cytotoxic) immunoglobulins, particularly IgA or IgG4 antibodies that are **not complement-fixing**.

G. Postoperative immunosuppressive therapy

1. **General principles**
   a. All transplant recipients require immunosuppressive therapy, which is directed primarily at blocking the induction or expression of cell-mediated immunity.
   b. The only **exception** to the need for immunosuppressive therapy is the case in which the donor and recipient are **identical twins**.

2. **Immunosuppressive drugs.** These agents and their mechanisms of action are discussed more fully in Chapter 6 II B.
   a. **Corticosteroids** are used for maintenance therapy or are given in a bolus at the time of a rejection crisis.
      (1) They are anti-inflammatory and also reduce the number of circulating lymphocytes.
      (2) Another action of corticosteroids is to interfere with the production of lymphokines, thus blocking the expansion of the immune response to the graft.
   b. **Antimetabolites** and **alkylating agents** exert their immunosuppressive effects by interfering with DNA and RNA function. This in turn causes death of rapidly dividing cells such as lymphocytes, particularly those undergoing immunologic induction.
      (1) **Azathioprine** is a commonly used antimetabolite. In the body, azathioprine is converted to the purine analog mercaptopurine.

    (2) Cyclophosphamide, a cyclized nitrogen mustard, is a popular alkylating agent.

  c. Cyclosporine (cyclosporin A), a cyclic peptide antibiotic produced by various fungi, is very effective in inhibiting the T cell component of the rejection process.

    (1) Cyclosporine binds to the active site of **cyclophilin,** a cellular enzyme that catalyzes the correct folding of proteins, and inhibits the transcription of the interleukin-2 (IL-2) gene.

    (2) In addition, cyclosporine blocks the secretion of **gamma interferon,** a lymphokine. This effect is important to graft survival because gamma interferon has several **anti-graft properties**:

      (a) It increases the expression of MHC (target) antigens on graft tissues.

      (b) It activates macrophages which participate in the rejection process.

    (3) Recently, **FK-506,** a macrolide antibiotic, has been shown to be a potent immunosuppressant that acts synergistically with cyclosporine to block T cell responses.

      (a) FK-506 blocks the transcription of genes for interleukins 2, 3, and 4, for gamma interferon, and for tumor necrosis factor.

      (b) It is currently undergoing clinical trials.

  d. Antibody preparations. Antilymphocyte globulin and **antithymocyte globulin** are capable of destroying human T cells by sensitizing them to phagocytosis or complement-mediated lysis.

    (1) These antisera are used most frequently as prophylaxis, given postoperatively for about 2 weeks to block the induction of graft sensitization.

    (2) They are also used in many centers in the management of acute rejection episodes.

3. Problems of postoperative management

  a. With the use of high doses of immunosuppressive drugs, **infection** often occurs. About 25% of the deaths that occur in kidney transplantations are due to sepsis.

  b. About 6% of all transplant patients develop a **malignancy.**

    (1) Some are common malignancies, such as carcinoma of the skin; however, about one-half of the malignancies are lymphomas or reticuloendothelial cell sarcomas.

    (2) This excessive susceptibility to malignancy may be explained by a drug-induced impairment in immunosurveillance (see Chapter 13 III B).

      (a) Ordinarily, the immune system is policing the body for mutated cancerous cells.

      (b) When the immune system is suppressed, these cells are allowed to escape and proliferate.

H. Special graft situations

1. Privileged tissues

  a. Types of privileged tissues. Immunologically privileged tissues are tissues from different anatomic locations that are not rejected no matter where they are transplanted.

    (1) Included among these tissues are **bone, cartilage, tendon,** and sections of **major blood vessels**. These tissues are probably "privileged" due to their low content of HLA antigens.

    (2) The **fetus** can also be considered privileged tissue, although the mechanisms for its survival are complex and ill-defined. In addition, the womb may represent a privileged site (see III H 2).

  b. Nonvascularized tissue as privileged tissue. The use of nonvascularized tissue as the graft ordinarily eliminates immune rejection.

    (1) For example, the **cornea** can restore vision when transplanted under acceptable surgical conditions and when the vascular bed is not damaged.

    (2) However, if the cornea is placed in vascularized tissue or if trauma at the transplantation site causes inflammation and vascularization, the grafted cornea is rejected.

2. Privileged sites

  a. Certain areas such as the **brain** and the **anterior chamber of the eye** (and the **cheek pouch** of hamsters) are regarded as privileged sites. These sites tolerate grafting without sensitization of the recipient.

  b. This is most likely due to the dearth or complete lack of lymphatic drainage in surrounding tissues.

3. Graft-versus-host disease
   a. Etiology and pathogenesis
      (1) GVH reactions are an expression of T cell function. When an **immunologically competent graft** is transplanted into an **immunologically compromised host,** the graft tissue can mount an immunologic attack on the recipient. This is termed **graft rejection of the host**.
      (2) The problem occurs when there is an antigenic difference between the donor and the immunologically compromised recipient.
   b. Tissues affected
      (1) GVH disease is a major factor in limiting allogeneic **bone marrow transplantation** in humans.
      (2) It can also involve grafts of the skin, alimentary tract, and liver if the engrafted tissue contains immunocompetent T cells.
      (3) It is not a consideration with heart or kidney transplantation.
   c. Clinical features. GVH disease is characterized by liver abnormalities, a measles-like skin rash, diarrhea, wasting, and death.
   d. GVH disease in bone marrow transplantation
      (1) GVH disease follows a bone marrow transplant when the recipient possesses specific histocompatibility antigens that are not present in the immunologically competent donor.
      (2) In this case, the transplanted bone marrow contains immunologically competent lymphocytes that become sensitized to the recipient's antigens and mount an immunologic attack.
      (3) Therefore, bone marrow transplantation should only be done between people who are histocompatible—preferably between histoidentical siblings.
      (4) If the T cells are removed from the bone marrow before bone marrow engraftment, for example, by use of antithymocyte serum plus complement, the incidence and severity of GVH disease can be markedly reduced.
      (5) Vigorous immunosuppression is employed in bone marrow recipients at the first sign of GVH.

STUDY QUESTIONS

Directions: Each of the numbered items or incomplete statements in this section is followed by answers or by completions of the statement. Select the **one** lettered answer or completion that is **best** in each case.

1. Several types of immunologic rejection reactions can occur following organ transplantation. The rejection reaction that is caused by the presence of preformed antibodies in the recipient is referred to as

(A) acute
(B) hyperacute
(C) chronic
(D) immediate
(E) accelerated

2. Class I HLA antigens can be best described as

(A) cell surface proteins that contain HLA-A, HLA-B, and HLA-C determinants
(B) substances involved in macrophage interactions with B cells
(C) complement components
(D) antigens involved in the inductive (sensitization) phase of cell-mediated cytolysis (CMC)
(E) antigens principally responsible for the graft-versus-host (GVH) reaction

3. As compared to T cells, B cell membranes are rich in which of the following types of antigens?

(A) Class I antigens
(B) Class II antigens
(C) Class III antigens
(D) HLA-B antigens
(E) Complement-activating antigens

4. Graft-versus-host (GVH) disease is LEAST likely to occur in which of the following conditions?

(A) Bone marrow transplant from father to daughter
(B) Bone marrow transplant from daughter to mother
(C) Bone marrow transplant from sister to sister
(D) Bone marrow transplant from mother to a daughter with a T cell immunodeficiency
(E) Kidney transplant from father to daughter

5 Antilymphocyte globulin and antithymocyte globulin are effective in suppressing allograft rejection because of their ability to

(A) suppress cell-mediated immunity
(B) suppress humoral immunity
(C) block lymphocyte transformation
(D) react with antigens in the graft
(E) mimic anti-idiotype antibodies induced during graft rejection

6. Efficient T cell–mediated killing of virus-infected cells requires that the T cells and the target cells be identical with respect to

(A) ABO blood group antigens
(B) Rh blood group antigens
(C) class I antigens
(D) class II antigens
(E) class III antigens

7. A test that can be used for typing of class I histocompatibility antigens is

(A) cell-mediated lympholysis (CML)
(B) donor–recipient mixed lymphocyte response
(C) primed lymphocyte typing
(D) mixed lymphocyte response with homozygous typing cells
(E) antibody- and complement-mediated cytotoxicity

8. Donor–recipient compatibility is determined through evaluation of all of the following antigenic systems EXCEPT

(A) class I HLA antigens
(B) class II HLA antigens
(C) class III HLA antigens
(D) ABO blood group
(E) antibodies to donor lymphocytes

1-B	4-E	7-E
2-A	5-A	8-C
3-B	6-C	

9. All of the following are considered to be privileged tissues for grafting EXCEPT the

(A) cornea
(B) bone
(C) bone marrow
(D) cartilage
(E) fetus

10. The β_2-microglobulin component of class I antigens resembles a

(A) light (L) chain
(B) heavy (H) chain
(C) both
(D) neither

11. An antibody response to foreign tissue is suppressed in which of the following phenomena?

(A) Immune tolerance
(B) Immune enhancement
(C) Both
(D) Neither

12. Chronic graft rejection may be caused by

(A) T cells
(B) antibodies
(C) both
(D) neither

ANSWERS AND EXPLANATIONS

1. The answer is B *[III E 2 a (1)]*.
Hyperacute rejection of a transplanted organ occurs when the recipient's preformed antibodies attack the donor organ, causing a rapid vascular spasm and vascular occlusion and lack of organ perfusion by the recipient's blood. This could occur in the case of an ABO blood group mismatch, in which a donor organ containing blood group A or group B antigens is transplanted into a patient who has preformed anti-A antibodies or anti-B antibodies. This eventuality is avoided by blood group matching prior to transplantation. A similar hyperacute rejection reaction can result with HLA antigen mismatch, in which the recipient has preformed antibodies to an HLA antigen in the donor organ.

2. The answer is A *[II C 1 a)]*.
Class I histocompatibility antigens are cell surface membrane proteins that contain HLA-A, HLA-B, or HLA-C determinants. These antigens are involved in the effector phase of cell-mediated cytolysis (CMC) and in graft rejection. In both these processes, class I antigens are the major antigens by which the effector cells, cytotoxic T (Tc) cells, recognize target tissues. Class II antigens are the histocompatibility antigens involved in the presentation of antigen to T cells and B cells by macrophages. By a principle referred to as major histocompatibility complex (MHC) restriction, the macrophage must bear a class II antigen identical to that expressed on the B cell membrane. Class III HLA antigens include, among other substances, complement components C2, C4, and factor B; Class III HLA antigens are not involved in histocompatibility.

3. The answer is B *[II C 2 b]*.
B cell membranes are rich in class II HLA antigens, which also are found in macrophage membranes and in the membranes of activated peripheral blood T cells. Class I HLA antigens, including HLA-B antigens, are found on all lymphocytes and macrophages—in fact, class I antigens are found on all nucleated cells except sperm and trophoblasts. Class III HLA antigens are not involved in histocompatibility but are complement components, specifically C2, C4, and factor B; class III genes also code for tumor necrosis factors α and β (TNF-α and TNF-β) and for cytochrome hydroxylases.

4. The answer is E *[III H 3 b (3)]*.
The kidney contains practically no T lymphocytes, and hence it would not be likely to induce graft-versus-host (GVH) disease. After the organ is removed from the donor, it is perfused to remove all donor blood in its vasculature before its implantation. The bone marrow cannot be similarly purged of donor blood and must instead be treated with antithymocyte serum to remove the immunologically reactive cells.

5. The answer is A *[III G 2 d]*.
Antilymphocyte and antithymocyte globulins destroy T cells, thereby suppressing cell-mediated immunity and thus promoting graft survival. Antilymphocyte serum might also suppress antibody formation. Lymphocyte transformation could actually be triggered by antilymphocyte serum (in the absence of complement) if the serum was directed to the proper membrane component [e.g., to the phytohemagglutinin (PHA) or lipopolysaccharide receptors]. Non–complement-fixing antibodies could react with transplantation antigens and block cytotoxic T (Tc) cell interaction with the grafted tissue.

6. The answer is C *[II C 4 a; Ch 5 IV E 2 e (3) (c)]*.
Class I histocompatibility antigens (i.e., HLA-A, -B, and -C) are involved in cell-mediated immune functions. In cell-mediated cytotoxicity (CMC), the target cell and the cytotoxic T (Tc) cell must be identical with regard to the HLA antigens coded at the A and B loci. The class I antigen in the membrane of the virally infected target cell is recognized as "self" by the CD8 molecule in the membrane of the Tc cell, thus allowing destruction of the altered host cell. This requirement for cellular recognition is known as major histocompatibility complex (MHC) restriction; it is important as it ensures that Tc cells will "home" into infected cells rather than attacking free virus particles that may be at a site distant from the source of the virus (or its antigens). Class II identity is a similar prerequisite for the cellular interactions that occur during the inductive (sensitization) phase of an immune response.

7. The answer is E *[III C 2]*.
Class I antigens are also called serologically defined antigens because they can be identified by serologic tests. Class I antigens are detected by incubating lymphocytes with antisera specific to particular HLA-A, -B, or -C antigens. In the presence of complement the antibody-sensitized cells will be killed and the resultant membrane changes can be detected by the uptake of eosin or trypan blue, both of which are excluded from live cells.

8. The answer is C *[II D 1; III C 2, 3].*
Class III HLA genes code for non-histocompatibility antigens such as C2 and C4 of the complement system. The ABO blood group antigens are significant in the determination of histocompatibility. ABO blood group compatibility must exist between donor and recipient; crossing the blood group barrier compromises graft survival and may lead to hyperacute rejection. Typing of class I and class II HLA antigens must also be performed in the evaluation of donor–recipient compatibility. This is done through cytotoxicity assays, including the lymphocytotoxicity test. In this test, cytotoxic antibodies in serum from a sensitized recipient will react with cell surface antigens on donor lymphocytes, so that the lymphocyte cell membrane disintegrates and the cell dies. The reaction is detectable because dye is specifically taken up by damaged and dying cells. Such a reaction would negate the use of that particular donor. In the blastogenesis assay, which is based on the mixed lymphocyte reaction, lymphocytes from both the prospective donor and the recipient are cultured and observed for reactions. Histocompatibility is assumed to exist if blastogenesis does not occur.

9. The answer is C *[III H 1].*
The cornea, bone, and cartilage are "privileged" tissues: they do not evoke an immune response in a graft recipient. The fetus does not induce an immune response in the mother during pregnancy, although it has been theorized that the induction of labor may be due to an immunologically based rejection episode. Bone marrow transplantation is especially difficult and dangerous due to the high probability of rejection, particularly from graft-versus-host (GVH) disease.

10. The answer is D *[II C 3 a (2); Figure 12-3].*
The β_2-microglobulin component of class I HLA antigens is a nonpolymorphic, 12-kDa protein that does not resemble either the light (L) or the heavy (H) chain of an immunoglobulin molecule. It is not coded for by the HLA complex, which is on chromosome 6; rather, it is determined by a gene on chromosome 15. The entire class I molecule is anchored in the membrane by the α chain.

11. The answer is A *[III F].*
In immunologic tolerance, an immunologically competent host does not react to specific antigens produced by the graft. In such situations, the graft can survive almost indefinitely. In contrast to immunologic tolerance, immunologic enhancement involves antibodies on cells in the graft that block efficient antigen presentation by the graft.

12. The answer is C *[III E 2 a (3)].*
Chronic graft rejection may be due to specific antibody, sensitized cytotoxic T (Tc) cells, or both. Rejection of the graft may be total or may be partial, with recovery of the graft. The antigens involved in chronic graft rejection are usually antigens in minor histocompatibility loci; that is, weak antigens not coded for by the HLA complex.

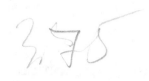

I. INTRODUCTION

A. Terminology

1. **Neoplasms** result from the new growth of cells (**neoplasia**) under conditions that would ordinarily not induce the multiplication of cells and the resultant growth of tissue.
2. Neoplasms are either benign or malignant.
   a. **Benign neoplasms** are characterized by slow growth and restricted anatomic location, and do not usually cause death.
   b. **Malignant neoplasms** may grow slowly or rapidly; they are characterized by **anaplasia** (in which cells lose their differentiating features; that is, they **dedifferentiate**), **invasion** of the body, and **metastatic spread;** and they can result in death.
3. A malignant neoplasm, or malignancy, is often referred to as **cancer** or a **tumor**. Strictly speaking, the term **tumor** refers to the swelling, or increase in tissue mass, that results from neoplasia, and thus could be either benign or malignant.

B. Cellular changes induced by malignancy

1. The progression from a normal cell to one with malignant potential is accompanied by many physiologic changes, such as dedifferentiation, acquisition of the potential for perpetual reproduction (i.e., tumorigenesis), loss of contact inhibition, and increased mitotic rate.
2. In addition, the antigenic composition of the cells is altered.

C. Evidence for an immune response to tumors

1. There is considerable clinical evidence suggesting that the human body responds immunologically to tumors.
   a. **Spontaneous regression** of human tumors (especially in malignant melanoma but also in neuroblastoma and other tumors) has been documented in over 100 published case reports.
   b. Certain tumors demonstrate **long-term indolence**. That is, some tumors grow very slowly or seem to be quiescent until suddenly they metastasize and kill the patient.
   c. The presence of a **mononuclear cell infiltrate** in situ in inflammatory carcinomas correlates with improved survival rates. For example, a person with a breast carcinoma accompanied by an inflammatory response seems to do better than someone whose carcinoma is not associated with an inflammatory process.
   d. Metastatic cells are commonly present in patients with cancer, but the frequency of their implantation and growth is low. Several findings demonstrate this:
      (1) After cancer surgery it is common to detect malignant cells in the blood; however, metastatic implantation is much more rare.
      (2) One can demonstrate malignant cells in regional veins draining a tumor in one-third of the cases; however, this incidence is much higher than the incidence of people with metastatic tumors.
   e. Autologous tumors fail to develop when malignant cells are transplanted from a primary tumor to subcutaneous sites.
   f. Cancer patients readily demonstrate immediate and delayed hypersensitivity to autologous tumor cell extracts in skin reaction tests.

2. Neuroblastoma, a malignancy that begins in utero and expresses itself early in infancy, has been a convenient model for the study of the immune responses of humans to their tumors.

    a. The lymphocytes of children with neuroblastoma are cytotoxic to the cells of this tumor but express no toxicity against normal cells or cells of other tumors.

    b. Lymphocytes from mothers of children with neuroblastoma demonstrate in vitro tumor-specific cytotoxicity toward neuroblastoma tumor cells but not toward other tumor cell types.

    c. In some neuroblastoma cases, both the child and the mother have antibodies that are cytotoxic for the neuroblastoma cells. In other cases of neuroblastoma, the serum does not kill the tumor cells but instead protects them via blocking factors such as antigen–antibody complexes.

II. TUMOR-ASSOCIATED ANTIGENS

A. General considerations

1. A distinct feature of tumor immunology is that the tumor-bearing host is interacting with a source of antigen that is constantly expanding. The quantity of tumor-associated antigen (TAA) increases proportionally with tumor growth and decreases with tumor response to treatment.

2. In addition, the antigenic profile of the cells is altered such that normally occurring antigens may be lost, while new epitopes emerge.

    a. These neoantigens may be found in the nucleus, in the cytoplasm, or as part of the cell membrane.

    b. Some neoantigens are excreted from the cell.

B. Types of tumor-associated antigens

1. TAAs may represent antigens **completely unique** to that particular tumor in that individual. **Carcinogen-induced cancers** are often accompanied by the emergence of completely unique TAAs.

    a. The carcinogen acts as a mutagen.

    b. The tumors induced in different individuals by a single carcinogen will not have similar antigens, as do malignancies of viral etiology, because of the random occurrence of the mutation.

2. More commonly, TAAs will be similar in all individuals carrying a particular tumor; such antigens are termed **tumor-specific antigens (TSAs).**

    a. It is perhaps a misnomer to consider any antigen as specific to a particular tumor type.

    b. However, there are antigens whose occurrence is highly correlated with certain tumors.

3. A subpopulation of TSAs can induce a protective immune response in the host. These are called **tumor-specific transplantation antigens (TSTAs).**

C. Tumor-specific antigens (TSAs). TSAs are found on the cell surface of tumors but are not present on normal cells of the same tissue origin. They may be oncofetal or viral in origin.

1. Oncofetal antigens

    a. General considerations

        (1) Oncofetal antigens are present during normal fetal development but are lost during differentiation of fetal tissue, and they are apparently not synthesized during adult life.

        (2) However, oncofetal antigens may reappear during regeneration of the appropriate tissue (e.g., liver) or as TAAs with the development of malignancy.

        (3) Two of the most widely studied oncofetal antigens are α-fetoprotein (AFP) and carcinoembryonic antigen (CEA).

    b. α-Fetoprotein

        (1) AFP is an alpha globulin that is synthesized and secreted by fetal liver cells.

            (a) It has 40% homology with serum albumin (i.e., 40% of its amino acid sequence matches that of albumin).

            (b) It reaches fetal concentrations of 3 mg/ml.

            (c) It can be detected in cord blood and, occasionally, in the mother's serum.

        (2) AFP is immunosuppressive, which may be important in the induction of neonatal tolerance to antigens. In cell culture, AFP has several effects on T cells.

            (a) It decreases helper T (Th) cell activity.

            (b) It enhances suppressor T (Ts) cell activity.

(3) Most but not all hepatomas secrete large amounts of AFP. However, its presence is not diagnostic of hepatoma, but is merely suggestive, since AFP has also been detected in other conditions.
  (a) AFP has been detected in the serum of patients with prostatic and gastric carcinomas, teratomas, and embryonal carcinoma of the testes.
  (b) It may also be found in certain nonmalignant conditions, such as cirrhosis of the liver and hepatitis.
(4) Monitoring the changes in the AFP content of a cancer patient's serum provides a prognostic index (or marker) after surgery or chemotherapy. For example, a dramatic increase in the serum concentration would signal recurrence of the malignancy.
c. Carcinoembryonic antigen
  (1) CEA is detected in the fetal gut, liver, and pancreas during the second trimester of pregnancy. It is found in low levels in the serum of normal adults.
  (2) CEA is associated with several types of cancer.
    (a) About 70% of patients with carcinoma of the colon have high serum levels of CEA.
    (b) An even higher association (90%) occurs in patients with pancreatic carcinoma.
    (c) CEA has also been detected in significant quantities in cancers of the lung, breast, and prostate.
  (3) CEA also occurs in several nonmalignant states.
    (a) Approximately 15% of heavy smokers have elevated serum CEA levels.
    (b) Serum CEA levels may also be elevated in cirrhosis of the liver and in chronic lung disease.
  (4) As in the case of AFP, the utility of CEA is in its prognostic potential.

2. Virus-induced TSAs
  a. General considerations
    (1) TSAs of viral origin are either viral component proteins or new enzymes induced in the cell to aid in the replication of the virus.
    (2) These viral "fingerprints" form a major part of the evidence linking viruses with human malignancy. However, the etiologic role of viruses is more complex than a simple cause-and-effect relationship, because the same viruses that have been detected in human tumors are also found in noncancerous tissues.
  b. Epstein-Barr virus antigens have been found in the cells of patients with Burkitt's lymphoma and nasopharyngeal carcinoma. These patients have high levels of specific antibodies to EBV antigens, further indicating that Burkitt's lymphoma and nasopharyngeal carcinoma are induced by a viral agent.
  c. Other RNA and DNA viruses (e.g., adenoviruses, papovaviruses, herpesviruses, and retroviruses) may also induce TSAs.

D. Tumor-specific transplantation antigens

  1. TSTAs occur on the membrane of the tumor cell.

  2. An appropriate immune response against these immunogens will favor the control of a malignancy and elimination of the cancer cells from the body.
  a. As a general rule, the cell-mediated immune response is the most efficient tumoricidal mechanism.
  b. Occasionally, cytocidal antibodies are also demonstrable in the host.

  3. Most human tumors of a given histologic type will have at least one TSTA in common.
  a. Thus, the lymphocytes and antibodies from neuroblastoma patient A will react with and try to destroy tumor cells from neuroblastoma patient B but not with other cells from patient B.
  b. They also will not react with tumor cells from patients suffering from other types of malignancies; that is, they have **immunologic specificity**.

III. IMMUNE RESPONSE TO TUMOR ANTIGENS

A. Overview

  1. The interaction between the host and a tumor that it harbors is extremely complex (Figure 13-1).
  a. Because the tumor cells have acquired new antigens, they are recognized by the host as foreign.
  b. The immune response therefore attempts to rid the body of the tumor cells.

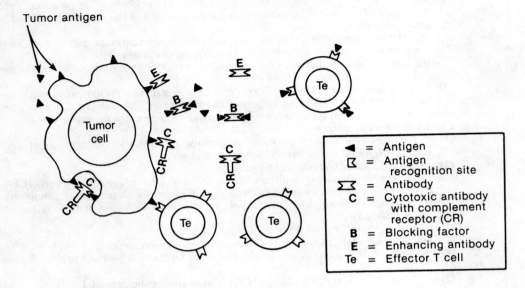

Tumor antigen

◄	= Antigen
ʁ	= Antigen recognition site
⋝⋜	= Antibody
C	= Cytotoxic antibody with complement receptor (CR)
B	= Blocking factor
E	= Enhancing antibody
Te	= Effector T cell

Figure 13-1. Potential host immune responses to tumors: those at the top half of the cell favor tumor growth; those at the bottom are cytotoxic. At the top of the figure, enhancing antibodies react with the tumor cell and protect it from cytotoxic antibodies or cells. Blocking factors and soluble tumor antigen can react with tumor-specific cytotoxic T (Tc) cells and cause premature release of cytotoxic mediators, thus protecting the tumor cell from cell-mediated destruction. At the bottom of the figure are shown the two antitumor cytotoxic reactions mediated by T effector cells (Te cells) and complement-activating antibodies.

    c. However, the tumor produces soluble antigens which tend to neutralize these protective responses.

    d. In addition, some antibodies may actually enhance tumor growth.

  2. The eventual outcome of the encounter is determined by factors that are poorly understood.

B. Immune surveillance and immunologic escape

  1. The realization that tumors are antigenic in the host and that an immune response against the tumor occurs very early in tumorigenesis led to development of the concept of **immune surveillance**.

  2. By this mechanism, the body is continuously purging itself of potentially cancerous cells, which are thought to arise frequently during a person's life span.

  3. Thus, cancer is an escape or bypass of this protective mechanism, and factors that decrease immune capabilities predispose an individual to malignancy.

C. Mechanisms of tumor rejection. Both specific and nonspecific immune responses—humoral and cell-mediated—are believed to be involved in the rejection of a tumor.

  1. Role of T cells. TSTA-specific sensitized T cells constitute the major immunologic barrier against cancer.

    a. Cytotoxic T (Tc) cells appear in response to antigens such as TSAs or viral antigens.

    b. Tc cells can kill tumor cells by direct contact, through the actions of several cytotoxic products (Table 13-1).

  2. Role of B cells. B cell involvement is manifested by the formation of specific **antibodies** that may help rid the body of tumor cells.

    a. The antibody that is formed can react with a tumor cell.

      (1) For example, antibody may play some role in the control of leukemia.

      (2) However, both experimental models and studies in humans demonstrate that antibody is not very effective in causing rejection of tumors, particularly solid tumors.

Table 13-1. Major Cytotoxic Products of Activated Tc Cells and NK Cells

Product	Effect on Tumor Cell
Perforins	Polymerize in the cell membrane to form polyperforin channels that allow cytosol out of and toxic molecules into the cell
Serine proteases	Degrade proteins in cell membrane
TNF-β	Depresses protein synthesis and causes production of toxic free radicals

NK cells = natural kilier cells; Tc cells = cytotoxic T cells; TNF = tumor necrosis factor (there are two: TNF-α and TNF-β; both seem to share some of the same activities).

    b. Complement-dependent cytotoxicity can be mediated by antibodies, particularly **IgM**. When antibody binds to the surface of a tumor cell, this triggers the classic complement pathway (see Chapter 4 II A 2), leading to the eventual destruction of the tumor cell.
    c. Antibody is also important in **antibody-dependent cellular cytoxicity (ADCC),** in which the effector cells are **natural killer (NK) cells**.
    d. The antibodies may also function by "arming" macrophages so that these cells can then react with and destroy the tumor cells (see III C 4 a).

3. Role of null (non-T, non-B) NK cells
    a. NK cells (see Chapter 1 II G 1) participate in the ADCC process.
    b. NK cells recognize malignant cells as targets and do not attack normal cells.
    c. The tumor cells are killed via a direct interaction between the NK cells and the tumor cells, by much the same mechanism as that used by Tc cells.
       (1) NK cells have an Fc receptor on the cell surface [FcγRIII, or CD16; see Chapter 3 II G 1 b (2)]; the antibody involved is IgG1 or IgG3.
       (2) When NK cells encounter a tumor cell that has IgG molecules on its surface, the NK cells will interact with the "sensitized" tumor cell and destroy it via release of cytotoxic molecules (see Table 13-1).
       (3) The ADCC process is independent of complement and requires much less antibody (i.e., several hundred-fold less) than does antibody-mediated complement-dependent cytolysis.
    d. NK cells can also be tumoricidal without prior sensitization by antibody.
    e. It is believed that NK cells are responsible for immune surveillance, the theory holding that malignant transformations occur continually but are prevented from being expressed—perhaps by the NK cells.

4. Role of macrophages. In their normal state, macrophages are not very cytotoxic. However, they can kill tumor cells when activated.
    a. Antibodies to TSAs may bind simultaneously to tumor cells and macrophages, through the antigen-binding site on the former and the FcγRI and FcγRII receptors [see Chapter 3 II G 1 b (2)] on the latter, thus forming a bridge that activates macrophage-mediated cytotoxicity, leading to death of the tumor cell.
    b. In vivo, sensitized T cells are triggered to release a lymphokine called **macrophage-activating factor (MAF)**. MAF interacts with macrophages, changing their metabolism and making them potent killers of tumor cells.
    c. Activated macrophages do not rely on interacting with any specific tumor antigen, but, like NK cells, do seem to distinguish malignant from normal cells.
    d. Macrophages produce many **antitumor products,** including:
       (1) Hydrolytic enzymes that degrade connective tissue and activate several complement components and coagulation factors
       (2) Alpha interferon, which acts indirectly by activating NK cells
       (3) Tumor necrosis factor α (TNF-α, cachectin), a protein that induces other cells to release interleukins 1, 6, and 8 and beta interferon
          (a) Locally, TNF-α increases T cell adhesion to the vascular endothelium and activates these cells to heightened cytotoxicity.
          (b) Systemically, TNF-α causes fever, synthesis of acute-phase proteins (see Table 5-3 footnote), intravascular coagulation, and suppression of hematopoiesis.

(4) Hydrogen peroxide and other **oxidative products** of the glycolysis that accompanies phagocytosis, which can be directly toxic to tumor cells by perturbing the cell membrane

(5) Complement components C1 to C5 and factors B, D, and P (properdin) of the alternative complement pathway, which can play a role in tumor cell lysis and also act as chemotaxins

IV. IMMUNOLOGIC FACTORS FAVORING TUMOR GROWTH

A. Tumor cell attributes often allow a tumor to escape immune destruction.

1. **Tumor heterogeneity** allows tumor survival more substantially than any other immunologic factor.
   a. During its growth, a tumor can change its antigens, its metastatic potential, or virtually any attribute of tumor biology that can be measured.
   b. Part of the reason for the change in antigens is the **antigenic modulation** phenomenon.
      (1) Modulation of tumor antigenicity (antigenic modulation) occurs when antibody to the tumor cell reacts with the appropriate antigens on the tumor cell surface.
      (2) If the antibody is cytotoxic, tumor cells expressing the homologous antigen will be destroyed. This favors the emergence of tumor cells whose membranes have a different antigenic mosaic.
   c. In addition, the tumor can change its antigenic makeup genetically.

2. **Rapid tumor growth** allows a tumor to outstrip the immune response, which is weak and slow by comparison.

3. Tumors release **immunosuppressive factors** such as AFP and prostaglandins. Many of the tumor-inducing viruses studied in animal models are immunosuppressive.

B. Blocking factors also may enhance tumor growth. The serum of cancer patients often contains soluble TSTA or TSTA–antibody complexes, which react with (i.e., "block") the tumor-specific receptors on sensitized T cells, thereby preventing their cytotoxic interaction with tumor cells.

1. **Free soluble tumor antigen**
   a. Ordinarily, free soluble TSTA interacts with the tumor antigen recognition site on the T cell surface. This triggers the cytotoxic activity of the T cell.
   b. However, if the T cell is triggered at a site away from the solid tumor, the lymphokines (e.g., lymphotoxin) will not have an opportunity to act on the tumor cell.
   c. Soluble TSTA can also react with cytotoxic antibody before the latter can attach to the tumor cell and sensitize it to ADCC or complement-mediated killing.
   d. Free tumor antigen also could mask the tumor antigen recognition site and actually not trigger the T cell, which would prevent the T cell from recognizing and attacking the tumor cell.

2. **Tumor-specific immune complexes**
   a. The most potent blocking factors in serum are the tumor-specific immune complexes that appear in the body.
   b. These antigen–antibody complexes act like free tumor antigen, masking the tumor recognition sites of T cells and thus preventing the T cells from recognizing and attacking the tumor cells.
   c. These complexes paralyze the T cells in a state of nonreactivity.

C. Specific antibodies in the serum may protect tumor cells from cell-mediated destruction.

1. This form of blocking is known as **immune enhancement,** and the effector antibodies are known as **enhancing antibodies**.

2. Enhancing antibodies are usually non–complement-fixing antibodies that react with TSTAs in the cell membrane and protect them from a cytotoxic interaction with complement-fixing antibodies, ADCC cells, or Tc cells.

D. Low numbers of Tc cells may result in immunostimulation of tumor growth, perhaps by stimulating cell division via cytokine action without sufficient cytotoxin release.

E. Suppressor cells (Ts cells or macrophages) serve as another mechanism promoting tumor growth.

1. Suppressor T (Ts) cells
  a. For some reason, tumor antigens are more conducive to the activation of Ts cells than to Tc cells.
  b. Ts cells can interact with Tc cell precursors and block their maturation, thus downregulating the immune response.
  c. Ts cells are abundant in tumor patients and may suppress the immune response to the point where it becomes ineffective in eliminating the tumor.

2. Suppressor macrophages
  a. These cells are poorly characterized but, like Ts cells, they appear to depress the T cell system.
  b. Certain immunostimulants [e.g., bacillus Calmette-Guérin (BCG) and *Corynebacterium parvum*] have been found to intensify macrophage-mediated suppression.

F. Immune selection also promotes tumor growth.

1. The immune response to tumor cells will eliminate those cells with the strongest antigen but will not be as effective against cells with lesser concentrations of antigen or with weaker antigens. Thus, the most antigenic cells will be killed off and the least antigenic will survive.

2. In certain cases, metastatic tumors will lack antigen, allowing a phenomenon termed **sneaking through** to occur.
  a. In its initial growth, the tumor only contains a few cells. The immune response to these cells is very small and somehow lags behind the responses necessary to kill the cells.
  b. As more cells appear, the immune response is still deficient and is never able to overcome and control the malignancy.

G. Other factors favoring tumor growth

1. Ontogenic status. The immune response is poorly developed or very weak at certain times of life, especially in the **neonatal period** and in **old age**. Indeed, at these extremes the incidence of malignancy is highest.

2. Immunologic deficiency. This may be hereditary or may be induced by such means as irradiation, infection [e.g., with the human immunodeficiency virus (HIV) that causes acquired immune deficiency syndrome (AIDS)], or immunosuppressive drugs. The incidence of malignancy is greatly increased in immunodeficient individuals.

V. IMMUNOTHERAPY

A. Principles of treating human tumors include the following:

1. Reduction of the tumor "load" by surgery, chemotherapy, or both

2. Modification of tumor cells to enhance their antigenicity and eliminate their viability

3. Activation of the immune response through the use of adjuvants

B. Immunotherapeutic modalities being tried for the treatment of human tumors include the following.

1. Injection of **tumor-specific monoclonal antibodies (MCAs)** that have been **conjugated to tumoricidal substances** such as radionuclides or toxins (e.g., diphtheria toxin or ricin): the MCAs carry the therapeutic agent directly to the tumor, thereby lowering toxicity to normal tissues.

2. Infusion of tumor-infiltrating lymphocytes (TILs; see Chapter 1 II G 4); these are lymphocytes that have been activated in vitro by cocultivation with tumor cells and interleukin-2 (IL-2).
  a. A bit of excised tumor is cultured in the presence of IL-2.
  b. Tumor-specific T cells proliferate and the tumor cells die.
  c. After 4 or 5 weeks in culture the Tc cells ($\sim 10^{11}$ cells) are injected back into the original patient.

3. **Administering macrophage-activating compounds.** Because activated macrophages are such potent killers (see III C 4), there is much interest at the clinical level in treating tumor patients with compounds known to activate macrophages. These include:
   a. **BCG,** the mycobacterial vaccine used to immunize against tuberculosis
   b. **Gamma interferon**
   c. **Muramyl dipeptide,** a synthetic peptide that mimics the action of mycobacteria

C. **Novel bifunctional antibody techniques** have been used to treat tumors successfully in experimental animals.

1. A monoclonal antibody against a TSTA is conjugated to a second monoclonal antibody that reacts with CD3, a surface marker protein on all Tc cells.
   a. The **anti-TSTA antibody** in the heteroduplex reacts with the tumor cell.
   b. The **anti-CD3 antibody** binds Tc cells to the tumor.
   c. The Tc cells are activated to cytotoxicity by aggregation of their CD3 membrane molecules.

2. A variant procedure links anti-TSTA antibody with an antibody that reacts with CD16 (FcγRIII), the Fc receptor for IgG1 and IgG3 [see III C 3 c (1)].
   a. CD16 is found on NK cells, granulocytes, and macrophages.
   b. Thus, cells bearing the TSTA are targeted for killing by these cells, most prominently by the NK cells.

STUDY QUESTIONS

Directions: Each of the numbered items or incomplete statements in this section is followed by answers or by completions of the statement. Select the **one** lettered answer or completion that is **best** in each case.

1. The strongest evidence for the role of the immune system in preventing the establishment of tumors (immune surveillance) is the

(A) hereditary pattern of malignancies
(B) peak incidence of malignancies in the age group 10 to 50 years
(C) rapid transformation of normal cells to malignant cells in vitro where the immune system is not available
(D) markedly increased incidence of malignancies in people with congenital or acquired immune deficiencies
(E) paucity of tumors in the very young

2. When viruses transform cells and cause tumors, new antigens appear in the tumor cells. Which one of the following statements best describes these antigens? They

(A) are found in the plasma membrane, cytoplasm, nucleus, or all of these locations
(B) are oncofetal antigens
(C) are tumor-specific transplantation antigens (TSTAs)
(D) will be a component of the mature virus
(E) will be unique to that tumor in that host

3. A unique tumor-specific antigen (TSA) is found in only a single tumor and is not present in any other tumor, whether of the same or different histologic type. This can best be explained by

(A) a viral etiology
(B) derepression of a fetal antigen
(C) a random mutational event
(D) immunosuppression in the host
(E) faulty immune surveillance in the host

4. All of the following are naturally occurring components of the immune response to malignancies EXCEPT

(A) a heightened general immune responsiveness
(B) specific cellular immunity via lymphocytes
(C) cytotoxic antibodies that destroy tumor cells
(D) enhancing antibodies that interfere with the immunologic attack on tumor cells
(E) modulation of tumor antigenicity

5. Which of the following substances secreted by tumor cells can favor tumor growth?

(A) Antibodies
(B) Interleukin-1 (IL-1)
(C) Muramyl dipeptide
(D) Tumor-specific transplantation antigens (TSTAs)
(E) Tumor necrosis factor (TNF)

6. Human malignancies associated with tumor-specific antigens (TSAs) include all of the following EXCEPT

(A) carcinoma of the colon
(B) neuroblastoma
(C) hepatoma
(D) Burkitt's lymphoma
(E) mammary carcinoma

7. All of the following statements about immunologic factors favoring tumor growth are true EXCEPT

(A) such factors may act by binding to tumor cells and protecting the cells from cytotoxic lymphocytes
(B) they may be composed of TSTA-antibody complexes
(C) they may act by inducing complement-activating antibodies
(D) they may act by binding to immune lymphocytes and neutralizing their action against tumor cells
(E) they may cause a change in the antigenic composition of the tumor

1-D   4-A   7-C
2-A   5-D
3-C   6-E

8. All of the following statements about oncofetal antigens are true EXCEPT that they are

(A) normal components of embryonic and regenerating tissues
(B) prognostic indicators used to follow patients undergoing therapy for certain malignancies
(C) found as membrane components of tumor cells
(D) diagnostic of malignancy
(E) sometimes secreted from cells

9. Prevention of, and recovery from, cancer may involve all of the following factors EXCEPT

(A) natural killer (NK) cells
(B) macrophages
(C) cytotoxic T (Tc) cells
(D) suppressor T (Ts) cells
(E) tumor-specific IgM antibodies

10. Immune responses favoring tumor growth include all of the following factors EXCEPT

(A) immunologic suppression
(B) blocking factors
(C) enhancing antibodies
(D) cellular immunity
(E) soluble tumor antigen

ANSWERS AND EXPLANATIONS

1. The answer is D *[I C; III B].*
Suppression of the immune system, whether congenital or induced by disease [e.g., acquired immune deficiency syndrome (AIDS)], irradiation, or chemotherapy, is associated with a high incidence of infections and malignancies. Neonates and the aged also have an elevated incidence of cancer (when compared to individuals in the 10- to 50-year-old age group), and these people are also somewhat deficient immunologically.

2. The answer is A *[II A 2, C 2].*
Virally induced tumor-associated antigens (TAAs) can occur anywhere in the cell. They are not oncofetal antigens in that they do not occur normally during fetal development. Some virus-induced TAAs are transplantation antigens, but those which occur inside the cell cannot play a role in tumor rejection. Most are components of the virus, but some may be early proteins used in viral synthesis or assembly. Antigens induced by chemical carcinogens are unique to each tumor as they are the result of a specific mutation. By contrast, the immunologic specificity of tumor antigens induced by viruses is controlled by the virus; hence they will be identical if the virus is the same, regardless of the host (or tumor).

3. The answer is C *[II B 1].*
A random mutation would result in a completely unique tumor-specific antigen (TSA). Virally induced tumors share antigens—that is, all tumors caused by a particular virus will have very similar antigens. Derepression of a gene that codes for a protein produced during fetal development would not lead to a unique antigen. Immune surveillance controls the development of malignant neoplasms; it does not control the immunologic specificity of the tumor.

4. The answer is A *[III A, B, C; IV A 1 b].*
As a rule, the development of malignancy is accompanied by a decrease in the immune responsiveness of the individual. Some tumors produce immunosuppressive compounds, such as the prostaglandins, which aid in the tumor's escape from host control. It has also been observed that immunosuppression favors the development of tumors, as evidenced by the increased incidence of cancer in transplant recipients and patients with immunodeficiency diseases.

5. The answer is D *[II D; IV B].*
Tumor-specific transplantation antigens (TSTAs) can interfere with the protective action of cytotoxic cells and complement-fixing antibodies. Antibodies are secreted by plasma cells, not tumor cells. Muramyl dipeptide is a synthetic compound that closely resembles an immunoaugmentor found in the cell wall of many bacteria (it is especially active in mycobacteria); it enhances macrophage activity. Interleukin-1 (IL-1), a monokine, triggers IL-2 production and proliferation of cells in the immune response. Tumor necrosis factor (TNF) is a macrophage product that helps rid the body of tumor cells.

6. The answer is E *[II C 2; II C 1 b, c, 2 b, D 3 a].*
Tumor-specific antigens (TSAs) are found on the cell surface of particular tumors; none has been described for breast cancer. Carcinoembryonic antigen (CEA) is an oncofetal antigen associated with carcinoma of the colon and pancreas. α-Fetoprotein (AFP) is another oncofetal antigen; it is found in fetal tissues and in the serum of most patients with primary carcinoma of the liver (hepatoma). It is also found in patients with prostatic carcinoma and other malignancies, and in those with hepatitis and cirrhosis of the liver. Patients with neuroblastoma usually have lymphocytes that are specifically cytotoxic for cells from their own tumor and from histologically similar tumors in others. This fact implies that these tumors also have specific antigens—in this particular case, a tumor-specific transplantation antigen (TSTA). Patients with Burkitt's lymphoma have high levels of specific antibodies to Epstein-Barr virus antigen, leading many investigators to speculate about the viral origin of this malignant neoplasm.

7. The answer is C *[III A, B, C].*
Activating complement would not be advantageous to the tumor cell. Factors favoring tumor growth can readily be demonstrated in vitro and, unfortunately, are usually effective in vivo as well. Such factors may coat tumor-specific transplantation antigens (TSTAs) and interfere with the antitumor effects of cytotoxic cells such as lymphocytes and macrophages. Similarly, they may compete with complement-fixing antibodies for TSTAs on the cell membrane. If these blocking factors react with cytotoxic cells at a site distant from the tumor, the antitumor action of these cells may be dissipated before it can exert a protective effect.

Chapter 13

8. The answer is D *[II C 1].*
Oncofetal antigens are induced by so many diverse factors (e.g., cigarette smoking) that they have little use in diagnosis: the number of false-positives is too great. Oncofetal antigens are normal components of developing fetal tissues that may reappear later in life as tumor-specific antigens (TSAs). As TSAs, these antigens may be excreted or may be components of the tumor cell itself. Their chief clinical value is as prognostic indicators of relapse after surgical or other therapeutic intervention.

9. The answer is D *[III C; IV E 1].*
Suppressor T (Ts) cells serve to down-regulate the immune response and would enhance tumor growth. IgM antibodies will fix complement, leading to tumor cell lysis. The effector cells of cell-mediated immunity, cytotoxic T (Tc) cells, are the major antitumor component of acquired immunity. Natural killer (NK) cells are responsible for the control of spontaneous mutations that could result in malignancy. They also are the cells of antibody-dependent cellular cytoxicity (ADCC). Like macrophages, NK cells are immune surveillance mechanisms of the body that are present without requiring antigenic exposure. Their antitumor function is enhanced by antibody, but does not require it.

10. The answer is D *[IV A–E].*
Intact cellular immunity, as expressed by the development of competent cytotoxic lymphocytes, acts to control tumor development, as do activated macrophages and cytotoxic (complement-fixing) antibodies. Similarly, suppression of the immune system would promote tumor growth. Enhancing (non–complement-fixing) antibodies and blocking factors [tumor-specific transplantation antigens (TSTAs) or TSTA–antibody complexes] favor tumor growth, as does immunologic anergy (a general depression of immune responsiveness).

Comprehensive
Exam

Introduction

One of the least attractive aspects of pursuing an education is the necessity of being examined on what has been learned. Instructors do not like to prepare tests, and students do not like to take them.

However, students are required to take many examinations during their learning careers, and little if any time is spent acquainting them with the positive aspects of tests and with systematic and successful methods for approaching them. Students perceive tests as punitive and sometimes feel that they are merely opportunities for the instructor to discover what the student has forgotten or has never learned. Students need to view tests as opportunities to display their knowledge and to use them as tools for developing prescriptions for further study and learning.

A brief history and discussion of the National Board of Medical Examiners (NBME) examinations are presented in this introduction, along with ideas concerning psychological preparation for the examinations. Also presented are general considerations and test-taking tips as well as how practice exams can be used as educational tools. (The literature provided by the various examination boards contains detailed information concerning the construction and scoring of specific exams.)

National Board of Medical Examiners Examinations

Before the various NBME exams were developed, each state attempted to license physicians through its own procedures. Differences between the quality and testing procedures of the various state examinations resulted in the refusal of some states to recognize the licensure of physicians licensed in other states. This made it difficult for physicians to move freely from one state to another and produced an uneven quality of medical care in the United States.

To remedy this situation, the various state medical boards decided they would be better served if an outside agency prepared standard exams to be given in all states, allowing each state to meet its own needs and have a common standard by which to judge the educational preparation of individuals applying for licensure.

One misconception concerning these outside agencies is that they are licensing authorities. This is not the case; they are examination boards only. The individual states retain the power to grant and revoke licenses. The examination boards are charged with designing and scoring valid and reliable tests. They are primarily concerned with providing the states with feedback on how examinees have performed and with making suggestions about the interpretation and usefulness of scores. The states use this information as partial fulfillment of qualifications upon which they grant licenses.

The author of this introduction, Michael J. O'Donnell, holds the positions of Assistant Professor of Psychiatry and Director of Biomedical Communications at the University of New Mexico School of Medicine, Albuquerque, New Mexico.

Students should remember that these exams are administered nationwide and, although the general medical information is similar, educational methodologies and faculty areas of expertise differ from institution to institution. It is unrealistic to expect that students will know all the material presented in the exams; they may face questions on the exams in areas that were only superficially covered in their classes. The testing authorities recognize this situation, and their scoring procedures take it into account.

The Exams

The first exam was given in 1916. It was a combination of written, oral, and laboratory tests, and it was administered over a 5-day period. Admission to the exam required proof of completion of medical education and 1 year of internship

In 1922, the examination was changed to a new format and was divided into three parts. Part I, a 3-day essay exam, was given in the basic sciences after 2 years of medical school. Part II, a 2-day exam, was administered shortly before or after graduation, and Part III was taken at the end of the first postgraduate year. To pass both Part I and Part II, a score equalling 75% of the total points available was required.

In 1954, after a 3-year extensive study, the NBME adopted the multiple-choice format. To pass, a statistically computed score of 75 was required, which allowed comparison of test results from year to year. In 1971, this method was changed to one that held the mean constant at a computed score of 500, with a predetermined deviation from the mean to ascertain a passing or failing score. The 1971 changes permitted more sophisticated analysis of test results and allowed schools to compare among individual students within their respective institutions as well as among students nationwide. Feedback to students regarding performance included the reporting of pass or failure along with scores in each of the areas tested.

During the 1980s, the ever-changing field of medicine made it necessary for the NBME to examine once again its evaluation strategies. It was found necessary to develop questions in multidisciplinary areas such as gerontology, health promotion, immunology, and cell and molecular biology. In addition, it was decided that questions should test higher cognitive levels and reasoning skills.

To meet the new goals, many changes have been made in both the form and content of the examination. These changes include reduction in the number of questions to approximately 800 on Parts I and II to allow students more time on each question, with total testing time reduced on Part I from 13 to 12 hours and on Part II from 12.5 to 12 hours. The basic science disciplines are no longer allotted the same number of questions, which permits flexible weighing of the exam areas. Reporting of scores to schools include total scores for individuals and group mean scores for separate discipline areas. Only pass/fail designations and total scores are reported to examinees. There is no longer a provision for the reporting of individual subscores to either the examinees or medical schools. Finally, the question format used in the new exams, now referred to as Comprehensive (Comp) I and II, is predominately multiple-choice, best answer.

The New Format

New question formats, designed specifically for Comp I, are constructed in an effort to test the student's grasp of the sciences basic to medicine in an integrated fashion. The questions are designed to be interdisciplinary. Many of these questions are presented as a vignette, or case study, followed by a series of multiple-choice, best-answer questions.

The scoring of this exam also is altered. Whereas, in the past, the exams were scored on a normal curve, the new exam has a predetermined standard, which must be met in order to pass. The exam no longer concentrates on the trivial; therefore, it has been concluded that there is a common base of information that all medical students should know in order to pass. It is anticipated that a major shift in the pass/fail rate for the nation is unlikely. In the past, the average student could only expect to feel comfortable with half the test and eventually would complete approximately 67% of the questions correctly, to achieve a mean score of 500. Although with the standard setting method it is likely that the mean score will change and become higher, it is unlikely that the pass/fail rates will differ significantly from those in the past. During the first testing in 1991, there will not be differential weighing of the questions. However, in the future, the NBME will be researching methods of weighing questions based on both the time it takes to answer questions vis à vis their difficulty and the perceived importance of the information. In addition, the NBME is attempting to design a method of delivering feedback to the student that will have considerable importance in discovering weaknesses and pinpointing areas for further study in the event that a retake is necessary.

Since many of the proposed changes were implemented in June 1991, specific information regarding actual standards, question emphasis, pass/fail rates, and so forth were unavailable at the time of publication. The publisher will update this section as information becomes available as we attempt to follow the evolution and changes that occur in the area of physician evaluation.

Materials Needed for Test Preparation

In preparation for a test, many students collect far too much study material only to find that they simply do not have the time to go through all of it. They are defeated before they begin because either they cannot get through all the material, leaving areas unstudied, or they race through the material so quickly that they cannot benefit from the activity.

It is generally more efficient for the student to use materials already at hand; that is, class notes, one good outline to cover or strengthen areas not locally stressed and for quick review of the whole topic, and one good text as a reference for looking up complex material needing further explanation.

Also, many students attempt to memorize far too much information, rather than learning and understanding less material and then relying on that learned information to determine the answers to questions at the time of the examination. Relying too heavily on memorized material causes anxiety, and the more anxious students become during a test, the less learned knowledge they are likely to use.

Positive Attitude

A positive attitude and a realistic approach are essential to successful test taking. If concentration is placed on the negative aspects of tests or on the potential for failure, anxiety increases and performance decreases. A negative attitude generally develops if the student concentrates on "I must pass" rather than on "I can pass." "What if I fail?" becomes the major factor motivating the student to **run from failure rather than toward success**. This results from placing too much emphasis on scores rather than understanding that scores have only slight relevance to future professional performance.

The score received is only one aspect of test performance. Test performance also indicates the student's ability to use information during evaluation procedures and reveals how this ability might be used in the future. For example, when a patient enters the physician's office with a problem, the physician begins by asking questions, searching for clues, and seeking diagnostic information. Hypotheses are then developed, which will include several potential causes for the problem. Weighing the probabilities, the physician will begin to discard those hypotheses with the least likelihood of being correct. Good differential diagnosis involves the ability to deal with uncertainty, to reduce potential causes to the smallest number, and to use all learned information in arriving at a conclusion.

This same thought process can and should be used in testing situations. It might be termed **paper-and-pencil differential diagnosis**. In each question with five alternatives, of which one is correct, there are four alternatives that are incorrect. If deductive reasoning is used, as in solving a clinical problem, the choices can be viewed as having possibilities of being correct. The elimination of wrong choices increases the odds that a student will be able to recognize the correct choice. Even if the correct choice does not become evident, the probability of guessing correctly increases. Just as differential diagnosis in a clinical setting can result in a correct diagnosis, eliminating incorrect choices on a test can result in choosing the correct answer.

Answering questions based on what is incorrect is difficult for many students since they have had nearly 20 years experience taking tests with the implied assertion that knowledge can be displayed only by knowing what is correct. It must be remembered, however, that students can display knowledge by knowing something is wrong, just as they can display it by knowing something is right. **Students should begin to think in the present as they expect themselves to think in the future.**

Paper-and-Pencil Differential Diagnosis

The technique used to arrive at the answer to the following question is an example of the paper-and-pencil differential diagnosis approach.

> A recently diagnosed case of hypothyroidism in a 45-year-old man may result in which of the following conditions?
>
> (A) Thyrotoxicosis
> (B) Cretinism
> (C) Myxedema
> (D) Graves' disease
> (E) Hashimoto's thyroiditis

It is presumed that all of the choices presented in the question are plausible and partially correct. If the student begins by breaking the question into parts and trying to discover what the question is attempting to measure, it will be possible to answer the question correctly by using more than memorized charts concerning thyroid problems.

- The question may be testing if the student knows the difference between "hypo" and "hyper" conditions.
- The answer choices may include thyroid problems that are not "hypothyroid" problems.
- It is possible that one or more of the choices are "hypo" but are not "thyroid" problems, that they are some other endocrine problems.
- "Recently diagnosed in a 45-year-old man" indicates that the correct answer is not a congenital childhood problem.
- "May result in" as opposed to "resulting from" suggests that the choices might include a problem that **causes** hypothyroidism rather than **results from** hypothyroidism, as stated.

By applying this kind of reasoning, the student can see that choice **A**, thyroid toxicosis, which is a disorder resulting from an overactive thyroid gland ("hyper") must be eliminated. Another piece of knowledge, that is, Graves' disease is thyroid toxicosis, eliminates choice **D**. Choice **B**, cretinism, is indeed hypothyroidism, but it is a childhood disorder. Therefore, **B** is eliminated. Choice **E** is an inflammation of the thyroid gland—here the clue is the suffix "itis." The reasoning is that thyroiditis, being an inflammation, may **cause** a thyroid problem, perhaps even a hypothyroid problem, but there is no reason for the reverse to be true. Myxedema, choice **C**, is the only choice left and the obvious correct answer.

Preparing for Board Examinations

1. **Study for yourself.** Although some of the material may seem irrelevant, the more you learn now, the less you will have to learn later. Also, do not let the fear of the test rob you of an important part of your education. If you study to learn, the task is less distasteful than studying solely to pass a test.

2. **Review all areas.** You should not be selective by studying perceived weak areas and ignoring perceived strong areas. This is probably the last time you will have the time and the motivation to review **all** of the basic sciences.

3. **Attempt to understand, not just memorize, the material.** Ask yourself: To whom does the material apply? When does it apply? Where does it apply? How does it apply? Understanding the connections among these points allows for longer retention and aids in those situations when guessing strategies may be needed.

4. **Try to anticipate questions that might appear on the test.** Ask yourself how you might construct a question on a specific topic.

5. **Give yourself a couple days of rest before the test.** Studying up to the last moment will increase your anxiety and cause potential confusion.

Taking Board Examinations

1. In the case of NBME exams, be sure to **pace yourself** to use time optimally. Each booklet is designed to take 2 hours. You should check to be sure that you are halfway through the booklet at the end of the first hour. You should use all your allotted time; if you finish too early, you probably did so by moving too quickly through the test.

2. **Read each question and all the alternatives carefully** before you begin to make decisions. Remember the questions contain clues, as do the answer choices. As a physician, you would not make a clinical decision without a complete examination of all the data; the same holds true for answering test questions.

3. **Read the directions for each question set carefully.** You would be amazed at how many students make mistakes in tests simply because they have not paid close attention to the directions.

4. It is not advisable to leave blanks with the intention of coming back to answer the questions later. Because of the way board examinations are constructed, you probably will not pick up any new information that will help you when you come back, and the chances of getting numerically off on your answer sheet are greater than your chances of benefiting by skipping around. If you feel that you must come back to a question, mark the best choice and place a note in the margin. Generally speaking, it is best not to change answers once you have made a decision, unless you have learned new information. Your intuitive reaction and first response are correct more often than changes made out of frustration or anxiety. **Never turn in an answer sheet with blanks.** Scores are based on the number that you get correct; you are not penalized with incorrect choices.

5. **Do not try to answer the questions on a stimulus–response basis.** It generally will not work. Use all of your learned knowledge.

6. **Do not let anxiety destroy your confidence.** If you have prepared conscientiously, you know enough to pass. Use all that you have learned.

7. **Do not try to determine how well you are doing as you proceed.** You will not be able to make an objective assessment, and your anxiety will increase.

8. **Do not expect a feeling of mastery** or anything close to what you are accustomed. Remember, this is a nationally administered exam, not a mastery test.

9. **Do not become frustrated or angry** about what appear to be bad or difficult questions. You simply do not know the answers; you cannot know everything.

Specific Test-Taking Strategies

Read the entire question carefully, regardless of format. Test questions have multiple parts. Concentrate on picking out the pertinent key words that might help you begin to problem solve. Words such as "always," "all," "never," "mostly," "primarily," and so forth play significant roles. In all types of questions, distractors with terms such as "always" or "never" most often are incorrect. Adjectives and adverbs can completely change the meaning of questions—pay close attention to them. Also, medical prefixes and suffixes (e.g., "hypo-," "hyper-," "-ectomy," "-itis") are sometimes at the root of the question. The knowledge and application of everyday English grammar often is the key to dissecting questions.

Multiple-Choice Questions

Read the question and the choices carefully to become familiar with the data as given. Remember, in multiple-choice questions there is one correct answer and there are four distractors, or incorrect answers. (Distractors are plausible and possibly correct or they would not be called distractors.) They are generally correct for part of the question but not for the entire question. Dissecting the question into parts aids in discerning these distractors.

If the correct answer is not immediately evident, begin eliminating the distractors. (Many students feel that they must always start at option A and make a decision before they move to B, thus forcing decisions they are not ready to make.) Your first decisions should be made on those choices you feel the most confident about.

Compare the choices to each part of the question. **To be wrong,** a choice needs to be incorrect for only part of the question. **To be correct,** it must be **totally** correct. If you believe a choice is partially incorrect, tentatively eliminate that choice. Make notes next to the choices regarding tentative decisions. One method is to place a minus sign next to the choices you are certain are incorrect and a plus sign next to those that potentially are correct. Finally, place a zero next to any choice you do not understand or need to come back to for further inspection. Do not feel that you must make final decisions until you have examined all choices carefully.

When you have eliminated as many choices as you can, decide which of those that are left has the highest probability of being correct. Remember to use paper-and-pencil differential diagnosis. Above all, be honest with yourself. If you do not know the answer, eliminate as many choices as possible and choose reasonably.

Vignette-Based Questions

Vignette-based questions are nothing more than normal multiple-choice questions that use the same case, or grouped information, for setting the problem. The NBME has been researching question types that would test the student's grasp of the integrated medical basic sciences in a more cognitively complex fashion than can be accomplished with traditional testing formats. These questions allow the testing of information that is more medically relevant than memorized terminology.

It is important to realize that several questions, although grouped together and referring to one situation or vignette, are independent questions; that is, they are able to stand alone. Your inability to answer one question in a group should have no bearing on your ability to answer subsequent questions.

These are multiple-choice questions, and just as is done with the single best answer questions, you should use the paper-and-pencil differential diagnosis, as was described earlier.

Single Best Answer—Matching Sets

Single best answer—matching sets consist of a list of words or statements followed by several numbered items or statements. Be sure to pay attention to whether the choices can be used more than once, only once, or not at all. Consider each choice individually and carefully. Begin with those with which you are the most familiar. It is important always to break the statements and words into parts, as with all other question formats. **If a choice is only partially correct, then it is incorrect.**

Guessing

Nothing takes the place of a firm knowledge base, but with little information to work with, even after playing paper-and-pencil differential diagnosis, you may find it necessary to guess the correct answer. A few simple rules can help increase your guessing accuracy. Always guess consistently if you have no idea what is correct; that is, after eliminating all that you can, make the choice that agrees with your intuition or choose the option closest to the top of the list that has not been eliminated as a potential answer.

When guessing at questions that present with choices in numerical form, you will often find the choices listed in an ascending or descending order. It is generally not wise to guess the first or last alternative, since these are usually extreme values and are most likely incorrect.

Using the Comprehensive Exam to Learn

All too often, students do not take full advantage of practice exams. There is a tendency to complete the exam, score it, look up the correct answers to those questions missed, and then forget the entire thing.

In fact, great educational benefits can be derived if students would spend more time using practice tests as learning tools. As mentioned earlier, incorrect choices in test questions are plausible and partially correct or they would not fulfill their purpose as distractors. This means that it is just as beneficial to look up the incorrect choices as the correct choices to discover specifically why they are incorrect. In this way, it is possible to learn better test-taking skills as the subtlety of question construction is uncovered.

Additionally, it is advisable to go back and attempt to restructure each question to see if all the choices can be made correct by modifying the question. By doing this, four times as much will be learned. By all means, look up the right answer and explanation. Then, focus on each of the other choices and ask yourself under what conditions they might be correct? For example, the entire thrust of the sample question concerning hypothyroidism could be altered by changing the first few words to read:

> "Hyperthyroidism recently discovered in . . . ."
> "Hypothyroidism prenatally occurring in . . . ."
> "Hypothyroidism resulting from . . . ."

This question can be used to learn and understand thyroid problems in general, not only to memorize answers to specific questions.

In the Comprehensive Exam that follows, every effort has been made to simulate the types of questions and the degree of question difficulty in the various licensure and qualifying exams (i.e., NBME Comp I and FLEX). While taking this exam, the student should attempt to create the testing conditions that might be experienced during actual testing situations.

Summary

Ideally, examinations are designed to determine how much information students have learned and how that information is used in the successful completion of the examination. Students will be successful if these suggestions are followed:

- Develop a positive attitude and maintain that attitude.
- Be realistic in determining the amount of material you attempt to master and in the score you hope to obtain.
- Read the directions for each type of question and the questions themselves closely and follow the directions carefully.
- Guess intelligently and consistently when guessing strategies must be used.
- Bring the paper-and-pencil differential diagnosis approach to each question in the examination.
- Use the test as an opportunity to display your knowledge and as a tool for developing prescriptions for further study and learning.

NBME examinations are not easy. They may be almost impossible for those who have unrealistic expectations or for those who allow misinformation concerning the exams to produce anxiety out of proportion to the task at hand. They are manageable if they are approached with a positive attitude and with consistent use of all the information the student has learned.

Michael J. O'Donnell

QUESTIONS

Directions: Each of the numbered items or incomplete statements in this section is followed by answers or by completions of the statement. Select the **one** lettered answer or completion that is **best** in each case.

1. A graft exchanged between brother and sister is called a

(A) xenograft
(B) isograft
(C) autograft
(D) allograft
(E) heterograft

Questions 2 and 3

An 18-year-old woman from a socially deprived background is admitted to the hospital in labor. On admission, she indicates that her pregnancy has been apparently normal despite her receiving essentially no prenatal care. Although she admits to having been sexually promiscuous, she has not observed the occurrence of a lesion suggestive of syphilis. Shortly after admission, she gives birth to an apparently healthy male infant.

2. At delivery, the procedure of choice for determining the presence of venereal disease in the mother would be a

(A) Coombs (antiglobulin) test
(B) flocculation test
(C) toxin–antitoxin reaction
(D) cell lysis test
(E) precipitation reaction

3. The mother's serum was positive for a diagnosis of syphilis. Although the infant remained asymptomatic, it was decided to monitor him carefully for possible congenital syphilis by testing his serum levels of

(A) IgA
(B) IgD
(C) IgE
(D) IgG
(E) IgM

4. Adjuvants are nonspecific substances that are sometimes used to

(A) enhance the immune response
(B) induce immune tolerance
(C) block mast cell release of histamine
(D) increase chemotaxis by neutrophils
(E) induce interferon production by fibroblasts

5. The receptor for complement component C3b on the macrophage is

(A) CR1
(B) CR2
(C) CR3
(D) CR4
(E) CR5

6. The HLA serologic typing on a particular family is as follows:

Father HLA-A10, A29, B5, B17, DR2, DR3
Mother HLA-A3, A10, B7, B44, DR2, DR4
Sib 1 HLA-A3, A10, B5, B7, DR2, DR4
Sib 2 HLA-A10, -, B5, B44, DR2, -

If sib 1 received a kidney from sib 2, what specific anti-HLA antibodies would sib 1 probably produce?

(A) anti-HLA-A3, B7, DR4
(B) anti-HLA-B44
(C) anti-HLA-A10, DR4
(D) anti-HLA-A10, B5, B44, DR2
(E) anti-HLA-A10, B5, DR2

7. Lymphokines play a mediator role in which of the following hypersensitivity disorders?

(A) Delayed hypersensitivity
(B) Serum sickness
(C) Atopy
(D) Hemolytic disease of the newborn
(E) Anaphylaxis

1-D   4-A   7-A
2-B   5-A
3-E   6-B

8. Unique amino acid sequences located in the variable (V) region of immunoglobulin molecules and associated with the antigen-binding capability of the molecule are called

(A) allotypes
(B) subclasses
(C) idiotypes
(D) domains
(E) isotypes

9. The test used to detect the presence of circulating nonagglutinating antibody is the

(A) liquid-phase radioimmunoassay (RIA)
(B) indirect Coombs test
(C) Rose-Waaler test
(D) Schick test
(E) complement fixation test

Question 10

The director of the hospital radioimmunoassay (RIA) laboratory needs an antiserum that will react specifically with gentamicin. He suggests the following protocol for production of the antiserum:

• Intramuscular injection of a rabbit with 5 mg of gentamicin dissolved in sterile physiologic saline
• Repetition of the injection 10 days later
• Bleeding the rabbit 10 days after the second injection
• Repetition of the three procedures listed above until a satisfactory immune response is obtained

10. The immunologist's recommendation to the laboratory director should include all of the following EXCEPT to

(A) chemically conjugate the antibiotic to a carrier molecule before injection
(B) use human erythrocytes as the test vehicle
(C) increase the number of animals
(D) adjust the route of administration and the dosage of the antibiotic
(E) culture lymphocytes from the immunized rabbit and obtain monoclonal antibodies

11. The most important antigenic system that must be evaluated for organ allotransplantation in humans is

(A) Rh
(B) ABO
(C) Gm
(D) HLA
(E) H-2

12. Although T cell and B cell membranes contain some shared receptors, only the B cell membrane has a receptor for

(A) bacterial lipopolysaccharide
(B) pokeweed mitogen
(C) phytohemagglutinin (PHA)
(D) sheep red blood cells (SRBCs)
(E) complement component C1q

13. Which of the following statements concerning a patient with an allergy to penicillin is true?

(A) He has produced T suppressor (Ts) cells that interfere with the antibiotic's action
(B) He has mast cells with IgE antibodies that are specific for the penicilloic acid moiety of the antibiotic molecule
(C) He has mast cells with IgD antibodies to the β-lactam ring portion of the penicillin molecule
(D) He can be treated with cephalosporin antibiotics
(E) He has mast cells with IgG antibodies to the β-lactam ring portion of the penicillin molecule

14. Immunopotentiating compounds that act as antigen depots include

(A) muramyl dipeptide
(B) polynucleotides
(C) aluminum hydroxide
(D) gamma interferon
(E) lipopolysaccharide

8-C	11-B	14-C
9-B	12-A	
10-E	13-B	

15. Recurrent pyogenic infections, defective processing of polysaccharide antigens, a T cell deficit, elevated levels of IgA and IgE, and depressed levels of IgM are characteristics of

(A) acquired immune deficiency syndrome (AIDS)
(B) chronic mucocutaneous candidiasis
(C) severe combined immunodeficiency (SCID)
(D) common variable hypogammaglobulinemia
(E) Wiskott-Aldrich syndrome

16. Bacterial products that enhance the immune response include

(A) interleukin-2 (IL-2)
(B) immunogenic RNA
(C) transfer factor
(D) endotoxin
(E) endogenous pyrogen

17. The diversity gene region, D, is present in

(A) δ domain DNA
(B) heavy (H) chain genes
(C) light (L) chain genes
(D) λ domain DNA
(E) κ domain DNA

18. In transfusion reactions that occur due to extravascular hemolysis of red blood cells, the hemolytic reaction almost invariably involves

(A) IgE
(B) complement
(C) anti-A antibodies
(D) anti-B antibodies
(E) anti-Rh antibodies

19. The delicate balance between effective chemotherapy and iatrogenic (physician-induced) disease is well exemplified in the treatment of human malignancies, where many of the therapeutic agents used to arrest the growth of the cancer cells will also cause

(A) hepatotoxic manifestations
(B) aplastic anemia
(C) immunosuppression
(D) drug allergies
(E) autoimmune diseases

20. DPT vaccine is used to induce protection against

(A) typhoid
(B) whooping cough
(C) dengue
(D) tularemia
(E) typhus

21. In bone marrow transplantation it is sometimes unfortunately true that the graft was a success but the patient died. This is because

(A) immunosuppressive therapy destroys both donor and recipient tissue
(B) the grafted tissue is accepted but not functional
(C) the grafted tissue contains mainly immature cells which fail to differentiate in the recipient
(D) the grafted cells attack the alimentary tract, skin, and liver of the recipient
(E) antibodies bearing the allotype of the donor attack the recipient cells

22. Class I major histocompatibility complex (MHC) restriction applies in which of the following types of interactions?

(A) Helper T (Th) cell–B cell interactions during the induction of antibody synthesis
(B) Th cell–macrophage interactions during the induction of antibody synthesis
(C) Cytotoxic T (Tc) cell–complement interactions during killing of virally infected cells
(D) Tc cell–target cell interactions during killing of virally infected cells

23. Epinephrine is valuable in the management of atopy through its ability to block mediator release by

(A) inhibiting phosphodiesterase
(B) inhibiting production of histamine
(C) inhibiting slow-reacting substance of anaphylaxis (SRS-A)
(D) stimulating production of adenylate cyclase
(E) stimulating release of lymphokines

15-E	18-E	21-D
16-D	19-C	22-D
17-B	20-B	23-D

24. Treatment of the IgG monomer with papain splits it into

(A) one F(ab')$_2$ fragment and one Fc fragment
(B) two Fab fragments and one Fc fragment
(C) two Fd fragments
(D) two Fc fragments
(E) one F(ab')$_2$ and two Fc fragments

25. Neuroblastoma is a malignancy that occurs predominantly in infants. Facts about the host response to neuroblastoma that suggest protective immune responses to malignancy include which of the following?

(A) The patient's lymphocytes are cytotoxic for that patient's neuroblastoma cells
(B) The patient's lymphocytes are cytotoxic for another patient's melanoma cells
(C) The fathers of patients commonly have lymphocytes that are cytotoxic for neuroblastoma cells
(D) The patient's serum protects the patient's tumor cells from cytotoxic lymphocytes
(E) The patient's serum is cytotoxic for another patient's normal red blood cells

26. In a child with severe combined immunodeficiency disease (SCID), the most important complication of treatment by bone marrow transplantation is

(A) malignant transformation of the transplanted cells
(B) failure to develop isohemagglutinins
(C) graft-versus-host (GVH) reaction
(D) rejection of the transplanted tissue
(E) lack of mature B cells in the bone marrow graft

27. The major antibody in immune globulin is

(A) IgA
(B) IgD
(C) IgE
(D) IgG
(E) IgM

28. The immunity that vaccines induce is

(A) active artificially acquired immunity
(B) passive artificially acquired immunity
(C) active naturally acquired immunity
(D) passive naturally acquired immunity

29. The initial laboratory workup of an immunodeficient pediatric patient reveals a positive mumps skin test, a positive Schick test (an inflammatory reaction at the site of diphtheria toxin injection), adequate chemotactic and intracellular killing activities, and serum that caused the hemolysis of antibody-sensitized erythrocytes. The child most likely has a defect in

(A) T cells
(B) B cells
(C) T cells and B cells
(D) complement
(E) phagocytes

30. A complement fragment that has chemotactic activity is

(A) C3a
(B) C4a
(C) C5a
(D) C2b
(E) C3b

31. B cells are involved in which of the following activities?

(A) Passive transfer of delayed hypersensitivity
(B) Production of lymphokines involved in poison ivy
(C) Secretion of interleukin-1 (IL-1)
(D) Development of atopic allergies
(E) Mitosis when mixed with phytohemagglutinin (PHA)

32. Which of the following vaccines could most safely be given to an immunosuppressed individual?

(A) Heptavax
(B) Sabin polio vaccine
(C) Yellow fever vaccine
(D) Rubella vaccine
(E) Mumps vaccine

33. Which of the following serologic tests would be the most useful for confirming a suspected case of infectious mononucleosis?

(A) Quantitative radial immunodiffusion
(B) Coombs test
(C) Sheep red blood cell (SRBC) agglutination
(D) Weil-Felix OX19 test
(E) Weil-Felix OX2 test

24-B	27-D	30-C	33-C
25-A	28-A	31-D	
26-C	29-B	32-A	

34. Delayed hypersensitivity (cell-mediated; type IV) reactions are suppressed by

(A) plasmapheresis
(B) complement depletion
(C) cortisone
(D) cromolyn sodium
(E) theophylline

35. Which one of the following statements best describes the idiotype of an antibody? It is

(A) determined by the amino acid residues in the framework region
(B) determined by the amino acid residues in the hypervariable region
(C) usually expressed on CD4 or CD8 molecules
(D) expressed by the B cell in response to antigen presentation by accessory cells

36. Immune tolerance can be induced by

(A) adult thymectomy
(B) neonatal thymectomy
(C) excess antibody
(D) excess antigen
(E) bursectomy

37. Toxoids are best described as being

(A) immunogenic and toxic
(B) nonimmunogenic and toxic
(C) immunogenic and nontoxic
(D) nonimmunogenic and nontoxic
(E) neither antigenic nor immunogenic

38. True statements describing cell-mediated immunity include which of the following?

(A) Antithymocyte serum suppresses its expression
(B) The cells have IgE antibody bound to the membrane
(C) Skin test results can be read in 30 to 45 minutes
(D) Cortisone enhances its expression
(E) Natural killer (NK) cells play a pivotal role in its expression

Questions 39 and 40

A 52-year-old man presents with the complaint of blood in his stools. He reports that he has experienced some changes in his bowel habits over the last 18 months and recently has become aware of the sensation that his evacuations are not complete. Proctoscopic examination reveals a large ulcerating mass in the descending colon. Biopsy results confirm the diagnosis of carcinoma of the colon, and the malignant mass is surgically removed. The patient is placed on appropriate chemotherapy and discharged 2 weeks later to be followed in the oncology clinic. Monthly blood specimens taken during the next year reveal the following carcinoembryonic antigen (CEA) levels:

	CEA (ng/ml)
Preoperative sample	50
Postoperative sample (day 1)	65
Month 1	15
Month 2	5
Months 3–9	<2.5
Month 10	10
Month 11	25
Month 12	40

39. The patient's serum CEA levels were assayed periodically because of the usefulness of CEA in

(A) localization of certain tumors in vivo
(B) diagnosing carcinoma of the colon
(C) diagnosing carcinoma of the pancreas
(D) diagnosing carcinoma of the prostate
(E) follow-up for the recurrence of certain malignancies

40. The CEA levels obtained during months 10 to 12 for this patient indicate that

(A) metastases have developed
(B) the initial diagnosis of colon cancer was incorrect
(C) surgical removal of the tumor was complete
(D) a revised diagnosis of carcinoma of the pancreas is warranted
(E) the patient is having an anamnestic response to the tumor

34-C 37-C 40-A
35-B 38-A
36-D 39-E

41. The predominant antibody in saliva is

(A) IgA
(B) IgG
(C) IgM
(D) IgD
(E) IgE

42. Under which of the following conditions do graft-versus-host (GVH) reactions occur?

(A) When the graft is contaminated with gram-negative microorganisms
(B) When tumor tissues are grafted
(C) When viable T cells are present in the graft
(D) When the graft has histocompatibility antigens not found in the recipient
(E) When the graft is pretreated with antilymphocyte serum

43. Immunodeficiency resulting in increased susceptibility to viral and fungal infections is due primarily to a deficiency in

(A) macrophages
(B) B cells
(C) T cells
(D) neutrophils
(E) complement

44. People with hereditary angioedema have a deficiency in

(A) C3b inactivator
(B) C1 esterase inhibitor
(C) C5 convertase
(D) properdin
(E) C3 activator

45. Agents used for nonspecific immunopotentiation include

(A) interleukin-2 (IL-2)
(B) anti-idiotypic antibody
(C) cortisone
(D) immunotoxins
(E) antithymocyte serum

46. Graft-versus-host (GVH) reactions are a major problem in bone marrow transplantation. Because these reactions require that the donor has mature T cells, one can conclude that

(A) the bone marrow contains stem cells capable of responding to host antigens
(B) a very young individual would be the best source of bone marrow for transplantation
(C) the host thymus must supply the donor stem cells with factors influencing T cell maturation
(D) it would be better to remove T stem cells from the marrow before transferring the cells
(E) bone marrow contains mature T cells

47. Anti-HLA antibodies are found in the serum of some humans because

(A) most humans have mounted an immune response to bacteria of their normal flora, and these bacteria may possess antigens cross-reacting with HLA antigens
(B) some humans make an immune response to HLA antigens during pregnancy or after receiving blood transfusions
(C) HLA antigens are sequestered during embryonic development and, when expressed during neonatal life, are seen as nonself by the immune system
(D) the childhood vaccinations we receive cause us to make anti-HLA antibodies
(E) anti-HLA antibodies are autoantibodies

48. Humoral factors contributing to innate immunity include

(A) lymphokine-activated killer (LAK) cells
(B) beta lysin
(C) antitoxin
(D) interleukin-1 (IL-1)
(E) cortisone

49. The receptor complex that recognizes an epitope associated with a class II major histocompatibility complex (MHC) molecule in the membrane of an antigen-presenting cell is the

(A) T cell receptor
(B) T cell receptor plus CD4
(C) T cell receptor plus CD3
(D) T cell receptor plus CD3 and CD4
(E) T cell receptor plus CD3, CD4, and CD8

41-A	44-B	47-B
42-C	45-A	48-B
43-C	46-E	49-D

50. A 7-month-old child was hospitalized for a yeast infection that would not respond to therapy. He had a history of acute pyogenic infections. Examination of the patient revealed lymphopenia, absence of a thymus shadow on x-ray, hypogammaglobulinemia, and lack of B cells. This history is most compatible with a diagnosis of

(A) acquired immune deficiency syndrome (AIDS)
(B) multiple myeloma
(C) chronic granulomatous disease (CGD)
(D) Bruton's X-linked hypogammaglobulinemia
(E) severe combined immunodeficiency disease (SCID)

51. Antigen-reactive lymphocytes that interfere with the development of a humoral immune response are called

(A) natural killer (NK) cells
(B) null cells
(C) suppressor cells
(D) contrasuppressor cells
(E) large granular lymphocytes

52. True statements concerning histocompatibility antigens include which of the following?

(A) They are composed of nucleic acids
(B) They are controlled by genes on autosomal chromosomes
(C) They do not induce a graft-versus-host (GVH) reaction
(D) They are located at the cell surface
(E) In humans, they are found in a segment of chromosome 17

53. In the generation of atopic hypersensitivity, fixation of IgE to mast cells and basophils occurs via the

(A) Fc fragment
(B) C1 domain
(C) Fab fragment
(D) C2 domain
(E) Variable (V) region

54. In the induction of delayed hypersensitivity, interaction between antigen-processing cells and T cells can only occur if the two participants

(A) possess Km markers
(B) possess class I major histocompatibility complex (MHC) antigens
(C) are idiotype-identical
(D) are MHC-identical
(E) are allogeneic

55. In the classic pathway of complement activation, C1 esterase mediates cleavage of

(A) C1
(B) C2
(C) C3
(D) C4
(E) C5

56. $Rh_o(D)$ immunoglobulin (RhoGAM) is used in human medicine to prevent

(A) erythroblastosis fetalis
(B) transfusion reactions
(C) hepatitis A in an exposed individual
(D) hepatitis B in an exposed individual
(E) graft-versus-host (GVH) disease in a bone marrow transplant recipient

57. Immune complexes in serum and other biological fluids can be detected by the

(A) Prausnitz-Küstner (PK) reaction
(B) radial immunodiffusion test
(C) radioallergosorbent test (RAST)
(D) C1q binding assay
(E) complement fixation test

50-E	53-A	56-A
51-C	54-D	57-D
52-D	55-D	

Questions 58 and 59

A 54-year-old pathologist was in good health until 12 days prior to hospital admission when, after receiving an influenza vaccination, he developed generalized malaise. The condition persisted for 6 days, and he became concerned that it was more than a mere vaccination reaction. Four days prior to admission he developed a severe headache with accompanying bone and muscle pain. Two days prior to admission he developed weakness of the extremities. On the day of admission he had been unable to get out of bed and was brought to the hospital by ambulance.

Physical examination revealed a well-developed, well-nourished white male in moderate respiratory distress with rapid, shallow breathing. Blood pressure was 160/120, pulse 86, and respirations 32/min. The remainder of the physical examination was unremarkable except for the muscular weakness and slight neurologic impairment. A lumbar puncture was performed and revealed the following: Opening pressure—normal; appearance—clear; sugar—60 mg/dl; chloride—120 mEq/L; leukocytes—absent; erythrocytes—3 to 4 per high-power field; protein—39 mg/dl. During the next 2 days, the patient's pulmonary capacity decreased from 3600 ml to 1000 ml. Blood gases at this time were Po_2—70; Pco_2—48; pH—7.41. A tracheostomy was performed, and the patient was placed on a respirator.

During the next 4 weeks, the patient's condition continued to deteriorate. His paralysis became almost complete. He developed pneumococcal pneumonia, which was treated successfully with penicillin. Seven weeks after admission he began to regain neurologic function. His muscular strength returned slowly, and his pulmonary function improved so that the respirator was discontinued on the sixty-third hospital day. He was discharged 2 weeks later and placed on an active physical therapy program. Recovery was complete, and 6 months after his initial illness the patient was able to return to work full-time.

58. The patient's symptoms were originally muscular and then became neurologic. Each of the following disorders is an autoimmune disease that would affect these tissues EXCEPT

(A) systemic lupus erythematosus (SLE)
(B) multiple sclerosis
(C) myasthenia gravis
(D) Guillain-Barré syndrome
(E) muscular dystrophy

59. The life-threatening component of the patient's symptomatology was pulmonary embarrassment. Why was a lumbar puncture performed? To

(A) rule out a brain abscess
(B) aid in administration of antibiotics
(C) confirm suspicion of increased intracranial pressure
(D) rule out encephalomyelitis
(E) rule out neuroblastoma

60. The major histocompatibility complex (MHC) of humans is composed of linked genes whose products show all of the following characteristics EXCEPT

(A) some are strong barriers to transplantation
(B) they include β_2-microglobulin and class I, class II, and class III molecules
(C) some are complement components
(D) their cellular distribution is diverse
(E) some are necessary for effective interaction between cells of the immune response

61. All of the following cell types participate in a humoral immune response to a thymus-independent antigen EXCEPT the

(A) T cell
(B) B cell
(C) macrophage
(D) antigen-presenting cell

62. Serum used for HLA typing by cytotoxicity assay is obtained from all of the following sources EXCEPT

(A) multiparous women
(B) rabbits immunized with human lymphocytes
(C) patients who have received many blood transfusions
(D) patients who have received and rejected transplanted grafts
(E) volunteers who have been HLA-sensitized

58-E   61-A
59-D   62-B
60-B

Questions 63–65

An acutely ill 3-year-old boy is brought to the emergency room. His breathing is extremely labored, and he is producing rust-colored sputum. A Gram stain of the sputum reveals numerous gram-positive cocci in random clusters. A diagnosis of staphylococcal pneumonia is made, and the child is hospitalized and placed on intravenous methicillin. The mother reports that the child has experienced several such episodes previously that were successfully controlled with antibiotics. Further discussion of the child's medical history reveals that he had experienced a normal recovery from measles approximately 6 months earlier.

63. The most probable diagnosis, based on this history, is

(A) DiGeorge syndrome
(B) Nezelof's syndrome
(C) Wiskott-Aldrich syndrome
(D) selective immunoglobulin deficiency

Leukocyte function studies are performed and indicate that phagocytosis, intracellular killing, and chemotactic responses are all within normal limits.

64. These features rule out defects in nonspecific resistance, a characteristic of all of the following disorders EXCEPT

(A) chronic granulomatous disease (CGD)
(B) lazy leukocyte syndrome
(C) Job's syndrome
(D) dysgammaglobulinemia

An immunoglobulin profile is ordered. The child has no detectable IgA or IgM in his serum. A small amount of IgG (30 mg/dl) is detected when the assay is repeated with low-level radial immunodiffusion plates.

65. Based on this information, the most probable diagnosis is

(A) selective immunoglobulin deficiency
(B) common variable hypogammaglobulinemia
(C) Wiskott-Aldrich syndrome
(D) Bruton's hypogammaglobulinemia
(E) transient hypogammaglobulinemia of infancy

66. Macrophages engage in all of the following activities EXCEPT

(A) processing antigen
(B) production of interleukin-2 (IL-2)
(C) presentation of antigen
(D) phagocytosis
(E) killing ingested bacteria

67. All of the following are goals in the immunotherapy of cancer EXCEPT

(A) reduction of the tumor burden to the lowest possible level by surgery, drugs, or irradiation
(B) use of modified tumor antigens to stimulate antibodies
(C) activation of macrophages and lymphocytes by adjuvants such as bacille Calmette-Guérin
(D) use of viable tumor cells for specific immunization of the patient
(E) bolstering immune function with substances such as interferon and interleukin-2 (IL-2)

68. The pharmacologically active mediators of anaphylaxis include all of the following EXCEPT

(A) serotonin
(B) histamine
(C) factor H
(D) serine protease
(E) platelet-activating factor (PAF)

69. Giving a person an injection of an antilymphocyte serum prepared in horses may cause all of the following EXCEPT

(A) serum sickness
(B) increased risk of malignancy
(C) increased susceptibility to opportunistic infections
(D) recurrence of latent viral infections
(E) rheumatoid arthritis

70. All of the following molecules are found in the B cell membrane EXCEPT

(A) concanavalin A (con A) receptors
(B) C3b receptors
(C) monomeric IgM
(D) class I major histocompatibility complex (MHC) molecules
(E) class II MHC molecules

63-D	66-B	69-E
64-D	67-D	70-A
65-D	68-C	

71. Macrophages secrete many antimicrobial factors, including all of the following EXCEPT

(A) cyclosporine
(B) tumor necrosis factor (TNF)
(C) interleukin-1 (IL-1)
(D) complement
(E) alpha interferon

72. T cells are involved in all of the following activities EXCEPT

(A) production of interleukin-2 (IL-2)
(B) acquired resistance to tuberculosis
(C) antibody response to polysaccharide antigens
(D) response to IL-1
(E) development of contact dermatitis

73. Processes that normally regulate the immune response include all of the following EXCEPT

(A) the idiotypic network
(B) major histocompatibility complex (MHC) restriction
(C) suppressor T (Ts) lymphocytes
(D) suppressor macrophages
(E) ionizing radiation

74. All of the following characteristics of tumor-specific transplantation antigens (TSTAs) are true EXCEPT that TSTAs may

(A) induce an antibody response
(B) have a viral etiology
(C) elicit cytotoxic T (Tc) cell responses
(D) induce suppressor T (Ts) cells
(E) be found in the nucleus of the cell

75. Factors that are chemotactic for neutrophils include all of the following EXCEPT

(A) C3b
(B) C5a
(C) histamine
(D) fibrinopeptides
(E) platelet-activating factor (PAF)

76. Patients receiving long-term immunosuppression commonly experience all of the following EXCEPT

(A) recurrence of herpes simplex and other viral infections
(B) decrease in antibody synthesis
(C) loss of T cell immunity
(D) enhanced suppressor T (Ts) cell activity
(E) infections with opportunistic pathogens

77. All of the following statements concerning antigen epitopes are correct EXCEPT

(A) the same epitope can be expressed multiple times in the molecule
(B) the epitope gives antigenic specificity to the molecule
(C) there can be several different types of epitopes in the molecule
(D) the valence of the molecule is the number of different antibody molecules that react with it
(E) the antigen's epitope reacts specifically with the antibody's paratope

78. All of the following are opsonins found in serum EXCEPT

(A) C3b
(B) antibody
(C) fibronectin
(D) tuftsin
(E) cachectin

79. All of the following tests measure phagocytic function EXCEPT

(A) chemiluminescence
(B) chemotaxis
(C) nitroblue tetrazolium (NBT) reduction
(D) microbicidal activity
(E) antibody synthesis

80. Hypervariable regions of IgG molecules exist on all of the folowing structures EXCEPT

(A) Fc fragments
(B) intact heavy (H) chains
(C) Fab fragments
(D) intact light (L) chains
(E) Fd fragments

71-A	74-E	77-D	80-A
72-C	75-A	78-E	
73-E	76-D	79-E	

81. Complement receptors that occur on the membranes of macrophages include all of the following EXCEPT

(A) CR1
(B) CR2
(C) CR3
(D) CR4

82. All of the following diagnoses are correctly matched with an immunologic test result that would support the diagnosis EXCEPT

(A) systemic lupus erythematosus (SLE)—antinuclear antibodies present
(B) multiple sclerosis—increase in spinal fluid IgG level
(C) myasthenia gravis—acetylcholine receptor antibodies present
(D) muscular dystrophy—antimyosin antibodies present
(E) Guillain-Barré syndrome—complement fixation

83. Immunoglobulin molecules contain all of the following structures EXCEPT

(A) heavy (H) and light (L) chains
(B) constant (C) domains
(C) variable (V) domains
(D) J chains
(E) hinge regions

84. True statements concerning antigens involved in transplantation include all of the following EXCEPT

(A) red blood cell (ABO) antigens appear on tissue cells; therefore, they can function as transplantation antigens
(B) HLA antigens appear on granulocytes, lymphocytes, and platelets; therefore, incompatibility of these antigens in certain recipients of whole blood can cause febrile transfusion reactions
(C) blood transfusion, pregnancy, and previous skin or organ transplants can sensitize individuals to histocompatibility antigens
(D) no immune response occurs in tissue transplants between identical twins
(E) graft-versus-host (GVH) reactions occur because the donor lymphocytes are rejected by the recipient

Questions 85 and 86

A boy scout troop in New Jersey is planning a summer trip to a remote region of Colorado. As a precaution, the boys receive booster shots for tetanus and typhoid fever. One week later, blood samples are drawn to determine whether the boys are responding to the vaccines.

85. Serologic techniques that could be used to detect antibodies to the tetanus toxin include all of the following EXCEPT

(A) toxin neutralization
(B) complement fixation
(C) agglutination
(D) enzyme-linked immunosorbent assay (ELISA)
(E) precipitation

86. Serologic techniques that could be used to detect antibodies to the typhoid bacillus include all of the following EXCEPT

(A) bacterial agglutination
(B) bactericidal assay
(C) complement fixation
(D) indirect immunofluorescence
(E) radial immunodiffusion

87. T cells produce all of the following cytokines EXCEPT

(A) interleukin-1 (IL-1)
(B) IL-2
(C) IL-3
(D) IL-4
(E) IL-5

88. The human major histocompatibility complex (MHC) has genes that code for all of the following EXCEPT

(A) antigens on the surface of B cells and macrophages
(B) tumor necrosis factors (TNFs)
(C) antigens that may elicit antibody formation in unrelated people
(D) variable domains of immunoglobulin molecules
(E) antigens on the surface of cytotoxic T (Tc) cells

81-B   84-E   87-A
82-D   85-C   88-D
83-D   86-E

89. Assays of immune competence involve the evaluation of all of the following EXCEPT

(A) T cells
(B) B cells
(C) neutrophils
(D) monocytes
(E) eosinophils

90. B cell membranes contain receptors for all of the following EXCEPT

(A) the Fc portion of immunoglobulin
(B) lipopolysaccharide
(C) endotoxin
(D) phytohemagglutinin (PHA)
(E) pokeweed mitogen

91. All of the following characteristics describe HLA-A and HLA-B antigens EXCEPT that they are

(A) class I antigens
(B) targets recognized by the host during graft rejection
(C) involved in major histocompatibility complex (MHC) restriction of cell-mediated cytolysis (CMC)
(D) composed of an α chain and a β chain both anchored in the cell membrane
(E) found on virtually all nucleated cells of the body

92. Termination of self-tolerance and resultant autoimmune disease could theoretically be triggered by all of the following EXCEPT

(A) excess of self-reactive helper T (Th) cells
(B) bypass of the need for self-reactive Th cell activity
(C) production of anti-idiotypic antibodies
(D) deficiency of suppressor T (Ts) cells
(E) release of sequestered self-antigen

93. A preparation of pooled human IgM injected into a rabbit may stimulate production of antibodies reactive with all of the following EXCEPT

(A) κ chain
(B) μ chain
(C) λ chain
(D) J chain
(E) α chain

94. Cells with antigen-specific receptors include all of the following EXCEPT

(A) macrophages
(B) B cells
(C) helper T (Th) cells
(D) cytotoxic T (Tc) cells
(E) suppressor T (Ts) cells

95. Immune response (Ir) genes can be described by all of the following statements EXCEPT that they

(A) are located within the major histocompatibility complex (MHC)
(B) encode the production of class I proteins
(C) specify the ability of an animal to recognize and respond to certain antigens
(D) exert their control through T lymphocytes
(E) are involved in immunoglobulin formation

96. Substances that are mitogenic for T cells include all of the following EXCEPT

(A) phytohemagglutinin (PHA)
(B) pokeweed mitogen
(C) specific antigen
(D) lipopolysaccharide
(E) concanavalin A (con A)

97. All of the following cellular changes are associated with the progression from normal to malignant EXCEPT

(A) increased mitotic rate
(B) acquisition of new membrane antigens
(C) loss of contact inhibition
(D) loss of membrane antigens
(E) decreased sensitivity to x-irradiation

98. All of the following statements about Km antigenic markers of immunoglobulin molecules are true EXCEPT that they are

(A) associated with κ chains
(B) genetically determined
(C) allotypic determinants
(D) associated with γ chains
(E) present in the constant domain

89-E	92-C	95-B	98-D
90-D	93-E	96-D	
91-D	94-A	97-E	

99. All of the following cells experience major histocompatibility complex (MHC) restriction EXCEPT

(A) helper T (Th) cells
(B) B cells
(C) macrophages
(D) cytotoxic T (Tc) cells
(E) natural killer (NK) cells

100. Antigens that can act as transplantation barriers include all of the following EXCEPT

(A) blood group A antigens
(B) class I antigens
(C) class II antigens
(D) class III antigens
(E) blood group O antigens

101. All of the following are present in the macrophage membrane EXCEPT

(A) IgE Fc receptors
(B) IgG Fc receptors
(C) IgM Fc receptors
(D) C3b receptors
(E) immune response–associated (Ia) antigens

Questions 102–106

102. Immunofluorescence examination of tissue from patients with Goodpasture's syndrome reveals linear deposits of immunoglobulin and complement on

(A) alveolar basement membrane
(B) glomerular basement membrane
(C) both
(D) neither

103. Immune complexes in serum could be detected by which of the following assays?

(A) Raji cell-binding assay
(B) C1q solid-phase binding assay
(C) Both
(D) Neither

104. Neutrophil membranes contain receptors for which of the following particles?

(A) Fc fragment of IgG
(B) C3b
(C) Both
(D) Neither

105. Properties of haptens include which of the following?

(A) Immunogenicity
(B) Reactivity
(C) Both
(D) Neither

106. Examples of cancer-associated antigens that probably arise from tissue dedifferentiation include

(A) carcinoembryonic antigen (CEA)
(B) α-fetoprotein
(C) both
(D) neither

Directions: Each group of items in this section consists of lettered options followed by a set of numbered items. For each item, select the **one** lettered option that is most closely associated with it. Each lettered option may be selected once, more than once, or not at all.

Questions 107–110

For each method of activating (fixing) complement listed, select the immunoglobulin most closely associated with that method.

(A) IgD
(B) IgA
(C) IgE
(D) IgG
(E) IgM

107. Fixes complement efficiently via the C_H2 domain

108. Fixes complement via the C_H3 domain

109. Fixes complement via the alternative pathway only

110. Fixes complement most efficiently in lytic reactions

99-E	102-C	105-B	108-E
100-D	103-C	106-C	109-B
101-A	104-C	107-D	110-E

Questions 111–113

For each situation listed below, select the adjective that best describes the type of antibodies involved.

(A) Autologous
(B) Allogeneic
(C) Cryptic
(D) Heterogenetic
(E) Idiotypic

111. Weil-Felix reaction

112. Administration of rabies immune globulin

113. Administration of tetanus antitoxin

Questions 114–117

For each person listed below, choose the vaccine which that person is most likely to receive.

(A) Diphtheria-pertussis-tetanus (DPT)
(B) Hepatitis B
(C) Meningococcal polysaccharide
(D) Measles-mumps-rubella (MMR)
(E) Pneumovax
(F) Rabies
(G) Sabin
(H) Salk

114. 24-year-old with AIDS-related complex (ARC)

115. Military recruit

116. Veterinary student

117. Dental student

Questions 118–125

For each immunologic characteristic stated below, select the disease most closely associated with it.

(A) Systemic lupus erythematosus (SLE)
(B) Pernicious anemia
(C) Myasthenia gravis
(D) Multiple sclerosis
(E) Rheumatoid arthritis
(F) Anaphylaxis
(G) Peptic ulcers
(H) Graves' disease
(I) Wiskott-Aldrich syndrome
(J) DiGeorge syndrome
(K) CREST syndrome

118. Antibodies to gastric parietal cell antigens

119. Immunoglobulins with a specificity for the Fc fragment of IgG

120. Antibodies to acetylcholine receptor

121. Glomerulonephritis triggered by deposition of DNA–antibody–complement complexes on vascular basement membrane

122. Elevated levels of antibodies to measles virus in serum and spinal fluid

123. Absence of T cells in peripheral lymphoid organs

124. Mediation by IgE antibodies

125. Antibodies to the centromere

111-D	114-E	117-B	120-C	123-J
112-B	115-C	118-B	121-A	124-F
113-B	116-F	119-E	122-D	125-K

Questions 126–128

For each function described below, select the cell with which it is most closely associated.

(A) Accessory cell
(B) B cell
(C) Macrophage
(D) Natural killer (NK) cell
(E) Eosinophil
(F) Fibroblast
(G) T cell
(H) Mast cell

126. Synthesizes immunoglobulin

127. Has a concanavalin A (con A) receptor

128. Expresses cytotoxicity without prior antigen exposure

Questions 129–133

Match the pathologic feature with the disorder with which it is most closely associated.

(A) Multiple myeloma
(B) Allergic rhinitis
(C) Arthus reaction
(D) Serum sickness
(E) Idiopathic thrombocytopenic purpura (ITP)
(F) Amyloidosis
(G) Multiple sclerosis
(H) Pernicious anemia

129. Strong hereditary association

130. Platelet-specific IgG antibodies

131. Local immune complex deposition

132. Systemic immune complex deposition

133. Bence Jones protein in the urine

Questions 134–137

For each type of transplant listed below, select the adjective that best describes it.

(A) Allogeneic
(B) Autologous
(C) Heterogeneic
(D) Idiotypic
(E) Syngeneic

134. Transfer of skin from the thigh to the face

135. Cadaver kidney transplant

136. Bone marrow transplant from mother to daughter

137. Bone marrow transfer between identical twins

Questions 138–141

Match the pathogenetic factor below with the disorder with which it is most closely associated.

(A) Angioneurotic edema
(B) Bruton's disease
(C) Chronic granulomatous disease (CGD)
(D) Graves' disease
(E) Poststreptococcal glomerulonephritis
(F) Sjögren's syndrome
(G) Waldenström's macroglobulinemia
(H) Hashimoto's thyroiditis

138. Immune complexes

139. Defective intracellular killing

140. Antibodies to thyrotropin receptors

141. Hypogammaglobulinemia

126-B	129-B	132-D	135-A	138-E	141-B
127-G	130-E	133-A	136-A	139-C	
128-D	131-C	134-B	137-E	140-D	

Questions 142–144

Match each characteristic of a laboratory technique below with the technique it best describes.

(A) Immunofluorescence
(B) Enzyme immunoassay
(C) Radioimmunoassay (RIA)
(D) Radial immunodiffusion
(E) Immunoelectrophoresis
(F) Agglutination
(G) Complement fixation
(H) Enzyme-linked immunosorbent assay (ELISA)

142. Requires the use of antibodies labeled with isotopes

143. Used to identify antigens in the cell wall or membranes

144. Used to quantitate immunoglobulin levels in serum

Questions 145–148

For each characteristic of a vaccine listed below, choose the vaccine or vaccine component that it best describes.

(A) Cholera toxin
(B) Hepatitis B
(C) Meningococcal polysaccharide
(D) Measles-mumps-rubella (MMR)
(E) Pneumovax
(F) Polyribose phosphate
(G) Rabies
(H) Salk

145. Product of recombinant DNA technology

146. Attenuated viral vaccine

147. Killed viral vaccine

148. Disappointing immunogenicity in infants under age 18 months

Questions 149–153

For each characteristic of a complement component listed below, select the component it best describes.

(A) C1qrs
(B) C3
(C) C3a
(D) C5b6789
(E) C3bB
(F) Properdin
(G) Bb
(H) Factor I

149. Destroyed by anaphylatoxin inactivator

150. Membrane attack complex

151. Binds to C4b2b complex

152. Cleaved by factor D

153. Activates macrophages and causes them to adhere to and spread on surfaces

Questions 154–157

Match the characteristic of a definable fragment of degraded immunoglobulin with the most appropriate fragment.

(A) Fab
(B) F(ab')$_2$
(C) Fc
(D) Fd
(E) FcεR

154. Monovalent fragment that binds antigen

155. Fragment that binds complement

156. Fragment formed by pepsin treatment

157. Fragment formed of V_H and C_H1 domains of the heavy chain

142-C	145-B	148-F	151-B	154-A	157-D
143-A	146-D	149-C	152-E	155-C	
144-D	147-H	150-D	153-G	156-B	

Questions 158–161

For each disorder listed below, choose the adjective that best describes the antigenic relationships involved.

(A) Autologous
(B) Allogeneic
(C) Xenogeneic
(D) Immunogenic
(E) Haptenic
(F) Syngeneic

158. Erythroblastosis fetalis

159. Asthma

160. Farmer's lung

161. Graves' disease

Questions 162–165

For each description listed below, select the cell with which it is most closely associated.

(A) Basophil
(B) B cell
(C) Neutrophil
(D) Macrophage
(E) Eosinophil
(F) Stem cell
(G) Monocyte
(H) T cell
(I) Mast cell
(J) Natural killer (NK) cell

162. IgM and IgD are present in the membrane

163. A major antigen-processing cell

164. Principally involved in graft rejection

165. Believed responsible for immune surveillance

ANSWERS AND EXPLANATIONS

1. The answer is D *[Ch 2 II B 2 c; Ch 12 I A].*
Grafts between members of the same species are termed allografts or homografts. Autografts involve the transfer of tissue from one location to another on the same individual (e.g., skin transplants). Isografts are grafts made between inbred animals and between identical twins, while xenografts cross species boundaries.

2 and 3. The answers are: 2-B *[Ch 8 II D 1, 2],* **3-E** *[Ch 3 III C 2 a].*
Syphilis serology, using serum specimens collected serially from pregnant women and from infants following delivery, is of value in diagnosing congenital syphilis. The syphilitic host develops, among other antibodies, an antibody (reagin) to a nontreponemal antigen (beef heart cardiolipin). Reagin may be found in both serum and spinal fluid and it forms readily visible clumps when it combines with cardiolipin in a flocculation test. Two such tests, the Venereal Disease Research Laboratory (VDRL) and rapid plasma reagin (RPR) tests, are practical and simple to perform. Although these useful tests are not specific for syphilis, they are extremely sensitive.
Since maternal IgM does not normally cross the placenta, the IgM level in the newborn is a reflection of antigenic stimulation during the intrauterine period. A pregnant woman with syphilis can transmit the causative microorganism, *Treponema pallidum,* to her fetus through the placenta beginning at about the tenth to sixteenth week of gestation. If therapy is not instituted the fetus may die in utero, the infected newborn may die shortly after delivery, or, as in the case presented in the question, the infant may survive but develop signs of congenital syphilis later. Rapid diagnosis of congenitally acquired syphilis in live newborns is essential, but it may be difficult if based only on clinical findings, since many infected infants may be asymptomatic at birth.
Certain intrauterine infections of the fetus, including syphilis, lead to elevated IgM levels in cord serum at birth or in the postnatal period. The normal IgM level in cord serum is approximately 10 mg/dl. Concentrations above about 20 mg/dl may be seen in syphilitic newborns who are totally asymptomatic at birth and remain so for variable periods. Screening of cord and newborn serum for IgM elevation can be of more diagnostic value in these types of infections than determination of VDRL titer. It should be emphasized, however, that an increase in IgM is not, per se, enough to establish the exact nature of the infection (i.e., the identity of the etiologic agent).

4. The answer is A *[Ch 6 IV B].*
Adjuvants are substances that enhance antibody synthesis nonspecifically. Adjuvants usually act as a depot for the slow release of antigen through the reticuloendothelial system (RES) of the animal being immunized. Some adjuvants have an irritant action that also enhances the immune response.

5. The answer is A *[Table 1-5; Ch 4].*
The complement receptors designated CR bind various complement components: CR1 binds components C3b, iC3b, and C4b; receptor CR3 binds iC3b; and receptors CR2 and CR4 bind iC3b and C3dg. There is no complement receptor designated CR5, although there are also receptors for other complement components. For example, a C3a receptor is present on mast cells; it is responsible for the initial event which triggers the release of mediators such as histamine when anaphylatoxin I (C3a) reacts with it.

6. The answer is B *[Ch 12 II B 2 a, c, d].*
The only antigen which sib 2 has that sib 1 lacks is HLA-B44. Sib 1 and 2 are a one-haplotype match, both having inherited the father's HLA-A10, B5, DR2 haplotype. This degree of matching currently enjoys a 1-year survival rate of 90% or better. This would be a fairly good tissue match, although the B and DR antigens seem to be the strongest in regard to graft rejection. If the graft went in the other direction (i.e., from sib 1 to sib 2), then sib 2 would recognize HLA-A3 and HLA- B7 as foreign.

7. The answer is A *[Ch 9 V B 3 e].*
In the manifestation of delayed hypersensitivity, binding of antigen to specific antigen-reacting T cells causes the cells to release various soluble mediators, or lymphokines, with various biological activities. Examples of lymphokines released are macrophage migration-inhibiting factor (MIF), macrophage-activating factor (MAF), macrophage chemotactic factor, and lymphotoxin.

8. The answer is C *[Ch 3 IV A 2].*
Idiotypes represent unique amino acid sequences in the variable (V) region of immunoglobulin molecules

which are associated with the antigen-binding capability of the molecule. They are usually specific for the individual antibody clone.

9. The answer is B *[Ch 8 III D 3, E 2].*
The indirect Coombs test is used to detect circulating nonagglutinating antibody; for example, it is valuable in detecting IgG-associated antibody in the serum of a woman who is believed to be sensitized to the Rh antigen and is at risk for carrying an erythroblastotic fetus. The Schick test is used to test for immunity to diphtheria. The complement fixation test, Rose-Waaler test, and liquid-phase radioimmunoassay (RIA) are different techniques used to measure antigen–antibody reactions.

10. The answer is E *[Ch 2 I B 2, 3; II B].*
Monoclonal antibodies are probably not needed in this instance; their production is laborious and time-consuming, and their monospecificity does not offer advantages sufficient to merit the extra effort and expense. The recommendations of the staff immunologist to the director of the radioimmunoassay (RIA) laboratory should include increasing the number of animals to at least three. Rabbits are random-bred animals and will not respond uniformly to an immunization procedure; increasing the number of animals improves the chances of finding one high responder. The route of administration and the dosage of the antibiotic are fine; if phagocyte interaction is deemed important, the intravenous route of injection would probably be more suitable because this route maximizes exposure to the entire reticuloendothelial system (RES) of the body, particularly the spleen, where much antibody is produced. Gentamicin is a hapten, and by itself is not likely to induce any immune response. The probability of its coupling to carrier proteins in the rabbit is extremely small. This problem could be bypassed by chemically conjugating the antibiotic to a carrier molecule before injection. Foreignness is important in immunogenicity; therefore, bovine serum albumin could be recommended as the carrier. An even better vehicle might be human erythrocytes. They are not only foreign to the rabbit but have the additional attributes of being more complex and phagocytizable.

11. The answer is B *[Ch 12 III A].*
The most important antigenic system in organ transplantation is the ABO system. An organ from a donor who has either the A or B antigens must not be transplanted to a recipient who has anti-A or anti-B isoagglutinins. This incompatibility causes hyperacute or accelerated graft rejection. In some instances, the graft will not even be vascularized. The HLA system is also important in evaluation for organ transplantation. Usually, there are not preformed antibodies against HLA antigens except in multiparous women and in people who may have received numerous transfusions or grafts at a previous time. Sensitization to these antigens is a slower process, and graft rejection may take weeks to months.

12. The answer is A *[Ch 4 V B 2 b (1); Ch 8 IV B 3 d (2) (b)].*
B cell membranes, but not T cell membranes, contain receptors for bacterial lipopolysaccharide. Pokeweed is mitogenic for both T and B cells; phytohemagglutinin (PHA) and concanavalin A (con A) are considered to be T cell–specific mitogens. When a mitogen reacts with the B or T cell, it induces mitosis. This can be quantitated by measuring the amount of radioactive thymidine which is incorporated into the DNA of the cell. T cells, but not B cells, have a membrane receptor for sheep red blood cells (SRBCs). B cells have a receptor for the C3b product of complement activation, but not for C1q.

13. The answer is B *[Ch 2 I B 3 b; Ch 9 II B 3].*
The antibodies on the mast cell are IgE. The patient may have IgG or IgD antibodies, but only IgE antibodies are involved in anaphylaxis. The most important antigenic determinant of the penicillin molecule appears to be the penicilloic acid moiety. It has been estimated that as many as 250 patients in the United States die each year as a result of penicillin-induced anaphylactic reactions induced by parenteral administration of the drug; in contrast, only 4 to 6 fatal cases are due to orally administered antibiotic. Certain cephalosporin antibiotics cross-react with the penicillins; hence these drugs cannot be categorically used in penicillin-allergic individuals. Some can, particularly the monobactams; however, there are reports of anaphylactic deaths resulting from the use of second- and even third-generation cephalosporins. T suppressor (Ts) cells would interfere with the immune response to the antibiotic, not with its antibacterial action.

14. The answer is C *[Ch 6 IV B 4 a].*
Alum-coprecipitated antigen and aluminum hydroxide-adsorbed antigen retard absorption from the site of injection. In this manner they extend the period of antigen exposure. They also are irritants and increase macrophage and lymphoid cell exposure to the antigen. Polynucleotides such as polyadenylate-uridylate (poly A:U) stimulate macrophage processing of antigens and also enhance helper T (Th) cell activity. Interferons are produced by various cells of the body; they increase proliferation and maturation of lym-

phoid cells. Interferons also activate macrophages and may induce interferon production. Muramyl dipeptide is a mycobacterial cell wall component active in complete Freund's adjuvant. Lipopolysaccharide is a polyclonal B cell mitogen that causes nonspecific expansion of B cell clones.

15. The answer is E *[Ch 11 V C].*
Wiskott-Aldrich syndrome consists of a triad of features: thrombocytopenia, which is usually present at birth; eczema, usually present at the age of 1 year; and recurrent pyogenic infection, starting after age 6 months. Immunologic abnormalities suggest combined B and T cell defects. The defect in antibody response to polysaccharide antigens renders the patients susceptible to infection with capsular polysaccharide–type organisms (e.g., *Streptococcus pneumoniae, Neisseria meningitidis,* and *Haemophilus influenzae*). Death is usually due to thrombocytopenia, sepsis, or both.

16. The answer is D *[Ch 5 IV F 2; Ch 6 IV B 6].*
Endotoxin, the lipopolysaccharide (LPS) component of the cell wall of most gram-negative bacteria, is immunopotentiating by virtue of its ability to induce proliferation in B cells. It acts as a polyclonal activator and can nonspecifically trigger humoral immune responses. Lymphokines are products of lymphocytes which have a positive effect on the immune response. Transfer factor is a soluble mediator of delayed hypersensitivity: it is released by specifically sensitized T cells and can confer identical reactivity to naive T cells. Immunogenic RNA is primarily a laboratory phenomenon wherein RNA extracted from lymphoid tissues of immunized animals will exhibit enhanced immunogenicity in a second experimental animal. Endogenous pyrogen is another name for interleukin-1 (IL-1), the cytokine released from antigen-processing cells that enhances T cell functions in the immune response.

17. The answer is B *[Ch 3 IV B 4 a].*
The organization of heavy (H) chain genes is similar to that of light (L) chain genes but is more complex in that three, not two, segments of DNA join together to generate the variable portion of the H chain. The additional segment is designated the diversity (D_H) gene region.

18. The answer is E *[Ch 9 III C 1 a (2) (b)].*
Transfusion reactions that are due to extravascular hemolysis are almost invariably involved with Rh incompatibility and are not complement-mediated. Extravascular destruction of the antibody-sensitized red blood cells is carried out primarily by the cells of the reticuloendothelial system (RES). Transfusion reactions that are due to intravascular hemolysis are characterized by anti-A or anti-B antibodies binding to complement, with almost immediate lysis of the transfused red blood cells. These immunologically mediated transfusion reactions are important clinical examples of cytotoxic (type II) hypersensitivity reactions. IgE is crucial to the pathogenesis of immediate hypersensitivity (type I) reactions; IgE is not involved in cytotoxic reactions.

19. The answer is C *[Ch 6 II B 1 c].*
Cancer chemotherapy involves the inhibition of cell division. Because immune responses depend upon the proliferation of lymphoid cells, drugs that block DNA replication or cause errors in the process will be immunosuppressive. This action will predispose the individual to infections, commonly by agents not normally considered to be pathogenic. These organisms often are normal flora or common environmental contacts and are known as opportunists because they take advantage of the depressed state of the host to invade, multiply, and produce disease.

20. The answer is B *[Ch 7 II A 3 a].*
Diphtheria-pertussis-tetanus (DPT) vaccine is used to protect against diphtheria, tetanus, and pertussis (whooping cough); it consists of toxoids of diphtheria and tetanus adsorbed to a carrier such as alum to enhance immunogenicity, combined with killed *Bordetella pertussis*. DPT vaccine is recommended for active immunization of children in a five-dose schedule at ages 2 months, 4 months, 6 months, 15 to 19 months, and 4 to 6 years (at school entry). Dengue is a mosquito-borne viral infection for which a vaccine has been prepared, but it is not included in DPT. A killed bacterial vaccine is used throughout the world to prevent typhoid fever. Tularemia vaccine is not included in DPT, nor is typhus vaccine; the latter is prepared from *Rickettsia prowazekii* grown in embryonated chicken eggs.

21. The answer is D *[Ch 12 III F].*
Bone marrow contains mature T cells which can mount an immunologic attack on the host. This may be so severe that, if not controlled by appropriate immunosuppressive measures, it can lead to the death of the recipient. This so-called graft-versus-host (GVH) reaction is minimized by treating the marrow with antithymocyte serum to purge it of these immunologically reactive cells. The stem cells that are trans-

ferred in the bone marrow will be tolerant of the host's HLA antigens because they will mature in their presence.

22. The answer is D *[Ch 5 III B; Ch 12 II A].*
Class I major histocompatibility complex (MHC) restriction affects cytotoxic T (Tc) cell–target cell interactions during killing of virally infected cells. There are two categories of MHC restriction. Class I restriction restricts the cytotoxicity of Tc cells to targets such as virally infected host cells, thus preventing Tc cells from releasing cytotoxins when they encounter free viral antigens in the body. Effective killing by Tc cells can only occur if these cytotoxic molecules are released in the immediate proximity of virally infected cells; class I MHC restriction ensures that this will occur. As practically all cells of the body carry class I MHC antigens, no tissue can serve as a sanctuary or protected haven for viruses. Class II restriction protects the body from unwanted autoimmune responses, because humoral immunity can only be initiated if the antigen is "presented" by a cell bearing a class II MHC gene product. Thus cells of the body such as erythrocytes or neurons cannot turn on antibody production.

23. The answer is D *[Ch 9 II D 3 c].*
One action of epinephrine is to stimulate adenylate cyclase, the enzyme responsible for converting adenosine triphosphate (ATP) to cyclic adenosine 3,5-monophosphate (cAMP). The latter blocks the release of mediators from mast cells and basophils. Theophylline, not epinephrine, inhibits phosphodiesterase, an enzyme that converts cAMP to AMP; thus, theophylline acts to preserve levels of cAMP essential for blocking mediator release. Epinephrine plays no significant role in inhibiting slow-reacting substance of anaphylaxis (SRS-A), in inducing release of lymphokines, or in stimulating production of histamine.

24. The answer is B *[Ch 3 II G 1].*
Treatment of the monomeric basic immunoglobulin unit with the enzyme papain splits the monomer into two monovalent Fab (antigen-binding) fragments and one Fc (crystallizable) fragment. Each Fab fragment contains the V_H and C_H1 domains of the heavy (H) chain (comprising the Fd fragment) and an entire light (L) chain, and each Fc fragment contains the carboxy terminal half of both heavy (H) chains.

25. The answer is A *[Ch 13 I C 2; II D 3].*
Neuroblastoma is a malignancy of infancy and early childhood. The lymphocytes of the patients (and sometimes those of their mothers) kill neuroblastoma cells but not cells from other malignancies. The patient's serum may contain enhancing factors such as non–complement-fixing antibodies or antigen–antibody complexes, or it may contain antibodies involved in cytotoxicity or the antibody-dependent cellular cytotoxic (ADCC) reaction.

26. The answer is C *[Ch 11 V A; Ch 12 III G, H 3].*
The major problem in bone marrow transplantation is the incorporation in the transplant of viable lymphoid cells, which could mount a graft-versus-host (GVH) reaction in the recipient. This is particularly true if the recipient's immune system is compromised, as in the case of a patient with severe combined immunodeficiency disease (SCID) or in the case of a transplant patient under immunosuppression.

27. The answer is D *[Ch 7 III B 2].*
Immune globulin, also called gamma globulin, is composed mainly of IgG antibodies against a number of different microorganisms. Immune globulin is prepared from pooled normal adult human plasma or serum by cold ethanol fractionation. Immune globulin is one of three basic types of serum preparations used to induce passive immunity artificially, the other two being antitoxin and specific immune globulin.

28. The answer is A *[Table 1-1; Ch 7 I B].*
Vaccines induce active artificially acquired immunity. An example of naturally acquired active immunity would be the immunity acquired as a result of recovering from disease. Passive artificially acquired immunity would result from administration of preformed antibody (e.g., antitoxin or antiviral antiserum), whereas naturally acquired passive immunity would be that gained by an infant via placental transfer of antibody from the mother.

29. The answer is B *[Ch 8 II C 1; Ch 11 I].*
A positive Schick test indicates that the patient is unable to mount a humoral immune response, which is a B cell immunodeficiency. If the patient had produced antibodies to the diphtheria toxin, the toxin would have been neutralized and no inflammatory reaction would have occurred at the site of injection. The presence of a positive mumps skin test suggests that the patient has intact T cell immunity. The ability of the serum to cause hemolysis of antibody-sensitized erythrocytes indicates that the complement system

is functioning. Phagocytic function tests of chemotaxis and intracellular killing suggest that the phago-cytes are also functioning normally in this patient.

30. The answer is C *[Ch 4 V B 1 d (1)].*
C5a acts to increase chemotaxis and chemokinesis of phagocytic cells. In addition, C5a, C3a, and C4a are all anaphylatoxins. These substances cause the contraction of smooth muscle and react with receptors on mast cell membranes, causing the release of mediators such as histamine. C2b is a serine protease which cleaves C3 into C3a and C3b. C3b is an opsonin.

31. The answer is D *[Ch 5 IV F 2; Ch 8 IV C 2; Ch 9 II B 3].*
B cells are the source of the IgE antibodies that cause atopic diseases. Delayed hypersensitivity is trans-ferred by T lymphocytes called Tdth cells. Tdth cells also produce the lymphokines that are responsible for the lesions of poison ivy. Monocytes and macrophages secrete interleukin-1 (IL-1). T cells are induced to go into mitosis when exposed to phytohemagglutinin (PHA) or concanavalin A (con A).

32. The answer is A *[Ch 7 II B 3, 6].*
Heptavax is a vaccine made from a viral subunit, rather than a live virus vaccine. It is used to prevent hepatitis B infection in individuals at high risk, such as dentists. All the other vaccines in the question (Sabin polio, yellow fever, rubella, and mumps vaccines) are live virus vaccines. Live virus vaccines are dangerous in individuals who have immunologic defects, particularly if these defects involve T cell func-tions.

33. The answer is C *[Ch 2 II B 3; Ch 8 III A 3 b, D 3].*
Infectious mononucleosis due to the Epstein-Barr virus can be diagnosed by the presence in the patient's serum of antibodies that agglutinate sheep red blood cells (SRBCs). These antibodies are directed to an antigen on the red cell that is very similar to one which is produced during infection by the Epstein-Barr virus. This is a heterophilic antigen relationship, and the test used to detect it is the Paul-Bunnell hemag-glutination procedure. A similar form of mononucleosis, caused by cytomegalovirus, another herpesvi-rus, is not accompanied by the production of SRBC agglutinins. Patients with rickettsial infections develop antibodies that agglutinate certain strains of *Proteus vulgaris*. This serologic reaction is termed the Weil-Felix test. Quantitative radial immunodiffusion is useful in determining hyper- or hypogammaglobuline-mic states. The Coombs test is used to detect antibodies to erythrocytes in conditions such as hemolytic disease of the newborn (erythroblastosis fetalis), autoimmune hemolytic disorders, and transfusion re-actions.

34. The answer is C *[Ch 9 V B 3, C 1].*
Cortisone administration causes a decrease in blood lymphocytes, with a significantly greater reduction of T cells than B cells. Delayed hypersensitivity, or cell-mediated tissue damage, results from the inter-action between sensitized T cells and specific antigen. This type of reaction is independent of antibody and complement but is primarily dependent upon $CD4^+$ cells. Complement depletion would not be ex-pected to affect cell-mediated reactions significantly. Plasmapheresis is used in the therapy of immune complex diseases and autoimmune phenomena. Theophylline is used in the treatment of asthma; it in-hibits phosphodiesterase, thus maintaining high levels of cyclic adenosine 3,5-monophosphate (cAMP) inside the mast cell. Cromolyn sodium stabilizes mast cell membranes and thereby inhibits mediator re-lease.

35. The answer is B *[Ch 3 IV A 2 a; Ch 5].*
The idiotype of an antibody is the sum of the idiotopes that the antibody possesses. The idiotopes are the epitopes that occur at the antigen-binding site (paratope) of the molecule or near it. Idiotopes—and hence idiotypes—are determined by the amino acid residues in the hypervariable region of the molecule, as this is what confers the specificity of the antibody. The framework regions in the variable portions of heavy (H) and light (L) chains will be similar from antibody to antibody. CD4 and CD8 are markers that occur in the membranes of helper T (Th) and suppressor T (Ts) cells, respectively. The B cell expresses its im-munologic commitment before exposure to the antigen.

36. The answer is D *[Ch 6 III B 2 b].*
There is an antigen threshold that must be reached before an immune response can be induced. There is also an upper limit, and if this is exceeded immune tolerance can result. The form of the antigen is also important. Aggregated antigens are usually quite immunogenic, whereas monomeric forms of the same protein are tolerogenic.

37. The answer is C *[Ch 7 II A 2 b].*
Toxoids are immunogenic and nontoxic preparations produced from toxins. The toxins of several bacteria can be converted into toxoids; heat or formalin can be used for their preparation. Toxoids make excellent vaccines for the purpose of inducing active antitoxic immunity.

38. The answer is A *[Ch 1 C 4 b; Ch 6 II B 2 a (2), c (2), d (1); Ch 8 IV C 2 a (1), (3)].*
Cell-mediated, or T cell, immunity can be suppressed by antithymocyte serum. Cell-mediated immunity is involved in tumor rejection. It is also involved in resistance to certain viral, fungal, and mycobacterial pathogens. Individuals who have a positive skin test to purified protein derivative (PPD) of the tubercle bacillus will react with an area of induration of 10 mm or greater 48 hours after exposure to that antigen. T cells do not have antibody bound to their membranes, and they are sensitive to cortisone suppression. Natural killer (NK) cells are lymphocytes that are neither B nor T cells; they are capable of killing cells without prior antigen exposure, and are not involved in cell-mediated immunity.

39 and 40. The answers are: 39-E *[Ch 13 II],* **40-A** *[Ch 13 II C 1 c].*
Carcinoembryonic antigen (CEA) is associated with carcinoma of the colon and pancreas; however, because CEA also occurs in nonmalignant conditions (e.g., as a result of cigarette smoking), it is not considered to be diagnostic of, but merely suggestive of, a cancerous condition. Assays for CEA show their greatest promise in monitoring for the recurrence of certain malignancies after surgery or chemotherapy.
The presence of CEA in the serum is correlated with the tumor burden of the host. The higher the level of CEA, the greater is the patient's tumor mass. Following surgical excision of the tumor, the CEA level should drop very low, perhaps even to indiscernible levels. If the CEA level rises again, it suggests that the tumor has metastasized and appropriate therapeutic or surgical intervention is indicated. The patient presented in the questions is gravely ill. Surgical removal of the tumor was incomplete, and metastases have developed, as indicated by the rise in CEA in months 10 to 12. The chemotherapeutic regimen should be reevaluated, and the patient should be thoroughly examined for possible radiologic and surgical treatment.

41. The answer is A *[Ch 3 III B 2].*
While some IgG and IgM can be found in gingival pocket fluid, IgA predominates in saliva. IgG is the major antibody in the serum. IgM is the first antibody synthesized in utero and during postnatal antibody responses. IgE is the immunoglobulin associated with anaphylaxis and atopic diseases such as asthma and hay fever. IgD occurs in large quantities on the B cell membrane and may be involved in B cell activation.

42. The answer is C *[Ch 12 III H 3].*
Graft-versus-host (GVH) reactions are an expression of T cell function, and elimination of the T cells by treatment with CD2 or CD3 antiserum before bone marrow engraftment should prevent a reaction from taking place. The presence of contaminating microbes in a graft would certainly contribute to the recipient's rejection of the graft but not to a GVH reaction, which is the graft's rejection of the recipient. Tumors are dedifferentiated tissues that cannot participate in GVH reactions. For a GVH reaction to occur, the recipient must have HLA antigens that are not found in the donor, not the other way around.

43. The answer is C *[Ch 11 IV A].*
Profoundly impaired T cell function, such as that seen in DiGeorge syndrome, manifests itself by recurrent infections with viruses, fungi, protozoa, and intracellular bacterial pathogens. Protection against such agents depends largely on intact cell-mediated immunity.

44. The answer is B *[Ch 4 IV B 1 c; Ch 11 VII A].*
Patients with hereditary angioedema have a deficiency of C1 esterase inhibitor, which leads to uncontrolled C1 esterase activity and resultant production of a kinin that increases capillary permeability. Hereditary angioedema is an inherited defect characterized by transient but recurrent edema of the skin, gastrointestinal tract, or respiratory tract.

45. The answer is A *[Ch 6 II B 2 d; Ch 7 IV A 5].*
Interleukin-2 (IL-2) stimulates the immune response nonspecifically by inducing the production of lymphokine-activated killer (LAK) cells and augmenting the activity of natural killer (NK) cells. Anti-idiotypic antibody and immunotoxins are used for antigen-specific suppression of the immune response. Cortisone and antithymocyte serum suppress T cell immunities.

46. The answer is E *[Ch 5 II B 3; III B; Ch 12 III F].*
Bone marrow contains stem cells; however, these are unable to respond to host antigens as they will be

rendered immunologically tolerant as they mature in the large antigen excess found in the host. The age of the donor has very little to do with suitability as a bone marrow donor because mature T cells capable of rejecting the recipient are present at a very early age, probably in utero. It is true that the host thymus must help the stem cells mature, but this is not important in graft-versus-host (GVH) reactions because of the excess that the cells will encounter during maturation. If it were possible, T stem cell removal before engraftment would be the ideal solution; however, this goal has proven elusive; removal of primordial stem cells would defeat the purpose of the graft. The T cells are not immunologically reactive until they mature. Hence, it can be concluded that there are some mature T cells in the bone marrow, as GVH reactions do occur in bone marrow transplantation. The purpose of the transplant is to supply stem cells which will mature into functional cells of the entire hematopoietic system.

47. The answer is B *[Ch 12 II A; III A 3].*
Humans will respond to foreign HLA antigens that they encounter in transfusions or as a result of pregnancy. The white blood cells are the major source of these antigens, as they are not found on erythrocytes. It is true that humans make an immune response to bacteria that colonize the upper respiratory, gastrointestinal, and genitourinary tracts, but, fortunately, these microbial antigens do not cross-react with HLA antigens.

48. The answer is B *[Ch 1 II F 2 d; Ch 5 IV G 3, B].*
The rather archaic term "humoral" means soluble or noncellular. While "humoral immunity" usually implies antibody-related or B-cell–mediated specific immunity, nonantibody humoral factors can also contribute to nonspecific, or innate, immunity. An example is beta lysin. This antibacterial protein is released from blood platelets when they rupture, as in clot formation, and it is active primarily against gram-positive bacteria. Antitoxin is a product of the adaptive immune response. Lymphokine-activated killer (LAK) cells are naturally occurring cytotoxic lymphocytes, not humoral factors. Interleukin-1 (IL-1) is a cytokine released from macrophages during the induction of an immune response. It stimulates T cells to proliferate and release other interleukins; thus, it contributes to specific, rather than to innate, immunity. Cortisone is a hormone released by the adrenal gland. Rather than contributing to the immune system, it is an immunosuppressant.

49. The answer is D *[Ch 5 III B 2 a (5), 3 b].*
Epitope recognition by a T cell occurs because of the unique structure of the T cell receptor: there is a T cell receptor for each possible epitope. The T cell receptor is noncovalently linked to the CD3 molecule, which is involved in transmembrane signals that initiate interleukin-2 (IL- 2) secretion and the maturational events that ensue. CD4 is the cell surface marker of helper T (Th) cells and plays a role in recognition of class II major histocompatibility complex (MHC) molecules.

50. The answer is E *[Ch 11 V A].*
Severe combined immunodeficiency disease (SCID) involves a combined defect in both humoral and cell-mediated immunity, as evidenced by lymphopenia, absence of a thymus shadow on x-ray, hypogammaglobulinemia, and lack of B cells or antibody response. Patients usually die within the first year or two of life from viral, bacterial, fungal, or protozoan infection.

51. The answer is C *[Ch 1 II G 1; Ch 6 C 1].*
Suppressor cells serve a negative control function in regulation of the immune response; contrasuppressor cells act to regulate the development of suppressor cells. Natural killer (NK) cells and other large granular lymphocytes are not antigen-reactive lymphocytes: they are normally present in the body without prior antigenic experience. They serve to protect the body from viral infections and cancers primarily. They are often called null cells because they do not have surface markers characteristic of B cells or the various T cell subsets.

52. The answer is D *[Ch 12 II B].*
In order to function in graft recognition, histocompatibility antigens must be accessible to the cells of the immune system (i.e., they must be located at the surface of the cell). Class I antigens are glycoproteins in noncovalent association with a β_2-microglobulin. They are found on all nucleated cells of the body. Class II antigens are found on the surfaces of macrophages, T cells, and B cells. They are composed of two membrane-inserted, glycosylated proteins, α and β, which are noncovalently bonded. The major histocompatibility complex (MHC) antigens in man are called human leukocyte antigens (HLAs) and are coded for by genes on chromosome 6.

53. The answer is A *[Ch 3 II C, D, E 1 a, b; III E 2 d; Ch 9 II B].*
In the generation of atopic hypersensitivity, antigen (allergen)-specific IgE is produced. IgE is described as homocytotropic due to its affinity for cells ("cytotropic") of the host species that produced it ("homo"), particularly for tissue mast cells and blood basophils. Cell adherence occurs via the Fc fragment (C3 and C4 domains).

54. The answer is D *[Ch 9 V B 3; Ch 12 II A 3].*
Delayed hypersensitivity involves the processing of antigen by macrophages and the consequent activation of T cells. Interaction between antigen-processing cells and T cells can only occur if the two participants are major histocompatibility complex (MHC)–identical; that is, only if both cell types possess identical surface antigens that are class II MHC determinants. Under the influence of immunogenic epitopes and MHC determinants, the T cells become antigen-reactive (activated, sensitized). Allogeneic refers to antigens that occur within a species but differ among members of that species.

55. The answer is D *[Ch 4 II B 2 a (3)].*
In the classic pathway of complement activation, the first component to bind is C1, which acquires esterase activity and is referred to as C$\overline{1}$ esterase. The latter then mediates cleavage of C4 into C4a and C4b. C4b can bind to cell membranes; C4a is released into the fluid phase and acts as an anaphylatoxin.

56. The answer is A *[Ch 6 II B 2 d (2); Ch 9 III C 1 b].*
Erythroblastosis fetalis can be prevented in a future pregnancy by injecting Rh_o(D) immunoglobulin (RhoGAM) into an Rh-negative mother shortly after delivery of an Rh-positive infant. RhoGAM is an antibody specific to the Rh_o(D) antigen—the antigen that induces erythroblastosis. If the mother is Rh-negative and carrying an Rh-positive fetus, some of the fetal red blood cells bearing the Rh_o(D) antigen enter the mother's circulation during delivery. Once sensitized, the mother will produce antibodies to the antigen, which can cross the placenta during a subsequent pregnancy and damage the fetus. RhoGAM blocks the induction of anti-Rh_o antibody production in the mother. RhoGAM cannot be given prior to delivery, as it would cross the placenta and cause damage to the fetus.

57. The answer is D *[Ch 8 VI A].*
Complement component C1q has an affinity for immune complexes. The many assays that are available for detecting immune complexes in serum can be divided into three types: solid-phase binding assays, fluid-phase binding assays, and cellular binding assays. The reaction of immune complexes with complement allows for many ways to detect immune complexes. For example, complement-fixing immune complexes can be detected by direct measurement of the binding of immune complexes to C1q; this can be done using a solid-phase or a fluid-phase binding assay. The interaction of complement-coated immune complexes with complement receptors on cells (e.g., Raji cells) also may be used; the Raji cell binding assay is an example of a cellular binding assay. The radioallergosorbent test (RAST) is used to assay specific IgE levels in vitro, the Prausnitz-Küstner (PK) reaction is an in vivo passive transfer test used to assay specific IgE in serum. Radial immunodiffusion is used to quantitate immunoglobulins and other proteins in serum or other biological fluids.

58 and 59. The answers are: 58-E *[Ch 10 II B, F, G, H],* **59-D** *[Ch 10 II F].*
Muscular dystrophy does not have any demonstrated autoimmune component, there are no major neurologic deficits, and patients do not recover. Systemic lupus erythematosus (SLE) is a possible diagnosis for the patient presented in the question. On occasion this disease can affect the central nervous system. However, the fact that the patient had been well up to the time of the present illness tends to rule out SLE, as does the predilection of the disease for young women. Myasthenia gravis and multiple sclerosis are possible diagnoses, although the rapid onset of a near-fatal disease tends to exclude these. The patient in this case has Guillain-Barré syndrome.

A lumbar puncture was performed to rule out encephalomyelitis. An elevated white blood cell count would suggest an infectious process, with neutrophils predominating if the cause is bacterial, and lymphocytes predominating if the cause is viral. Also, glucose levels usually are depleted if the disease is of bacterial origin. An elevated protein content coupled with otherwise normal cerebrospinal fluid findings is suggestive of Guillain-Barré syndrome. Lumbar puncture should not be done in the case of a brain abscess as the intracranial pressure could be great enough to cause downward displacement of the brain.

60. The answer is B *[Ch 12 II D 1 b].*
The β_2-microglobulin is not encoded by the major histocompatibility complex (MHC) of humans; it is a product of a gene on chromosome 15 in humans and chromosome 2 in mice. The MHC of humans encodes class I and class II human leukocyte antigens: the HLA-A, HLA-B, and HLA-C regions encode

class I molecules; the HLA-D region encodes class II molecules. The MHC also encodes certain other proteins such as complement components C2 and C4 as class III products. Class I antigens are found on all nucleated cells of the body except spermatozoa and trophoblasts; class II antigens are found only on macrophages, helper T (Th) cells, B cells, and activated cytotoxic T (Tc) cells. Class I antigens are involved in Tc cell recognition of tumor cells or virally infected cells; class II antigens play a central role in cellular collaboration during the induction of a humoral immune response. Both class I and II antigens are transplantation barriers.

61. The answer is A *[Ch 5 IV D 1 a].*
The cell that would not be needed in a thymus-independent immune response is the thymus-derived helper T (Th) cell. Antibodies are produced by B cells, so these cells must always participate in humoral immune responses. Macrophages, or some other antigen-presenting cells such as the Langerhans cells in the skin, are normally required to "process" and "present" the antigen to lymphocytes, although in some instances highly polymeric antigens can cross-link epitope receptors and initiate an immune response.

62. The answer is B *[Ch 12 II C 1].*
The serum employed in the cytotoxicity test used to identify HLA antigens is obtained from multiparous women, patients who have received and rejected allografts, patients who have received multiple transfusions, and volunteers who have been HLA-sensitized by blood transfusions, white cell inoculations, or tissue grafts. All of these people would be sensitized to HLA antigens, the antigens being unique to the fetus, the graft, or the transfused lymphocytes. Such sensitization would result in the production of antibodies specific for the particular HLA antigen to which the person has been exposed. Rabbits immunized with human lymphocytes would produce an array of antibodies to lymphocytes, which would not have the epitope specificity needed for the cytotoxicity assay.

63–65. The answers are: 63-D *[Ch 11 III D 2; IV A 2; V B, C],* **64-D** *[Ch 11 II B 1, 5, 6; III D],* **65-D** *[Ch 11 III A 2, B 1, C 1, D 2; V C].*
Normal recovery from viral diseases suggests an intact thymus-dependent immune system, thus eliminating DiGeorge, Nezelof's, and Wiskott-Aldrich syndromes, all of which feature variable or total deficits in T cell immunity. Selective immunoglobulin deficiency could be considered as a possible diagnosis due to its characteristic of normal T cell function.

Dysgammaglobulinemia is a selective immunoglobulin deficiency, in which one or more, but not all, immunoglobulins show a decrease in serum levels; nonspecific immunity is normal in this disorder. Normal leukocytic function would not be characteristic of chronic granulomatous disease (CGD) [impaired intracellular killing], Job's syndrome (faulty chemotactic response), or the lazy leukocyte syndrome (defective chemotactic response and abnormal inflammatory response).

The patient has Bruton's hypogammaglobulinemia. The presence of a small amount of IgG is consistent with this diagnosis. Common variable hypogammaglobulinemia resembles Bruton's disease, except that symptoms first appear in patients age 20 to 30 years. Selective immunoglobulin deficiency is characterized by a decrease in serum levels of one or more immunoglobulin classes; in selective IgA deficiency, the most common form, there is little serum IgA but normal or increased levels of IgG and IgM. Wiskott-Aldrich syndrome features low IgM levels, elevated IgA and IgE, but normal IgG levels. Transient hypogammaglobulinemia of infancy is self-correcting by age 30 months, and thus would be an unlikely diagnosis by age 3 years.

66. The answer is B *[Ch 5 III A; IV A 2, D 1 b; Table 5-3].*
Macrophages do not produce interleukin-2 (IL-2). They produce IL-1, a hormone-like substance that induces helper T (Th) cell proliferation. Th cells release IL-2, which stimulates other T cells to proliferate. IL-2 also induces the production of other interleukins, which cause proliferation of many different cells in the body, including B cells. The macrophage also serves as an antigen-processing cell. After ingesting and processing an antigen, the macrophage presents the antigen to the B cell, and if the appropriate Th cell is present, the B cell matures and differentiates into a plasma cell. Macrophages also function as phagocytes: they recognize, engulf, and destroy bacteria and other antigenic materials.

67. The answer is D *[Ch 13 V A].*
The principles of immunotherapy of human tumors include the reduction of tumor load by surgery, chemotherapy, or both; modification of tumor cells to enhance antigenicity and eliminate viability; and activation of the immune response via adjuvants. The use of viable tumor cells for specific immunization of the patient should not be attempted, as the possible presence of oncogenic viruses in the vaccine presents a major threat to the recipient.

68. The answer is C *[Ch 4 IV B 2; Ch 9 II B 4].*
Factor H is not involved in type I hypersensitivity. It acts in concert with factor I to cleave and thereby inactivate complement component C3b. Immediate hypersensitivity reactions (e.g., anaphylaxis or atopic allergies) are initiated by the interaction between antigens and cell-bound antibody—usually IgE. (Antigens that preferentially induce the production of IgE are known as allergens.) The bridging of adjacent membrane-bound IgE molecules by allergen initiates the degranulation of mast cells and basophils, causing the release of several pharmacologically active mediators or their precursors from storage in these cells. Among the various mediators are eosinophil chemotactic factor of anaphylaxis (ECF-A), histamine, platelet-activating factor (PAF), slow-reacting substance of anaphylaxis (SRS-A), serotonin, and prostaglandins. Serine protease activity is seen in anaphylactic reactions and is also common to several of the complement proteins.

69. The answer is E *[Ch 6 II C 3; Ch 9 IV C 2; Ch 10 II A].*
The administration of foreign serum will not cause rheumatoid arthritis. However, it may cause the development of an immune complex disease called serum sickness. Because the foreign serum is an effective immunosuppressant, it can predispose the patient to infections by organisms that are members of the normal flora or are innocuous agents in the environment. Latent infections may reappear in immunosuppressed individuals, and such patients have a heightened likelihood of developing cancer.

70. The answer is A *[Ch 4 V B 2 b (1) ; Ch 8 IV B, C].*
Concanavalin A (con A) receptors are found in the T cell membrane; B cells have receptors for bacterial lipopolysaccharide, complement component C3b, and the Fc fragment of immunoglobulin molecules. Monomeric IgM is the first antibody to appear in the B cell membrane. Both class I and class II major histocompatibility complex (MHC) proteins are found in the B cell membrane.

71. The answer is A *[Ch 6 II B 2].*
Cyclosporine is an antibiotic produced by several fungal species; a potent immunosuppressant, it specifically interferes with interleukin-2 (IL-2) activities. Macrophages secrete tumor necrosis factor (TNF), IL-1, complement, and alpha interferon, as well as many other substances. Enzymes such as cathepsins and phosphatases are released, as are compounds which influence cell differentiation, such as colony-stimulating factor (CSF). The secreted substances are called "monokines" because they are the products of mononuclear cells, either blood monocytes or tissue macrophages.

72. The answer is C *[Ch 5 IV D 1 b, F 5; Ch 9 V C 1 c (1)].*
Although humoral immune responses usually do require the helper T (Th) cell, the immune response to most carbohydrate antigens is thymus- independent and only requires a B lymphocyte plus a macrophage as accessory cell. T cells are involved in contact dermatitis and are effector cells in tuberculosis immunity. In addition, T cells respond to interleukin-1 (IL-1) produced by antigen-presenting cells and will produce IL-2 in response to that hormonal signal.

73. The answer is E *[Ch 5 IV D; Ch 6 II A 2, B 2 a].*
Ionizing radiation does not regulate the immune response: it inhibits all phases of the immune response, even intracellular killing within phagocytic cells. The idiotypic network has been proposed as a control mechanism; major histocompatibility complex (MHC) restriction plays a role in control of autoimmunity. Suppressor T (Ts) cells function in the down-regulation of immune responses, as do suppressor macrophages. The latter have been demonstrated in vitro as highly activated phagocytic cells from infected or tumor-bearing hosts that inhibit immune reactions by releasing products of arachidonic acid metabolism (prostaglandins) or toxic oxygen radicals.

74. The answer is E *[Ch 13 II D].*
Tumor-specific transplantation antigens (TSTAs) are found on the membranes of tumor cells. Tumors may have unique antigens in the nuclear membrane but they will not function as transplantation antigens because the immune effectors [antibodies and cytotoxic T (Tc) cells] cannot interact with them. TSTAs may be viral in origin. They may induce an antibody response in the host, and may induce the development of Tc cells or suppressor T (Ts) cells.

75. The answer is A *[Table 1-5; Ch 4 II B, C].*
C3b is a split product of complement which acts as an opsonin, not as a chemotactic agent. CR1 receptors on the phagocytic cell surface react with the C3b molecule, and this enhances the interaction between the cell and the particle to be engulfed.

76. The answer is D *[Ch 6 II B 1 c; Ch 11 I A 1; Table 11-1].*
Both cytotoxic T (Tc) and suppressor T (Ts) cells may be depressed in individuals under long-term immunosuppression. In addition, patients suffering from autoimmune disease and transplant recipients receiving immunosuppression commonly suffer from recurrent herpes simplex infections, as well as manifestations of other viral diseases. They also will have a decrease in total antibody synthesis and will have depression of cell-mediated immune responses. These patients commonly have infections caused by opportunists of the normal flora. Factors that decrease immune capabilities predispose an individual to malignancy.

77. The answer is D *[Ch 2 I C 3; Ch 3 II F].*
The epitope is the antigenic determinant site on an antigen molecule; it is the site that interacts specifically with its homologous paratope on an antibody molecule. The valence of an antigen is the sum of all the epitopes possessed by that molecule, the internal epitopes as well as the ones accessible on the surface. The valence would be inaccurate if it were inferred from the number of antibody molecules that react with the antigen, because that number would underestimate both the internal epitope composition and the interference that occurs due to spatial competition for reaction sites. A single antigen can have, and usually does have, multiple copies of several different types of epitopes. The larger the molecule, the greater will be the number of types and the number of copies. An increase in chemical complexity increases the number of different epitopes as well.

78. The answer is E *[Ch 1 II D 6 b, E 2; Ch 13 III C 4 d].*
Cachectin, also known as tumor necrosis factor α (TNF-α), is not an opsonin; it is a protein secreted from macrophages that has antitumor activity. Cachectin was originally described as a substance found in patients with malignancies and in experimental animals with heavy parasitic infestations. It had a profound effect on cellular metabolism and was responsible for the weight loss seen during infections or malignancies. Opsonization is a process in which a substance coats or binds to a foreign particle, so that the end result is an enhancement of phagocytosis. The coating substance is known as an opsonin. C3b, antibody, fibronectin, and tuftsin are all opsonins—they enhance the interaction of the phagocytic cell with the particle to be engulfed. Other enhancers of phagocytosis, such as C5a, are not opsonins but chemotactic factors, which attract phagocytes to areas of inflammation. Some leukotrienes are opsonins, and some are chemotactic; since leukotrienes are lipoxygenase metabolites of arachidonic acid, they may also increase the rate of phagocytosis due to their vasodilatory effect, which would increase the blood flow in the area.

79. The answer is E *[Ch 8 IV A, B 2 a].*
Antibody synthesis is a function of B cell activity, not phagocytic activity, although phagocytic cells do participate indirectly by serving as antigen processors. Phagocytic chemotaxis can be assayed by separating the phagocyte from a chemotactic stimulus by a micropore membrane or in an agar menstruum. Chemiluminescence is used to measure the light produced by singlet oxygen, a microbicidal compound generated by oxygen-dependent mechanisms within the phagocyte's lysosomal granules that are responsible for destroying foreign particles. Nitroblue tetrazolium (NBT) is a yellow water-soluble dye that converts within cells to formazan, a purple water-insoluble compound, when phagocytizing neutrophils produce hydrogen peroxide and superoxide anion during the phagocytic process. The microbicidal activity of phagocytic cells can also be measured by direct plate counting of mixtures of microorganisms and cells, or by the use of supravital stains such as acridine orange to assess the viability of engulfed microbes.

80. The answer is A *[Ch 3 II D 1 b, G 1 b].*
Fc fragments contain the carboxy terminal (i.e., constant) portion of immunoglobulin heavy (H) chains, and thus do not contain hypervariable regions. Rather, hypervariable regions occur in the variable (V) regions of H and light (L) chains. These areas of high variability [also called "hot spots" or complementarity-determining regions (CDRs)] are most intimately involved in formation of the antigen-binding site. The V_H region has four CDRs, and the V_L region has three. Fab fragments are so named because they are **a**ntigen **b**inding. They are composed of the entire L chain [V_L and the constant region (C_L)] and the amino terminal half of the H chain. The Fd fragment is the H chain portion of the Fab fragment and consists of the V_H domain and the first constant (C_H) domain.

81. The answer is B *[Table 1-5; Table 4-4].*
CR2 is found on B, T, and natural killer (NK) cells, but not on macrophages. The potent opsonin C3b and two of its degradation products, iC3b and C3d, react with complement receptors CR1, CR3, and CR4 in the membrane of phagocytic cells to enhance engulfment. CR1 also binds C4b. C3aR is found on phagocytes and also occurs on basophils and mast cells; its interaction with the anaphylatoxin C3a results in degranulation and release of mediators from these cells.

82. The answer is D *[Ch 10 II B, G, H].*
Antimyosin antibodies have not been demonstrated in muscular dystrophy; no autoimmune phenomena have been noted in this disorder.

A positive test for antinuclear antibodies is necessary, but not sufficient, for the diagnosis of systemic lupus erythematosus (SLE). Antinuclear antibodies can also be present in patients with other diseases, such as rheumatoid arthritis and scleroderma, and in cases in which there is a history of ingestion of certain drugs, so obviously these factors must first be ruled out.

The diagnosis of multiple sclerosis is contingent upon the clinical features of the disease. However, most patients with multiple sclerosis will have abnormalities on laboratory tests; one of the most dependable findings is an increase in IgG in the patient's spinal fluid. IgG values often are normal early in the course of multiple sclerosis. The increase in spinal fluid IgG is highest in cases of the greatest duration and in patients with severe neurologic deficits.

The most important autoimmune feature of myasthenia gravis is the presence of antibodies to the human acetylcholine receptor. Approximately 80% to 85% of patients with myasthenia gravis have high serum levels of these antibodies.

Autoantibodies to nervous tissue can be detected in the serum of patients with Guillain-Barré syndrome by complement fixation test procedures.

83. The answer is D *[Ch 3 II A 2, D 1, H].*
Not all immunoglobulin classes have J chains, only IgA and IgM polymeric forms (e.g., δ IgA, pentameric IgM). All classes (isotypes) of immunoglobulins contain heavy (H) and light (L) chains, constant (C) and variable (V) domains, and hinge regions.

84. The answer is E *[Ch 12 II A 1, 3, 4; III C 1, H 3].*
The ABO blood group antigens are very potent transplantation antigens, and incompatibility between donor and recipient can result in hyperacute rejection if the recipient has preformed isoagglutinin antibodies. The presence of HLA antigens on white blood cells and platelets can cause HLA sensitization and febrile reactions upon secondary exposure. In graft-versus-host (GVH) reactions, the graft tissue mounts an immunologic attack on the recipient. Such reactions occur when a graft containing immunocompetent T cells is implanted into an immunocompromised recipient and the T cells reject their new host.

85 and 86. The answers are: 85-C *[Ch 7 II A 3 c; Ch 8 II B 3, C; III A 1, C, D 1, F],* **86-E** *[Ch 7 II A 3 e; Ch 8 II B 4].*
Agglutination would not be of any value for detecting tetanus antitoxin because the toxin is excreted and is not cell-bound. However, passive hemagglutination, in which the antigen (as tetanus toxoid) is adsorbed to a red blood cell carrier, would be an excellent assay. Other tests that could be used to detect tetanus antitoxin include toxin neutralization, complement fixation, enzyme-linked immunosorbent assay (ELISA), and precipitation. Toxin neutralization requires the use of animals or tissue cultures and hence may be beyond the means of many laboratories. Complement fixation is an acceptable alternative; however, it requires the pretitration of the component reagents, which would necessitate the purchase of a standardized tetanus antitoxin. The simplest assay, although not the most sensitive, would be precipitation, either in solution or in an agar medium; the advantage of the latter is economy of reagents, as several serum samples could be assayed against the same toxoid preparation in an Ouchterlony plate technique.

Radial immunodiffusion requires soluble antigens such as serum proteins and would not be useful to detect antibodies to typhoid bacilli. Antibodies to this organism are conveniently titrated by tube or slide agglutination procedures. A classic application of the agglutination reaction is the Widal test, used in the diagnosis of typhoid fever. Bactericidal assay, complement fixation, and indirect immunofluorescence could also be employed; however, all of these procedures are considerably more complex and time-consuming and none would be the test of choice.

87. The answer is A *[Table 5-3].*
Interleukin-1 (IL-1) is released by macrophages, B cells, and natural killer (NK) cells, but not by T cells. When antigen-presenting macrophages secrete IL-1, T cells respond by producing IL-2. T cells also produce interleukins 3, 4, 5, 6, 9, 10 and other cytokines such as interferons. Cytokines are soluble mediators with hormone-like actions; those produced by lymphocytes are called lymphokines.

88. The answer is D *[Ch 12 II C 4, D 1, 2].*
The immunoglobulin variable (V) domains are coded for by genes on chromosomes 2, 14, and 22. The human major histocompatibility complex (MHC) is composed of a cluster of genes located on chromo-

some 6, which code for three (and possibly four) distinct classes of molecules. Class I and class II MHC molecules are important for controlling immunologic defense. The MHC-encoded class I antigens (HLA-A, HLA-B, and HLA-C) can be expressed on all human nucleated cells. MHC-encoded class II antigens (HLA-D region antigens), which are also called immune response–associated (Ia) antigens, can be expressed on the surface of immunocompetent cells, principally B cells and macrophages. Class II antigens are important in the cellular recognition that permits the cellular interaction needed to induce an immune response. Class III molecules are certain complement components (C4, C2, factor B of the alternative pathway), tumor necrosis factors (TNFs), and cytochrome hydroxylases encoded by genes in the MHC.

89. The answer is E *[Ch 8 IV].*
Eosinophils are involved in allergic reactions such as asthma and hay fever, and eosinophilia is seen in allergies and certain parasitic diseases, but eosinophil involvement is secondary to the immune response of the host. T cells, B cells, and phagocytic cells (neutrophils and monocytes) are all evaluated in order to assess immune competence. Phagocytic cells are analyzed by testing for the metabolism and generation of toxic molecules, the ingestion and killing of microorganisms, and chemotaxis. Analysis of B cells and T cells involves their enumeration and the enumeration of pre-B cells and T cell subsets as well, and determining whether all these cells are functional.

90. The answer is D *[Ch 8 IV B 3 d].*
Receptors for concanavalin A (con A) and phytohemagglutinin (PHA) are contained in the T cell membrane but not in the B cell membrane. B cell membranes contain receptors for pokeweed mitogen, as well as for lipopolysaccharides such as the endotoxin of gram-negative bacteria. These molecules will induce mitosis in the B cell. This mitosis can be quantitated by measuring the incorporation of tritiated thymidine into the DNA of the cells. Thus, the amount of B cell activity can be quantitated. B cells also contain an Fc receptor in the membrane.

91. The answer is D *[Ch 12 II C 1, 2 a, 4 a, b].*
HLA antigens that are coded for by the A, B, and C loci are class I antigens. Their specificity is determined by polymorphism in the α chain, which is combined with a nonpolymorphic β2-microglobulin (the β chain) on the cell membrane. Only the α chain has a hydrophobic transmembrane segment. HLA-A and HLA-B are involved in the phenomenon known as major histocompatibility complex (MHC) restriction: interactions between cytotoxic T (Tc) cells and target cells can only occur if the class I antigens of the two types of cells are homologous.

92. The answer is C *[Ch 6 I C 2; Ch 10 I A 3].*
Anti-idiotypic antibodies are thought to be a mechanism of control of the immune response. They are of the same reactivity as the original epitope and can theoretically down-regulate the B and T cells by reacting with the surface-bound immunoglobulin or T cell receptor and blocking the "triggering" signal normally delivered by epitope-specific ligand interaction. An excess of self-reactive helper T (Th) cell activity may be produced by altered forms of self-antigen triggered by virus (e.g., influenza) coupling to the self-antigen (the presumed mechanism of acute disseminated encephalomyelitis). There is convincing evidence that certain polyclonal B cell activators (e.g., bacterial lipopolysaccharide) may precipitate autoantibody production by bypassing the need for self-reactive Th cell activity. If a population of suppressor T (Ts) cells is involved in down-regulating the immune response to self, then a deficiency of such cells may terminate self-tolerance. Indeed, mice of the NZB/NZW strain, which spontaneously develop a disease resembling systemic lupus erythematosus (SLE), show a deficiency of Ts cells. Autoantibody production has also been demonstrated following the release of sequestered antigen (e.g., autoantibody formation against sperm after vasectomy).

93. The answer is E *[Ch 3 II B 1 b; Table 3-1].*
The α chains are the heavy (H) chains of IgA molecules, and are not found in IgM. IgM molecules contain μ H chains and either κ or λ light (L) chains. IgM has a pentameric structure consisting of five basic monomeric units linked by J chain and by disulfide bonds at the Fc fragment. A preparation of pooled human IgM injected into a rabbit would be expected to be antigenic and to induce the formation of rabbit antibodies reactive with the individual immunoglobulin components.

94. The answer is A *[Ch 5 III A 1, B 2, 3 a, b, d].*
Macrophages participate in the immune response in a nonspecific manner. They possess receptors for the Fc portion of immunoglobulins and for complement component C3b, and they will attempt to phagocytize any particle that has either of these molecules on its surface. The B cell membrane contains

epitope-specific receptors, namely IgD and monomeric IgM. Helper T (Th) cells, cytotoxic T (Tc) cells, and suppressor T (Ts) cells also have epitope specificity; therefore, they also must have an antigen-recognition mechanism. This is provided by the T cell receptor for antigen, a heterodimer on the T cell surface that has marked structural homology with the Fab portion of the antibody molecule, although it is not a partial antibody molecule.

95. The answer is B *[Ch 12 II D 2].*
Immune response (Ir) genes code for the production of class II major histocompatibility complex (MHC) antigens referred to as immune response–associated (Ia) antigens. Ir genes are important in the interaction of the antigen-presenting macrophage with the antigen-specific B cell. The macrophage and lymphocyte must share the same class II (Ia) antigen in order to have effective interaction.

96. The answer is D *[Ch 8 IV B 3 d].*
Mitogens are substances that induce cells to undergo mitosis. Lipopolysaccharide, the endotoxin from gram-negative bacteria, is mitogenic for B cells but not for T cells. Phytohemagglutinin (PHA) and con-canavalin A (con A) are specific mitogens for T cells; pokeweed is mitogenic for both T and B cells. Specific antigens will induce mitosis in cells that bear homologous receptors in their membranes.

97. The answer is E *[Ch 13 I B].*
All cells that are rapidly dividing (as are cancer cells) will be susceptible to radiation damage. Malignant cells are usually dedifferentiated, have the potential for uncontrolled growth (i.e., they are immortal), and do not demonstrate growth inhibition when they come in contact with other similar cells. They usually acquire new epitopes, not uncommonly at the expense of preexisting antigens in differentiated tissues.

98. The answer is D *[Ch 3 IV A 1 a, b, c (3)].*
Allotypic markers designated Km are found in κ light (L) chains, not in IgG heavy (H) chains (γ chains). Allotypes are genetic markers on H and L immunoglobulin chains, usually localized in the constant region; they are inherited in a mendelian fashion.

99. The answer is E *[Ch 1 II G 1 c (3); Ch 5 IV D 1, 2; Ch 12 II C 4].*
In order for effective induction of an immune response to occur, the cells involved (macrophages, T cells, and B cells) must be identical at the class II major histocompatibility complex (MHC) locus. Cytotoxic T (Tc) cells have class I MHC restriction. Natural killer (NK) cells do not have any MHC restriction.

100. The answer is D *[Ch 12 II C 4 b (2); III B 1].*
The chief transplantation antigens that function as barriers to the acceptance of a graft in humans include class I and class II HLA antigens of the major histocompatibility complex (MHC) and the antigens of the blood group ABO system. Class III HLA antigens are not transplantation antigens but are serum proteins; specifically, the complement factors C2 and C4, factor B of the alternative complement pathway, tumor necrosis factors (TNFs) α and β, and two cytochrome hydroxylases.

101. The answer is A *[Figure 1-1; Ch 12 II C].*
Macrophage and neutrophil membranes contain receptors for the Fc fragment of IgG and IgM (but not IgE) as well as for the complement activation product C3b. These receptors are involved in the process of opsonization (i.e., sensitization of foreign material to phagocytosis). In addition, the macrophage membrane contains molecules referred to as immune response–associated (Ia) antigens. These are products of genes that occur in the major histocompatibility complex (MHC) and are involved in interaction of the macrophage with lymphoid cells in the immune response; most particularly, the interaction between the macrophage as the antigen-processing cell and the B cell as the precursor of the antibody-producing plasma cell. In the human, they are referred to as class II antigens and are coded for by genes occurring at the HLA-D region.

102. The answer is C *[Ch 10 II L 2 a].*
In Goodpasture's syndrome, the deposits of immunoglobulin (usually IgG) on alveolar and glomerular basement membranes represent antibody specific for antigen shared by the kidneys and lungs. Symptoms are referable to both the lungs (pulmonary hemorrhage, hemoptysis) and kidneys (glomerulonephritis, hematuria). The prognosis for patients is poor.

103. The answer is C *[Ch 8 VI].*
Either a cell-binding assay or the C1q solid-phase binding assay could be used to detect immune complexes. Both solid-phase and liquid-phase procedures are available for evaluating the affinity of com-

plement component C1q for immune complexes. Raji cells, a human lymphoblastoid cell line, are used in the cell-binding assay, which is based on the ability of immune complexes to bind to the Raji cells through C3 receptors. The immune complexes bound to the surface of the Raji cells can be assayed by the addition of radiolabeled anti-IgG antibody.

104. The answer is C *[Ch 3 III A 2 f; Ch 4 V B 2 b (1); Table 4-4].*
Neutrophil membranes contain receptors for the Fc fragments of IgG and IgM and also for complement component C3b. C3b molecules are opsonins: they enhance the phagocytosis of foreign materials such as bacterial cells. An antibody that has reacted on the surface of a bacterium would have the Fc fragment pointing away from the organism. If complement were activated, the C3b molecule would also be attached to the bacterial cell surface. The neutrophil membrane receptors interacting with the Fc fragment, the C3b molecule, or both would then be in firm union with the particle to be engulfed.

105. The answer is B *[Ch 2 I B].*
Haptens are reactive but not immunogenic: haptens by themselves are unable to induce an immune response. They gain immunogenicity when they interact with a carrier molecule (usually an antigen itself). Haptens do possess the ability to react with their homologous antibody or T lymphocyte, although this reactivity may not yield a visible manifestation. For example, simple haptens react with their homologous antibody, but the reaction cannot be visualized because no lattice structures are built up; the hapten is monovalent. It will occupy both antigen-reactive sites on the antibody molecule, and will interfere with the antibody's precipitating capabilities. Simple hapten–antibody reactions can be visualized, then, because the hapten is able to block the precipitation of hapten–carrier complexes by the same antibody. Haptens are usually low-molecular-weight compounds and hence have a relatively simple chemical composition and a small size.

106. The answer is C *[Ch 13 II C 1].*
Carcinoembryonic antigen (CEA) and α-fetoprotein are both antigens which are common in dedifferentiated tissues. They are found in the fetus and in certain malignancies. CEA is associated with cancer of the colon. α-Fetoprotein is associated with primary hepatic carcinoma. Other conditions will cause these antigens to appear in the serum (e.g., pregnancy, heavy cigarette smoking, and various infectious diseases). Consequently, they cannot be used diagnostically for the detection of cancer.

107–110. The answers are: 107-D *[Ch 4 II B 1 b]*, **108-E** *[Ch 4 II B 1 b]*, **109-B** *[Ch 3 III B 1 b (1); Ch 4 II C 1]*, **110-E** *[Ch 3 III C 2 c].*
The complement system, which plays a major role in host defense and the inflammatory process, can be activated (fixed) via the classic or alternative pathways. Activation of the pathways may occur via antigen–antibody complexes or by aggregated immunoglobulins. IgG molecules (mainly the IgG1 and IgG3 subclasses) are capable of fixing complement. Activation of the classic pathway follows binding of complement to the C_H2 domain on the Fc fragment of IgG. Serum IgA fixes complement via the alternative pathway only. Activation of this pathway can be triggered immunologically primarily by IgA (and to a lesser degree by some IgG). IgM is the most efficient immunoglobulin at activating complement via the classic pathway. Only one molecule of IgM is required to react with complement. Activation of the classic pathway follows binding of complement to the C_H3 domain on the Fc fragment of IgM.

111–113. The answers are: 111-D *[Ch 2 II B 3 a (2) (c)]*, **112-B** *[Ch 2 II B 2 c; Ch 7 II B 3 a (5); Ch 9 IV C 2]*, **113-B** *[Ch 2 II B; Ch 7 IV A 2 c; Ch 9 IV C 2].*
The Weil-Felix test employs heterogenetic (heterophile) antibodies to obtain serologic "clues" to infections caused by certain rickettsiae. The rickettsial agents produce serious diseases, such as Rocky Mountain spotted fever in the United States (over 1000 cases/year, with 20 to 40 fatalities) and epidemic typhus in other parts of the world. The latter disease was of major concern in World War I, being the cause of death for over 3,000,000 Russians alone. During the course of the rickettsial disease, the patient produces antibodies that cross-react with the O (somatic carbohydrate) antigens (termed OX antigens) of certain *Proteus vulgaris* strains. The simple Weil-Felix agglutination test detects these heterophile antibodies to *P. vulgaris* strains OX2, OX19, and OXK. Because *Proteus* can be pathogenic in its own right, causing urinary tract and wound infections and pneumonia, primarily nosocomially as an opportunistic pathogen, it is important to confirm the proteus agglutination results in the Weil-Felix test by using rickettsial antigens in a specific serologic procedure such as complement fixation.

Rabies antiserum and tetanus antitoxin are specific immune globulins obtained from human volunteers and as such are alloantigenic products. (Rabies antiserum is usually obtained from veterinary students who are immunized during their schooling and are tested by the Centers for Disease Control to assure successful vaccination.) Equine-derived antiserum is not recommended for clinical use because the greater foreignness of the gamma globulin increases immunogenicity, making the likelihood of anaphylaxis or serious serum sickness much greater.

114–117. The answers are: 114-E *[Ch 7 II A 3 f]*, **115-C** *[Ch 7 IV B 1 e]*, **116-F** *[Ch 7 II B 3 a (5)]*, **117-B** *[Ch 7 II B 3 a (6)]*.
Patients with AIDS-related complex (ARC) have evidence of human immunodeficiency virus (HIV) infection and show some signs of immunologic abnormality, but they do not have full-blown AIDS. Individuals with ARC should be vaccinated against diseases that are likely to become problems as their immunodeficiency develops. The most appropriate vaccine among those listed in the question would be Pneumovax, which protects against pneumococcal pneumonia. Patients with ARC should probably not receive live virus vaccines.

Meningococcal disease may become epidemic among military recruits; hence, the vaccine made from the meningococcal polysaccharide capsule antigen is recommended.

Veterinary students are routinely immunized against rabies, as this is a serious occupational threat. For similar reasons, dental students receive hepatitis B vaccine.

118–125. The answers are: 118-B *[Ch 10 II M 2]*, **119-E** *[Ch 10 II A 2 a (3)]*, **120-C** *[Ch 10 II H 2 b]*, **121-A** *[Ch 10 II B 2 b (2) (b)]*, **122-D** *[Ch 10 II G 2 a (2)]*, **123-J** *[Ch 11 IV]*, **124-F** *[Ch 9 II A, B 1]*, **125-K** *[Ch 10]*.
Pernicious anemia results from defective red blood cell maturation due to faulty absorption of vitamin B$_{12}$. Normally, dietary B$_{12}$ is transported across the small intestine as a complex with intrinsic factor (synthesized by parietal cells in the gastric mucosa). In pernicious anemia, the process is blocked due to the presence of antibodies to parietal cells and to intrinsic factor.

Rheumatoid arthritis is a chronic inflammatory joint disease; joint deformity is common. A hallmark of the disease is the presence, in serum and synovial fluid, of rheumatoid factors, which are antibodies (mainly IgM) with a specificity for the Fc fragment of IgG. Complexes composed of rheumatoid factor, IgG, and complement in the joint fluid attract neutrophils which damage the synovium by discharging their lysosomal contents.

Myasthenia gravis results from faulty neuromuscular transmission triggered by depletion of acetylcholine receptors at the myoneural junction. Autoantibody binds to acetylcholine receptors at the myoneural junction, causing the endocytosis of receptors. Complement-activating immune complexes may cause further problems at the junction.

Systemic lupus erythematosus (SLE) is a chronic multiorgan (systemic) disease characterized by the production of a variety of autoantibodies against, for example, DNA, RNA, red cells, platelets, and ribosomes. The anti-DNA antibodies are most closely associated with active disease and the glomerulonephritis triggered by deposition of DNA–antibody–complement complexes on the basement membrane of blood vessels of renal glomeruli.

Multiple sclerosis is a relapsing neurologic disorder associated with lesions (plaques) confined to the central nervous system and consisting of mononuclear cell infiltrates and demyelination. The cause is unknown. Patients tend to have elevated levels of antibodies to measles virus in their serum and spinal fluid, but the exact role of measles virus is unknown. Other viral agents may also be involved.

DiGeorge syndrome is a T cell immunodeficiency disorder caused by a failure of development of the third and fourth pharyngeal pouches. Infants with DiGeorge syndrome have no T lymphocytes.

Anaphylaxis is a type I (IgE-mediated) hypersensitivity reaction. It results when an allergen reacts with and cross-links two IgE molecules on a basophil or mast cell, causing the cell to release vasoactive mediators. The consequences depend on the target organ affected, which varies from species to species; in humans the primary target organ is the lung, and the most serious consequence is potentially fatal bronchoconstriction.

The CREST syndrome is a form of progressive systemic sclerosis (systemic scleroderma) which is named for its pentalogy of symptoms: calcinosis (nodular calcium deposition in various body tissues), Raynaud's phenomenon (intermittent painful ischemia in the fingers, toes, and sometimes the nose and ears), esophageal dysmotility, sclerodactyly (scleroderma in the fingers and toes), and telangiectases (small local skin lesions due to permanently dilated small blood vessels). Patients produce a unique antinuclear antibody that reacts with a protein in the centromere. It is detected by an indirect immunofluorescence technique in which only the mitotic plate of dividing cells is stained.

126–128. The answers are: 126-B *[Ch 3 I B]*, **127-G** *[Ch 5 III B 2; Table 5-1]*, **128-D** *[Ch 1 II G; Ch 13 III C 3 a]*.
Although most antibody is secreted by plasma cells, B cells also produce immunoglobulin, inserting it into the B cell membrane, where it is accessible to antigen. Some B cells excrete immunoglobulin as well.

Concanavalin A (con A) is a T cell–specific mitogen. It reacts with a receptor in the T cell membrane and induces proliferation of the T cells. Mitosis is identified by pulse-labeling the cells for 24 hours with tritiated thymidine.

Natural killer (NK) cells are non-B, non-T (null) lymphocytes that are distinct in their ability to express cytotoxicity against targets such as tumor cells, virally infected autologous cells, and transplanted tissues without any previous exposure to these foreign materials. NK cells have a membrane receptor for the Fc portion of antibody but will also kill targets in the absence of antibody.

129–133. The answers are: 129-B *[Ch 9 II B 5 a, b]*, **130-E** *[Ch 9 III C 2 c; Ch 10 II O]*, **131-C** *[Ch 9 IV C 1]*, **132-D** *[Ch 9 IV C 2]*, **133-A** *[Ch 9 VI B 1 b]*.

Allergic rhinitis (hay fever) is an atopic allergy. Atopic allergies show a strong hereditary association: if both parents are atopic, it is probable that their children also will be atopic. Atopic allergies are type I (immediate) hypersensitivity reactions due to IgE antibodies.

In idiopathic thrombocytopenic purpura (ITP), platelet-specific IgG antibodies are found on platelet surfaces, and patients show profoundly suppressed peripheral blood platelet counts and various bleeding problems. ITP is a cytotoxic (type II) hypersensitivity reaction. Cytotoxic reactions are initiated by IgG or IgM antibody reacting with antigenic determinants on cell membranes or tissues. The ultimate effect of these reactions is lysis or inactivation of target cells.

The Arthus reaction and serum sickness are classic examples of immune complex–mediated (type III) hypersensitivity reactions: they are associated, respectively, with local and systemic deposition of immune complexes. In type III reactions, antigen–antibody (immune) complexes form locally or in the circulation and are deposited in vascular or glomerular basement membrane, where they cause inflammation. The Arthus reaction is induced in rabbits by repeated subcutaneous injections of antigen. It is characterized by local foci of erythema, edema, and necrosis at injection sites, which are related to a vasculitis caused by immune complex deposition on vascular basement membrane. Serum sickness is a syndrome that follows injection of foreign serum in humans. It is characterized by fever, rash, splenomegaly, arthritis, and glomerulonephritis; the primary damage, as in the Arthus reaction, appears to be a vasculitis associated with destruction of vascular basement membrane.

Bence Jones protein, a dimer of immunoglobulin light (L) chains, is found in the urine in about 10% of patients with multiple myeloma. Multiple myeloma, the most common of the plasma cell dyscrasias, is a plasma cell tumor in bone marrow that overproduces a single class of monoclonal immunoglobulins. The most characteristic feature of multiple myeloma is the demonstration of an abnormal protein (M component) in blood, urine, or both. The M component usually consists of any one or a combination of heavy (H) chains, L chains, or intact IgG or IgA. In 25% of cases, the M component consists only of L chains and only appears in the urine.

134–137. The answers are: 134-B *[Ch 2 II B; Ch 12 I A]*, **135-A** *[Ch 2 II B; Ch 12 I A]*, **136-A** *[Ch 2 II B; Ch 12 I A]*, **137-E** *[Ch 2 II B; Ch 12 I A]*.

The transfer of skin from thigh to face in the same person is an autograft, which involves the transfer of autologous tissue; that is, tissue moved from one part of the body to another. Autografts are done in plastic surgery to repair burn wounds, for example. Bone is also commonly employed in autograft procedures to promote healing of nonunited fractures, to restore structural integrity to the skeleton, and to facilitate cosmetic repair, as in facial reconstruction where pieces of bone from the hip are used to rebuild portions of the face damaged by accident or malignancy. Allogeneic bone grafts are also performed; these involve the transfer of bone between genetically dissimilar members of the same species. For this purpose the bone is aseptically removed, sterilized by ethylene oxide or gamma irradiation, and frozen. Freezing is used for all bone tissue transplants except fresh autografts because it reduces immunogenicity.

Transplanting of a cadaver kidney is a relatively standard procedure that employs allogeneic tissue to replace a patient's diseased organs. Individuals awaiting a cadaver kidney transplant often receive blood transfusions to treat anemia and to increase graft survival. Untransfused patients have approximately 40% to 50% graft function after 2 years, while patients who have received transfusions have a 60% to 80% chance of long-term graft function. Mechanisms of this transfusion effect include the elimination of immunologic responders who will demonstrate donor-specific cytotoxic antibodies in the pre-graft screening, the development of suppressor T (Ts) cells, and the generation of blocking or anti-idiotypic antibodies.

A bone marrow transplant from mother to daughter is allogeneic: the mother's bone marrow is antigenically different (alloantigenic) and will be recognized by the daughter's immune system and rejected as foreign. This is unfortunate and necessitates immunosuppression of the bone marrow recipient to prevent rejection of the graft. To accomplish this the daughter would be treated with immunosuppressive drugs and, probably, with irradiation before the transplant was performed. Strict isolation procedures would have to be maintained as she would be very susceptible to nosocomial infections. A second threat to the recipient would be graft-versus-host (GVH) disease, in which mature lymphocytes in the grafted tissue (bone marrow) mount an immunologic attack on the recipient, with devastating results. Management following an allograft procedure includes monitoring for GVH, and prompt and vigorous immunosuppression at the first sign of trouble. Because of the potential difficulties of allografts, bone marrow autografts have been employed in the treatment of some malignancies, notably acute myelogenous leukemia, which has a mortality rate of over 90% in adults. In this instance the patient's own bone marrow is removed during remission, treated with cyclophosphamide to kill residual leukemic cells, and frozen. The patient is then vigorously treated with antineoplastic drugs and re-infused with the stored marrow.

Identical twins are syngeneic antigenically. They behave immunologically just like inbred animals and do not reject grafted tissues. This is clinically fortunate, because it obviates the need for immunosuppression of the bone marrow recipient, as is done in homografts to prevent the host from rejecting the graft.

138–141. The answers are: 138-E *[Ch 9 IV C 3]*, **139-C** *[Ch 11 II B 1]*, **140-D** *[Ch 10 II J]*, **141-B** *[Ch 11 III A]*.

Immune complex–mediated (type III) reactions are initiated by antigen–antibody complexes that form locally or in the circulation and deposit on vascular or glomerular basement membranes, where they cause inflammation. Glomerulonephritis is an example of systemic immune complex disease. This disease can occur in association with persistent infections or with the acute release of bacterial products, as in the case of poststreptococcal glomerulonephritis.

Chronic granulomatous disease (CGD) develops because neutrophils and macrophages fail to generate toxic oxygen metabolites during phagocytosis and are therefore unable to kill ingested microorganisms. Patients with CGD are characterized by repeated infections with various bacterial agents.

Patients with Graves' disease (thyrotoxicosis) develop antibodies that react with the thyrotropin receptor on the thyroid cell membrane. These antibodies are known as thyroid-stimulating antibodies because they cause the overproduction of the thyroid hormone thyroxine.

Bruton's X-linked hypogammaglobulinemia is a B cell deficiency disorder. Patients with this hereditary disorder are unable to produce immunoglobulins because they lack B cells, germinal centers, and so forth. Therefore they suffer from recurrent bacterial infections, beginning at about age 6 months, the time when maternal antibodies have waned to nonprotective levels.

142–144. The answers are: 142-C *[Ch 8 III E 1 a]*, **143-A** *[Ch 8 III B]*, **144-D** *[Ch 8 II B 4]*.

Radioimmunoassay (RIA) procedures are extremely sensitive measures of either antigen or antibody. It is the coupling of a radioactive isotope [commonly, iodine-125 (^{125}I)] to the compound being detected that gives these procedures such great sensitivity, allowing minute amounts of antigen or antibody to be detected.

In the immunofluorescence technique, antibody to a particular bacterium, cell membrane, or cytoplasmic constituent is labeled with a fluorescent dye, usually fluorescein. Once the antibody has reacted with the organism or tissue component, the excess antibody is removed by washing the slide, which is then examined in an ultraviolet-light microscope. Fluorescein, when excited by ultraviolet rays, emits light in the green wavelengths, so that wherever a fluorescein molecule is (i.e., where the antibody is), an apple-green appearance will be seen in the darkfield microscope.

Radial immunodiffusion is used to quantitate serum levels of immunoglobulins or other serum proteins such as complement components or α_1-trypsin inhibitor. In this procedure, the antigen in question diffuses out into an agar menstruum, which is impregnated with specific antibodies. When the antigen meets its homologous antibody, a precipitant ring develops. The diameter of the ring is directly proportional to the amount of antigen placed in the well, so that it is possible to quantitate the amount of a serum protein in an unknown specimen.

145–148. The answers are: 145-B *[Ch 7 II B 3 a (6)]*, **146-D** *[Ch 7 II B 3 a (1), (3)]*, **147-H** *[Ch 7 II B 3 a (4) (a)]*, **148-F** *[Ch 7 II A 3 h; IV B 2 h]*.

Hepatitis B viral vaccine is commercially prepared as a subunit viral product by recombinant DNA techniques. Measles-mumps-rubella (MMR) vaccine contains attenuated measles, mumps, and rubella viruses. The Salk poliomyelitis vaccine contains three types of poliovirus, but they have been killed by mild formaldehyde treatment. It is the Sabin oral poliomyelitis vaccine that contains live, attenuated poliovirus. The rabies vaccine used for humans is also a killed viral agent; the preparation used for animals is a live, attenuated agent. Unfortunately, very young children (under 18 months of age) do not respond well to the polyribose phosphate capsule of *Haemophilus influenzae;* however, this carbohydrate vaccine is an excellent immunogen in older children and affords protection against meningitis in children of about 2 years of age.

149–153. The answers are: 149-C *[Ch 4 IV A 2]*, **150-D** *[Ch 4 III B 3 b]*, **151-B** *[Ch 4 II B 2 d]*, **152-E** *[Ch 4 II C 2 c]*, **153-G** *[Ch 4 V E 2]*.
In the classic pathway of complement activation, circulating C3 binds to the C4b2b complex (C3 convertase) and is cleaved into two fragments, C3a and C3b.

In the alternative pathway of complement activation, the complex C3bB is susceptible to enzymatic cleavage by factor D. The Ba fragment is released and the C3bBb complex becomes a C3 convertase. C3a, along with C5a and C4a, are anaphylatoxins which cause release of vasoactive amines from mast cells and basophils. Their biological activity is enzymatically destroyed by anaphylatoxin inactivator.

Bb, a factor generated by the alternative but not the classic pathway of complement activation, activates macrophages and causes them to adhere to and spread on cell surfaces. It is a component of the C3bBb complex (C3 convertase), and its dissociation from the complex is slowed by properdin.

Assembly of the membrane attack complex is triggered by cleavage of C5. The larger cleavage product, C5b, forms a trimolecular complex with C6 and C7. The membrane-bound C5b67 complex then binds C8 and C9. The C5b6789 complex (the membrane attack complex) induces the formation of hollow cylinders in the cell membrane, leading ultimately to osmotic lysis of the cell.

154–157. The answers are: 154-A *[Ch 3 II G 1 a (2)]*, **155-C** *[Ch 3 II G 1 b (1)(a)]*, **156-B** *[Ch 3 II G 2]*, **157-D** *[Ch 3 II G 1 a (1)]*.
Treatment of the monomeric basic immunoglobulin unit with papain splits it into two monovalent Fab (antigen-binding) fragments and one Fc (crystallizable) fragment. Pepsin treatment of the immunoglobulin molecule digests away most of the Fc fragment, leaving two Fab fragments and the hinge region, termed an $F(ab')_2$ fragment, which is bivalent. The Fc fragment that is produced by papain digestion of immunoglobulin contains the carboxy terminal half of the heavy (H) chain. It is the site for complement binding. Each Fab fragment derived from papain digestion of immunoglobulin contains an entire light (L) chain plus the V_H and C_H1 domains of the H chain (the Fd fragment). FcεR is the receptor on mast cells that binds IgE to the cell membrane and gives the cell its allergen specificity.

158–161. The answers are: 158-B *[Ch 2 II B; Ch 9 III C 1 b]*, **159-C** *[Ch 2 II B; Ch 9 II]*, **160-C** *[Ch 2 II B; Ch 9 V C 3; Table 9-5]*, **161-A** *[Ch 2 II B; Ch 10 II J]*.
Erythroblastosis fetalis, or hemolytic disease of the newborn, is caused by the mother's immune response to an antigen on the infant's erythrocytes, usually the Rh antigen D (approximately 85% of people are Rh-positive). The D antigen is found on most human red blood cells and as such is an alloantigen. It is also found on the red cells of Rhesus monkeys (hence the term Rh) and as such is actually a xenogeneic antigen for humans.

Asthma is an example of Gell and Coombs type I hypersensitivity reaction and is mediated by IgE antibodies induced by various allergens. The offending antigens can be extremely diverse, including such materials as house dust, animal dander, pollens, molds, and foods. These antigens are certainly well removed from man phylogenetically and hence are xenogeneic.

Farmer's lung is a form of hypersensitivity pneumonitis and thus is a Gell and Coombs type IV (T cell–mediated) allergic disease. Hypersensitivity pneumonitis affects the lung interstitium and is induced by inhaled allergens, most commonly bacteria or fungal spores. Farmer's lung is caused by inhalation of thermophilic actinomycetes, which are in the plant kingdom and hence are xenogeneic antigens in humans.

Graves' disease (hyperthyroidism) involves autologous antigens, since it is caused by the production of autoantibodies to thyrotropin receptors. The autoantibodies mimic the action of the thyroid-stimulating hormone produced in the pituitary; the result is the overproduction of thyroid hormone.

162–165. The answers are: 162-B *[Ch 3 III C, D; Ch 5 III C]*, **163-D** *[Ch 5 IV A 2]*, **164-H** *[Table 5-2; Ch 12 II C 4; III E]*, **165-J** *[Ch 1 II G 1; Ch 13 III B, C 2, 3]*.
IgM and IgD are the first antibodies made in utero. Mu heavy (H) chains first can be seen in the cytoplasm of pre-B cells. Later in development, IgM and IgD appear as a part of the B cell membrane. They are the external expression of the immunologic commitment (specificity) of the cell. T cells are the cells primarily involved in graft rejection. Human leukocyte antigens HLA-A, HLA-B, and HLA-DR are the principal antigen products of the major histocompatibility complex (MHC) recognized by the host during the process of graft rejection. In cell-mediated cytolysis (CMC), the in vitro correlate of graft rejection, HLA-A and HLA-B antigens are the target antigens recognized by the cytotoxic T (Tc) cells. The macrophage is the major antigen-processing cell. Before an antigen can be recognized by T cells, the antigen must be processed by an antigen-processing cell and then presented to the T cell in conjunction with the appropriate MHC molecule. This requirement is known as MHC restriction. Natural killer (NK) cells are believed to be involved in surveillance against malignancy.

Index

Note: Page numbers in *italics* denote illustrations; those followed by (t) denote tables; those followed by Q denote questions; and those followed by E denote explanations.

A

ABO blood group antigens, 182
 as transplantation antigens, 220Q, 229Q, 237E, 247E
ABO blood group compatibility, 187
ABO blood group incompatibility, 136
ABO blood group system, genetics of, 187–188, 187(t)
Accelerated rejection, 189
Accessory cell(s), in immune response, 70–71, 70(t)
N-Acetyl-muramyl-L-alanyl-D-isoglut-amine, as adjuvant, 95
Acetylcholine receptor, in myasthenia gravis, 137, 157
Acid(s)
 bile, mechanisms of action, 3(t)
 fatty, mechanisms of action, 3(t)
 nucleic, immunogenicity of, 16
 organic, mechanisms of action, 3(t)
 sialic, 31
Acquired hypogammaglobulinemia, 170(t), 171
Acquired immune deficiency syndrome (AIDS), 174, 179E
Acute rejection, 189
Addison's disease, tissue involvement in, 153(t)
Adjuvant(s), 14
 defined, 87, 94, 219Q, 236E
 directional influence of, 95
 Freund's, 95
 of immune response, 94–95
 for immunization, 100
Affinity, defined, 21, 26E
Agammaglobulinemia, Bruton's, *see* Bruton's hypogammaglobulinemia; Hypogammaglobulinemia, Bruton's
Age, and immunity, 3
Agglutination, 111–112
 bacterial, 112(t)
 passive, 117–118
 procedures involving, 117–118
 sheep red blood cell, 222Q, 240E
Agglutinin, defined, 111
AIDS, *see* Acquired immune deficiency syndrome
AIDS-related complex, Pneumovax in, 232Q, 251E
Aldrich syndrome, 227Q, 244E
Alkylating agents
 immunosuppressive effects of, 90
 in transplantation, 190–191
Allele exclusion, 42
Alleles
 MHC, diseases associated with, 186, 187(t)
 O, 188

Allergens, 35, 131–132, 227Q,245E
Allergic reactions, *see also* Hypersensitivity reactions
 atopic, 146Q, 148E, 233Q, 252E
 to food, 133, 149E
 genetic factors in, 133–134
 to penicillin, 220Q, 237E
 skin, incidence of, 134(t)
 to vaccine, 106
Allergic rhinitis, incidence of, 134(t)
Allergic urticaria, 149E
Alloantigen(s), 15
 HLA, in cell-mediated cytotoxicity, 186
Allogeneic antigen(s), 15, 25E
Allogeneic graft, 181
 bone, 233Q, 252E
Allograft, 15, 181
 defined, 219Q, 236E
Alloreactivity, 190
Allotypes
 immunoglobulin, 35
 markers for, 35
Alpha-fetoprotein, 198–199, 207E, 231Q, 250E
Alpha interferon, 8
 as macrophage antitumor product, 201
Alternative pathway, 54–56, *55*
 amplification in, 56
Alum, as adjuvant, 95
Aluminum hydroxide, as adjuvant, 95
Ameboid movement, 5
Amplification, in complement activation, 56
Amyloidosis, 145
 primary, 146Q, 148E
Anamnesis, 67, 84E
Anaphylactic shock, 134
 incidence of, 134, 134(t)
Anaphylatoxins, cleavage products of, 60
Anaphylatoxin inactivator, 58, 62Q, 64E
Anaphylaxis, 232Q, 251E
 eosinophil chemotactic factor of, as mediator of atopic disease, 133(t)
 features of, 134
 incidence of, 134(t)
 mediators of, 227Q, 245E
 passive cutaneous, 124
 slow-reacting substance of (SRS-A), 132, 133(t)
Anaplasia, 197
Anemia
 hemolytic
  cold-antibody, 160
  warm-antibody, 160, 164E
 pernicious, 159–160, 232Q, 251E
 tissue involvement in, 153(t)
 vitamin B$_{12}$ for, 153

Angioedema, hereditary, 174–175, 224Q, 241E
Ankylosing spondylitis, incidence of, 152(t)
Antibiotics, in immunodeficiency disorders, 167
Antibody(ies), *see also* Immunoglobulin(s)
 anti-CD3, for tumors, 204
 anti-HLA, 224Q, 242E
 anti-idiotypic, 36–37, 224Q, 241E
  in immune regulation, 88
  in immune response, 230Q, 248E
  production of, *36*
  for vaccines, 105
 anti-TSTA, for tumors, 204, 207E
 antigens and, *see* Antigen–antibody complex
 antinuclear, 117
  in autoimmune diseases, 154(t)
  in SLE, 155, 229Q, 247E
 CD16, for tumors, 204
 cell-bound, 118
 in cell-mediated immunity, 144
 circulating nonagglutinating, Coombs test for, 118
 cytotoxic, anti-idiotypic, in immune tolerance, 93
 defined, 27
 diversity of, 35–43
  mechanisms contributing to, 41
  somatic mutation theory of, 41
 Donath-Landsteiner, 160, 162Q,164E
  in paroxysmal cold hemoglobinuria, 164E
 enhancing, 202
 fluorescent monoclonal, for T-cell subsets, 122, 122(t)
 human acetylcholine receptor, 229Q, 247E
 in humoral immune response, 226Q, 244E
 idiotype of, 223Q, 240E
 in immune globulin, 222Q, 239E
 immunologic effects, 90
 measurement of, 127Q, 128E
 monoclonal
  versus anti-idiotypic antibody vaccines, 125
  fluorescent, for T-cell subsets, 122, 122(t)
  production by murine hybridoma technique, 125–126
  tumor-specific, 203
  uses of, 125
  for vaccines, 105
 and opsonization, 7
 in rabies immune globulin, 102, 232Q, 250E

255

K

Kallikrein, 51, 132
Keratoconjunctivitis sicca, in Sjögren's syndrome, 155, 164E
Kidney failure, in SLE, 155
Killer (K) cells, natural, *see* Natural killer cells
Km markers, immunoglobulin, 230Q, 249E
Kupffer cells, 4

L

Lactoferrin, 6, 8
  mechanisms of action, 3(t)
Lactoperoxidase, 8
Langerhans cells, in humoral immune response, 226Q, 244E
Latex agglutination test, 117
Lazy leukocyte syndrome, 169, 227Q, 244E
Le gene, 188
Leprosy, lepromatous, immunosuppression in, 91
Leukocyte(s), polymorphonuclear, 4, 5(t)
Leukocyte adhesion deficiency, 169–170
Leukocyte-inhibiting factor, 141(t), 142
Leukotriene(s), 246E
  C5a and, 60
  as mediator of atopic disease, 133(t)
  as opsonins for phagocytosis, 7
Levamisole, 144
  experimental use of, 103
Light (L) chains
  hypervariable regions of, 228Q, 246E
  immunoglobulin, 27–28, *28*, 29(t)
Lipids, immunogenicity of, 16
Lipopolysaccharide, 16, 230Q, 238E, 248E
  for B cells, 121
  mitogenicity of, 230Q, 249E
Lipopolysaccharide endotoxin, 17
Lipoprotein(s), 16
Lumbar puncture, in Guillain-Barré syndrome, 226Q, 243E
Lupus erythematosus (LE) cell phenomenon, 155
Lymph nodes, B and T cell areas of, 70
Lymphocyte(s)
  B, *see* B cell(s)
  bone marrow-derived, *see* B cell(s)
  granular, 225Q, 242E
  in immune response system, 68, *69*
  T, *see* T cell(s)
  tumor-infiltrating, 9, 203
    development of, 103
Lymphocyte proliferation assays
  for B cells, 121
  for T cell subsets, 122–123
Lymphocytotoxic agents, 89
Lymphocytotoxicity test, 186, 188
Lymphoid organs, 68, *69*
  removal of, and immune responsiveness, 88
Lymphoid system, 67–70
Lymphoid tissue, 68, *569*
  peripheral, removal of, and immune responsiveness, 88
Lymphokine(s), 73, 73(t)
  as adjuvant, 95
  in delayed hypersensitivity, 141–142, 141(t), 219Q, 236E
  in immune response, 221Q, 239E

Lymphokine-activated killer cells (LAK), 9
Lympholytic agents, 89
Lymphoma
  Burkitt's, immunoglobulin gene rearrangement and, 43
  follicular, immunoglobulin gene rearrangement and, 42–43
  immunosuppression in, 91
Lymphotoxin, 141(t), 142
Lysin
  beta, 8, 224Q, 242E
  defined, 111
Lysis
  in antigen–antibody reactions, 112–113
  red blood cell, in cytotoxic reactions, 136
  white blood cell, in cytotoxic reactions, 137
Lysosomal granules, 5
Lysosome, 5
  defined, 5
Lysozyme, 6, 8, 11E, 12E
  epitopes on, *14*

M

M component, 144
Macroglobulinemia, Waldenström's, 144, 149E
Macrophage(s), 4, 235Q, 254E
  activating factor (MAF), 141, 141(t), 201, 204
  in delayed hypersensitivity, 140
  alveolar, immunologic function of, 11E
  antigen presentation by, 76
  antimicrobial products of, oxygen-dependent, 10Q, 12E
  characteristics and functions of, 70–71, 70(t), 227Q, 230Q, 231Q, 244E, 248E–249E, 249E
  complement receptors on, 229Q, 246E
  in humoral immune response, 226Q, 244E
  secreted products of, 6–7, 10Q, 12E, 228Q, 245E
  suppressor, 203, 207E
  in tumor rejection, 201–202
  viral infection effects on, 91(t)
Magnesium ions, for C4b2b complex, 62Q, 64E
Major histocompatibility complex (MHC)
  alleles associated with, 186, 187(t)
  characteristics of, 181
  in epitope presentation, 76–77
  and histocompatibility genes, 182–186, *183*, *185*
  restriction, 67, 184, 186, 221Q, 231Q, 235Q, 239E, 249E, 254E
  anamnestic, 87
  in cell-mediated cytolysis, 186
  in immune response system, 76–77, 87
  and T-cell receptor complex, interaction between, *72*
Major histocompatibility complex (MHC) genes, 229Q, 247E
  characteristics of, 226Q, 243E–244E
Malignancy, *see also* Cancer
  cellular changes in, 197, 230Q, 249E
  chemotherapy for, immunosuppressive effects of, 89
  immunoglobulin gene rearrangement and, 42–43

Malnutrition, immunosuppression in, 91
Measles, immunosuppression in, 91, 174
Measles immune globulin, 102, 109E
Measles-mumps-rubella vaccine, 234Q, 253E
Measles vaccine, 101
Membrane(s), cell
  complement regulatory proteins in, 62Q, 64E
  regulatory proteins in, 59
Membrane attack complex
  effect on cell membrane, *58*
  formation of, 57
Membrane attack pathway, in complement activation, 56–57
Memebrane cofactor protein, 59
Meningococcal disease, vaccines in, 232Q, 251E
MHC, *see* Major histocompatibility complex
Microbicidal assay, 120, 228Q, 246E
Migration-inhibiting factor (MIF), 141, 141(t)
Minor histocompatibility antigens, 182
Mitogens, 230Q, 249E
Mixed lymphocyte reaction, 123, 186, 188–189
Molecular mimicry, 151
Molecule(s)
  B-cell, 227Q, 245E
  CD3, 224Q, 242E
  CD4, 224Q, 242E
  IgG, hypervariable regions of, 228Q, 246E
  insulin, forces of antigen–antibody attraction in, 21
  size of, in immunogenicity, 16–17, 17(t)
Monoclonal antibodies, *see* Antibody(ies), monoclonal
Monoclonal gammopathy(ies), 131
  benign, 145
Monocytes, 4
Monokines, 245E
Mononucleosis
  infectious, heterophile antibody response for, 15
  sheep red blood cell agglutination for, 222Q, 240E
Mucus, function of, 3, 3(t), 11E
Multiple myeloma, 144, 148E
  Bence Jones protein in, 233Q, 252E
Multiple sclerosis, 151, 226Q, 232Q, 243E, 251E
  causes of, 157
  diagnosis of, 229Q, 247E
  HLA alleles and, 187(t)
  incidence of, 152(t)
  symptoms of, 157
  tissue involvement in, 153(t)
Mumps vaccine, 101
Muramyl dipeptide, 238E
  for tumors, 204
Muscular dystrophy, 226Q, 243E
Myasthenia gravis, 226Q, 232Q, 243E, 251E
  acetylcholine receptors in, 137, 157
  anticholinesterase agents in, 153
  diagnosis of, 229Q, 247E
  features of, 157–158
  HLA alleles and, 187(t)
  tissue involvement in, 153(t)